T0332620

# Syntactic Pattern Recognition

# Series in Computer Vision

ISSN: 2010-2143

**Series Editor:** C H Chen *(University of Massachusetts Dartmouth, USA)*

In recent years, there has been significant progress in computer vision in theory and methodology and enormous advancement on the application front, accompanied by rapid progress in vision systems and technology.

It is hoped that this book series in computer vision can capture most of the important and recent progress and results in computer vision. The target audiences cover researchers, engineers, scientists and professionals in many disciplines including computer science and engineering, mathematics, physics, biology, and medical areas, etc.

Topics include (but not limited to)

- Computer vision theory and methodology (algorithms)
- Computer vision applications in biometrics, biomedicine, etc
- Robotic vision
- New vision sensors, software and hardware systems and technology

*Published*

*Forthcoming*

More information on this series can also be found at http://www.worldscientific.com/series/scv

Series in Computer Vision - Vol. 6

# Syntactic Pattern Recognition

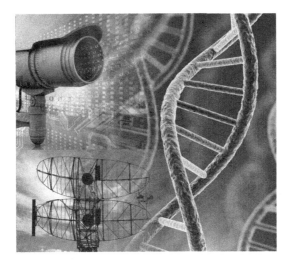

## Mariusz Flasiński

Jagiellonian University, Poland

**World Scientific**

NEW JERSEY · LONDON · SINGAPORE · BEIJING · SHANGHAI · HONG KONG · TAIPEI · CHENNAI · TOKYO

*Published by*

World Scientific Publishing Co. Pte. Ltd.

5 Toh Tuck Link, Singapore 596224

*USA office:* 27 Warren Street, Suite 401-402, Hackensack, NJ 07601

*UK office:* 57 Shelton Street, Covent Garden, London WC2H 9HE

**British Library Cataloguing-in-Publication Data**
A catalogue record for this book is available from the British Library.

**Series in Computer Vision — Vol. 6**
**SYNTACTIC PATTERN RECOGNITION**

ISBN 978-981-3278-46-2

For any available supplementary material, please visit
https://www.worldscientific.com/worldscibooks/10.1142/11216#t=suppl

Printed in Singapore

The book is dedicated to the memory of Professor King-Sun Fu (1930–1985)

# Preface

*Syntactic pattern recognition* is a research field of computer science which develops and applies models of the general theory of formal languages and automata to classify and characterize objects, systems, processes, phenomena, etc. which can be represented as structural patterns. The *general* theory of formal languages and automata means here an extension of the (standard, i.e., string) theory of formal languages and automata to include tree and graph languages. In general, three formal tools are investigated in syntactic pattern recognition: generative grammars, formal automata (and their algorithmic specifications in the form of syntax analyzers) and language inference algorithms. (Syntax analyzers are used for the recognizing and characterizing of structural patterns in syntactic pattern recognition systems, whereas language inference algorithms are applied for the constructing of learning modules in these systems.) Hence, three basic parts (II, III and IV) of this book are devoted to string-, tree-, and graph-based models. Each basic part contains a chapter which presents automata/syntax analyzers (Chaps. 3, 7 and 10) and a chapter which presents language inference algorithms (Chaps. 5, 8 and 11). The important issue of the enhancing of string grammars is discussed in Chap. 4.

Research into syntactic pattern recognition has delivered a variety of efficient methods for pattern recognition applications since the early 1960s, when Robert S. Ledley and his collaborators developed the FIDAC system for karyotype analysis. (The term *bioinformatics* had not yet been coined.) Then, fundamental models were developed and applied for the constructing of many syntactic pattern recognition systems by King-Sun Fu and his collaborators until his untimely death. Indeed, his contribution to the field is monumental. (More than 60 seminal publications authored and co-authored by K. S. Fu are included in the bibliography to this book.) Nowadays, the number of syntactic pattern recognition applications is really impressive. These applications include shape and image analysis, optical character recognition (OCR), structure analysis in bioinformatics, scene analysis, analysis of medical signals and images, speech recognition, natural language processing (NLP), analysis of visual events and activities, signal analysis for industrial process monitoring and control, fingerprint identification, radar signal analysis, architectural object analysis, computer aided design and manufacturing (CAD/CAM), signal analysis in seismology, structure analysis in chemistry and geology and time-series analysis in finance and economics. The three surveys of the applications of string-, tree-, and graph-based models, presented in Chaps. 6, 9 and 12, contain more than 1000 carefully selected sources. Thus, dozens of papers on syntactic pattern recognition have been published every year from the 1960s to date. This means that this approach has enjoyed unabated popularity for almost sixty years.

The introductory issues are discussed in Part I. Paradigmatic considerations on syntactic pattern recognition are included in Chap. 1, whereas the general methodology of syntactic pattern recognition is presented in Chap. 2. The last part of the book, Part V, contains a summary of the research results, a list of the open problems (Chap. 13) and the methodological principles recommended (Chap. 14). Selected notions on the theory of formal languages and automata are presented in Appendix A.

The most recent monograph on syntactic pattern recognition – the classic and nonpareil book *Syntactic Pattern Recognition and Applications* by King-Sun Fu – was published by Prentice Hall in 1982. Then, the excellent collection *Syntactic and Structural Pattern Recognition - Theory and Applications*, edited by Horst Bunke and Alberto Sanfeliu, was published by World Scientific in 1990. In 2015 Prof. Chi-Hau Chen asked me to write a chapter on syntactic pattern recognition for the renowned *Handbook of Pattern Recognition and Computer Vision* (World Scientific, 5th Edition, 2016) edited by him. In writing the chapter, I realized the need for a new, updated monograph on syntactic pattern recognition.

I would like to thank Professor Chi-Hau Chen for his encouragement to write the book.

*Kraków, December 2018*                    *Mariusz Flasiński*

# Nomenclature

$2^A$      power set of $A$, page 120

$\circ$      max-min composition, page 75

$\cong$      graph isomorphism, page 327

$\delta$      state-transition function, page 324

$\Gamma$      graph edge labels, page 327

$\lambda$      empty word, page 321

$\Longrightarrow$      derivational step, page 322

$\mathbb{N}$      nonnegative integers, page 180

$\mathbb{N}_+$      positive integers, page 180

$\mathbb{R}_{\geq 0}$      nonnegative reals, page 80

$\mathcal{F}$      string (tree) transformation, page 77

$\mathcal{I}$      interpretation, page 250

$\mathcal{O}(\cdot)$      computational complexity (big O notation), page 324

$\mathfrak{S}$      relational structure, page 248

$|\cdot|$      string length, page 321

$\|\cdot\|$      sum of lengths of strings, page 124

$\mu$      membership function, page 72

$\partial_u Y$      Brzozowski derivative of $Y$ with respect to $u$, page 124

$\rho(\cdot, \cdot)$      distance function, page 77

$\rightarrow$      production arrow, page 322

$\Sigma$      alphabet, page 321

$\Sigma^*$      Kleene star on $\Sigma$, page 321

$\Sigma^+$      Kleene plus on $\Sigma$, page 321

$\Sigma^\oplus$      multisets over $\Sigma$, page 117

$\Sigma_N$      nonterminal symbols, page 322

$\Sigma_T$      terminal symbols, page 322

$\simeq$      matrix row compatibility, page 133

$\vdash$      automaton transition, page 324

$D_t$      domain of $t$, page 181

$f|_A$      restriction of $f$ to $A$, page 187

$F$      final states, page 324

$F_A$    accepting final states, page 123
$F_R$    rejecting final states, page 123
$L(A)$   language accepted by automaton $A$, page 324
$L(G)$   language generated by grammar $G$, page 323
$P$      grammar productions, page 322
$Q$      automaton states, page 324
$q_0$    initial state, page 324
$r(\cdot)$    rank mapping, page 180
$S$      start symbol, page 322
$S_+$    positive sample, page 123
$S_-$    negative sample, page 123
$t/x$    subtree of $t$ at $x$, page 181
$T_\Sigma$    trees over $\Sigma$, page 181
$u^R$    reverse of $u$, page 62
$\mathcal{L}(\cdot)$    class of languages, page 33
$\vdash^*$    reflexive and transitive closure of $\vdash$, page 324
$\xRightarrow{+}$    transitive closure of $\Longrightarrow$, page 323
$\xRightarrow{*}$    reflexive and transitive closure of $\Longrightarrow$, page 322

# Contents

## GRAPH-BASED MODELS                                        229

## FUTURE OF SYNTACTIC PATTERN
## RECOGNITION                                               301

# PART 1
# INTRODUCTORY ISSUES

# Chapter 1

# Paradigmatic Considerations on Syntactic Pattern Recognition

Recognition is considered to be a basic human mental ability in psychology [Myers and DeWall (2018); Reisberg (2013)]. It consists of identifying the objects (systems, processes, etc.), which stimulate our senses, by *recalling information* stored in memory. (The word *recognition* comes from the Latin *recognoscere* meaning "recall to mind", "cognise again", from *re-* "again" and *cognoscere* "cognise", "to know".) Computer pattern recognition systems just simulate this human ability. Since this human skill is one of the fundamental components of intelligence, the research into pattern recognition is one of the most important areas of Artificial Intelligence (AI) [Flasiński (2016a); Russell and Norvig (2009); Winston (1993)].

Pattern recognition systems are constructed in order to analyze, identify, classify and, sometimes, characterize/interpret objects (systems, processes). Of course, objects cannot actually be processed. Therefore their patterns are defined. A *pattern* is the description of an object which is used as its model. (The word *pattern* comes from Middle English *patron* meaning "something that is used as a model".)[1]

The pattern recognition methods are grouped into two main approaches according to the nature of the representational patterns used. In the *decision-theoretic approach* [Bishop (1995, 2006); Duda *et al.* (2001); Fukunaga (1990); Jain *et al.* (2000); Koutroumbas and Theodoridis (2008); Marques de Sá (2001); Ripley (2008); Schalkoff (2005); Vapnik (1998); Webb and Copsey (2011)] the pattern takes the form of a collection of features, whereas within the *syntactic* (or *structural*) *approach* [Bunke and Sanfeliu (1990); Fu (1974, 1977, 1982); Gonzales and Thomason (1978); Pavlidis (1977)] this manifests itself as structural characteristics.[2] Considerations on the structural nature of physical and abstract objects are contained in the next section. In Section 1.2 we introduce the notion of *syntax* as rules for the arrangement of well-formed structures. The discussion on when and why the syntactic pattern recognition approach is recommended is included in the last section.

---

[1]Thus, patterns are analogous to mental representations of objects as considered in some theories of cognitive psychology and philosophy of mind.

[2]These approaches will be characterized in the following sections.

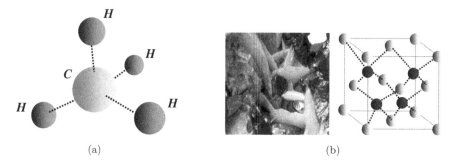

Fig. 1.1  Examples of structures of natural objects at various levels of the physical world. (a) Molecule (methane) composed of atoms. (b) Chemical compound (the mineral sphalerite) composed of molecules and its crystal structure. (Photo courtesy of Dr. B. Gołębiewska, Department of Mineralogy, Petrography and Geochemistry, AGH University of Science and Technology, Cracow.)

## 1.1   Structure - Property of Natural Objects and Artifacts

*Structure* is an arrangement of the parts of a complex object (a whole). A structure is described by defining the component parts and their relationships.

Let us note that natural (complex) objects are structural. Atoms may be viewed as structures which are composed of subatomic particles. Compositions of simple molecules formed out of atoms are represented by structural formulas. (For example, the methane molecule ($CH_4$) is represented by the structure shown in Fig. 1.1a.) Natural chemical compounds, e.g., minerals, have also specific structures. (The example of the mineral sphalerite (zinc sulphide, $ZnS$) and its crystal structure is shown in Fig. 1.1b.) Objects considered at the levels of biochemistry and molecular biology are structural, and so on. (The structure of adenine, one of the nucleobases used in forming the nucleotides of DNA, is illustrated in Fig. 1.2a, whereas the structure of DNA is shown in Fig. 1.2b). Obviously, physical (complex) artifacts such as buildings, cars, airplanes, computers etc., are also structural, i.e., they consist of interrelated functional components.

The human view of the world is *structure-oriented*, and it is independent of geographic and cultural areas. Indeed, the issues of: part-whole relationship, the nature of relations, kinds of relations, the metaphysics of structure and the like have been studied in all the great philosophical traditions. Let us give a few examples.

The assumption of the structural order of the universe is characteristic of holistic-oriented *Chinese Philosophy*. According to the Confucius', Kǒng Fūzǐ (551-479 BC), concept of harmony, cosmic structures should find their reflection within social relations. Deng Xi (c. 546-501 BC), a founder of the School of Names, Míngjiā (the logicians), claimed that the structures of the universe relate to human cognitive/mental structures. Huì Shī (370-310 BC), another representative of this school, studied the paradoxes which concern relations (e.g., spatial and temporal).

In *Ancient Western Philosophy*, Plato (427-347 BC) discussed the problem of the structural nature of complex objects in his dialogues. In view of his theory

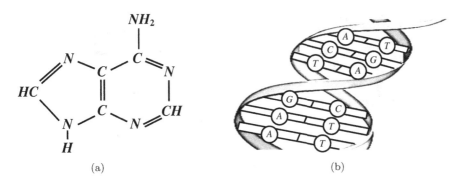

Fig. 1.2 Examples of structures of natural objects at various levels of the physical world - cont. (a) Nucleobase adenine. (b) DNA double helix.

of parts and wholes, the structures of objects are both irreducible and intelligible. He considered relations that are polyadic (i.e., $n$-ary relations, $n > 1$). Aristotle (384-322 BC) established the systematic mereology[3] which consists of a set of fundamental principles (e.g., the properties of wholes are not necessarily reducible to the properties of their parts).

The Huayan school of (*Chinese*) *Buddhist Philosophy* stressed the importance of interrelations among things. Du Shun (557-640) proposed a solution of the reductionism[4]-essentialism[5] dilemma of the part-whole relationship. The solution was based, among others, on the assumption that the boundaries of things are fuzzy.[6]

In the philosophical treatises of Adi Śaṅkara (788-820), the consolidator of the Advaita Vedānta school of *Indian Hindu Philosophy*, the phenomenal world seems to be like the network (structure) which consists of relationships. The structure-oriented ontological view of the world is also characteristic of the Vaiśeṣika school with this being especially visible in Udayana's (c. 1050) *Laksanavali*. Raghunātha Śiromani (c. 1477-1547), a representative of the logical/epistemological Nyāya school, analyzed the nature of relations.[7]

Al-Fārābī (c. 870-950), the great thinker of *Islamic Philosophy*, claimed that hierarchical structures of the world not only relate to notions ingrained in human minds, but also to the grammatical categories of natural languages. Thus, there exists a universal structure of both thought and language which reflects the structure of the world.

According to Maimonides (Mōšeh bēn-Maymōn, Rambam, 1135-1204), the great representative of *Jewish Philosophy*, objects are described by their relations to other objects. The universe may be viewed as a unified system. Both the nature of the elements of the universe and their interrelations are comprehensible.

---

[3]That is, the theory of parthood relations.

[4]Here, *reductionism* means the view that the whole can be reduced to its parts.

[5]According to *essentialism* the essence of the whole cannot be reduced to its parts.

[6]We make this assumption introducing e.g., fuzzy languages in syntactic pattern recognition.

[7]He introduced the important distinction between inherence relations and collecting relations (i.e., the relations concerning those objects which are treated collectively).

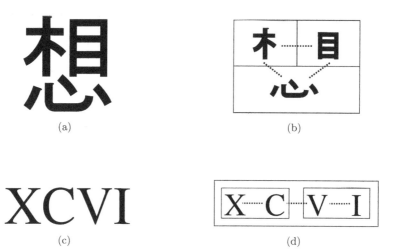

Fig. 1.3   Examples of representational structures of mathematical/linguistic objects.  (a) The Chinese character *think*.  (b) Structural composition of the character *think* from the composite characters: *tree/wood*, *eyes* and *heart*.  (c) Number *96* written with Roman numerals.  (d) Structural composition of *96*.

Thomas Aquinas (1225-1274), one of the greatest scholars of *Medieval Western Philosophy*, considered relations to be a condition *sine qua non* for both thought and action. He recognized, following Aristotle, a distinction between real relations[8] and logical relations (relations of reason).[9]

The structural view of the world is common in modern/contemporary philosophy (e.g., the epistemic structural realism of Bertrand Russell) as well as in sciences like linguistics (e.g., in Ferdinand de Saussure) and anthropology (e.g., the works of Claude Lévi-Strauss).

The fact that human thinking is structure-based may also be noticed if we look at *abstract* concepts and systems created by humans, like, for example, the characters used in some natural languages or symbolic representations as they appear in mathematics. Chinese characters are a good example, since some of them are structural compositions which are composed of simpler characters themselves. The Chinese character shown in Fig. 1.3a means *to think*. It consists of three simple characters, shown in Fig. 1.3b, which mean: *tree/wood* (top-left), *eyes* (top-right) and *heart* (bottom). Let us note that this structure is of a graph-like form. *Roman numerals* are also defined as structures.[10] The number *96* written in the Roman numeric system is shown in Fig. 1.3c, whereas its structural composition is shown in Fig. 1.3d.

---

[8]These relations concern real things.

[9]These relations are the result of mind activity.

[10]Of course, *Hindu-Arabic numerals* are also structural compositions. In this case the structure is linear and positional.

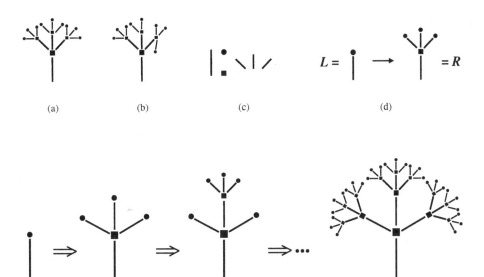

Fig. 1.4   Defining the syntax for branching plant structures.

## 1.2   Syntax - Rules to Arrange Well-Formed Structures

If a set of structures is given, we can try to define the syntax for this set. *Syntax* means here the set of (syntax) rules for constructing the well-formed structures considered.

For example, we can analyze the sentences of some natural language by asking whether their grammatical structures are correct (in the given language). For this purpose we use the syntax of this language, meaning the rules of creating well-formed sentences. For instance, $<S> \rightarrow <NP> <VP>$, where $<S>$ means a (well-formed) simple sentence, $<NP>$ means a noun phrase and $<VP>$ means a verb phrase, is one of the rules inherent within English language syntax.[11] Let us give other examples of defining a syntax.

Let us assume that we want to model and analyze the growth processes of plant development.[12] Let the (idealized) regular branching structure of the plant under study be of the form shown in Fig. 1.4a. This form will be treated as a well-formed structure. (The example of an ill-formed structure is shown in Fig. 1.4b.) Firstly, we define a set of elementary simple patterns, called *primitives* in syntactic pattern recognition, which are used for constructing structural patterns. They are shown in Fig. 1.4c. The small square represents the branching point while the dot represents

---

[11]The formal grammar model as the set of (generative) rules was introduced by Noam Chomsky for English language syntax in the 1950s.

[12]This application area of formal grammar-based models (L-systems) was originated and developed by Aristid Lindenmayer in the 1960s.

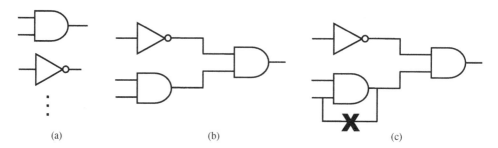

Fig. 1.5   Combinational logic circuits as structural patterns. (a) Primitives. (b) The structure which is consistent with the syntax rules. (c) The structure which is not consistent with the syntax rules.

the end of the branch (i.e., it is a potential branching point).

Now, we can define the syntax for our structures. This is described by the (syntactic) rule shown in Fig. 1.4d. The left-hand side of the rule (denoted with $L$) represents the substructure which is to be replaced in the transformed (constructed) structure. The right-hand side of the rule (denoted with $R$) represents the substructure which is to be put in the place of $L$ within the transformed structure. Syntactic rules which are interpreted in this way are called *generative rules*, since they allow one to "generate" (well-formed) structures. Additionally, let us assume that we start constructing any structure from $L$. The example of constructing a well-formed structure is shown in Fig. 1.4e.

We define also syntax rules in the case of (structural) artifacts. Combinational logic circuits are a good example of artifactual structures. Their structural patterns are represented by circuit diagrams. The graphical symbols of the gates are used as pattern primitives (see Fig. 1.5a) and the lines represent wires connecting the gates. In this case the syntax is defined with the following well-known rules.
• An output wire from a gate can be used as input to another gate.
• Combining two input wires is forbidden.
• An input wire can be split into two wires and used as an input for two separate gates.
• The output of a gate cannot eventually feed back into that gate.
For example, the circuit shown in Fig. 1.5b is consistent with these syntax rules, whereas the circuit shown in Fig. 1.5c is not because the last rule is violated.

## 1.3   Syntactic Pattern Recognition: When and Why

As we have already stated, pattern recognition methods are grouped into two main complementary approaches: the *decision-theoretic* approach and the *structural/syntactic* approach. (The latter is further divided into the *structural* approach and the *syntactic* approach, as we will see later.) The choice of the approach which is adequate for solving a given practical problem is the fundamental issue here. We discuss this here in this section in order to determine the conditions under which the use of the syntactic pattern recognition approach is appropriate. Let us begin with introducing the problem of pattern recognition more formally. At the minimum it may be defined as a classification problem in the following way: let $\mathcal{U}$ be a nonempty set of objects (events, processes, etc.), called a *universe*. Let us assume that each object of $\mathcal{U}$ belongs to one of $C$ classes:

$$\omega^1, \omega^2, \ldots \omega^C.$$

The classification problem is to assign any object $u \in \mathcal{U}$ to the proper class $\omega^i$, $i \in \{1, 2, \ldots, C\}$. As we have mentioned, since objects of $\mathcal{U}$ cannot really be processed, their patterns are defined for this purpose. Now, the pattern classifier (pattern recognizer) $R$ is defined as follows. If $p'$ is the pattern defined for some $u' \in \mathcal{U}$, then

$$R(p') = k \quad \text{iff} \quad u' \text{ belongs to } \omega^k, \ k \in \{1, 2, \ldots, C\}.$$

The form (nature) of the patterns defined for the objects is the key factor that decides which approach should be chosen. Now, we will discuss the following four issues (premises) which determine the choice of the appropriate approach.

(1) Structure-based distinguishability of objects.
(2) Reusability of structural subpatterns.
(3) Hierarchy-oriented multilevel recognition.
(4) Requirement of structure-based interpretation.

As we will see, the first premise determines the choice of the structural/syntactic approach (i.e., the rejection of the decision-theoretic one). The premises 2, 3 and 4 are indications for the use of the syntactic approach.

### 1.3.1 *Structure-Based Distinguishability of Objects*

For the object $u \in \mathcal{U}$, its pattern $p$ has been defined above as the description of $u$. This description is in the form of the *composition of the features* that are characteristic of the object $u$.

Let us assume that the object $u$ belongs to the class $\omega'$. If $u$ can be characterized by the quantitative features: $X_1, X_2, \ldots, X_n$ which are mutually independent then the decision-theoretic approach is used and the composition of the features is defined as the *feature vector*. That is, the object $u$ is described by the pattern $p = \mathbf{X} = (x_1, x_2, \ldots, x_n)$, where $x_k$ is the value of the feature $X_k$, $k = 1, 2, \ldots, n$.

Of course, the phrase *the object $u$ can be characterized* means here *the object $u$ can be characterized so $u$ is distinguishable from any object $u'$ which does not belong to the class $\omega'$*. However, if objects of $\mathcal{U}$ are structural substantially, we are not able to characterize them with compositions of independent quantitative features. Then, the use of structural patterns is *necessary* and the structural/syntactic approach is applied as a consequence.

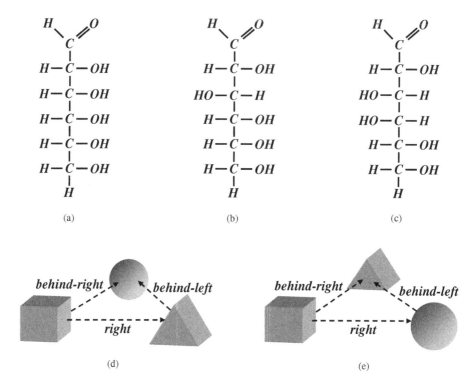

Fig. 1.6    The structures of the exemplary aldose monosaccharides (hexoses, $C_6H_{12}O_6$). (a) Allose. (b) Glucose. (c) Galactose. (d)-(e) The structures of simple scenes.

We illustrate this issue with the problem of the recognition/identification of aldose monosaccharides. (Each aldose monosaccharide structure has an aldehyde functional group, i.e., the substructure -$CHO$ shown in Figs. 1.6a, b and c "at the top".) For example, let us analyze the aldose monosaccharides with six carbon atoms, called hexoses (see Figs. 1.6a, b and c). Various hexoses cannot be distinguished from each other on the basis of quantitative features, like, for example, the numbers of: carbon atoms ($C$), oxygen atoms ($O$) and hydrogen atoms ($H$) because these quantities are the same for each hexose. (That is, any hexose has the chemical formula $C_6H_{12}O_6$.) These can be distinguished from each other only on the basis of the structural configurations of the component atoms as is shown in Figs. 1.6a, b and c.[13]

In the area of computer vision an analogous situation takes place for the problem of scene analysis.[14] In order to distinguish the scene shown in Fig. 1.6d from the one shown in Fig. 1.6e we have to represent them with their structural patterns.

As we have shown above, there are some categories of objects considered in the

---

[13]The same holds for other groups of monosaccharides, e.g., trioses ($C_3H_6O_3$), tetroses ($C_4H_8O_4$) etc.

[14]The purpose of *scene analysis* can be defined here as a holistic (visual) understanding of a physical scene which consists of the objects and their spatial inter-relations.

area of pattern recognition which are inherently structural. That is, they cannot be represented by patterns which are the compositions of quantitative features but structural patterns have to be used. In that case the decision-theoretic approach is not appropriate.

In the examples considered above the use of the structural/syntactic approach seems to be *necessary*. Such a case, in which one has to use structural patterns, should not be mistaken with those cases when the use of structural patterns is just *convenient* or simply *possible*. Then, one should analyze the advantages and disadvantages of applying the structural/syntactic approach and the decision-theoretic one. In the following sections we shall discuss the premises which can determine the proper choice.

### 1.3.2 *Reusability of Structural Subpatterns*

Firstly, we introduce the distinction between the structural approach and the syntactic one. Although the use of structural patterns is a fundamental assumption in both approaches[15] they differ in the generic technique of recognition observed.

*Pattern matching* is the main recognition technique in the *structural approach*. Each class is represented by a finite set of reference structural patterns in a pattern recognition system.[16] During a recognition process an unknown pattern is compared to these reference patterns in order to find the one that is the most similar. Defining a similarity measure which is adequate for this purpose is a key issue here. For example, if structural patterns are symbolic strings (like the words of a language), then we can define a similarity measure in the form of the "distance" between two strings.[17] This "distance" can be computed as the number of characters in an unknown pattern which are not compatible with the corresponding characters of a reference pattern. If we compare e.g. the (unknown) string *fundimental* with the reference string *fundamental*, then the distance is 1. (Let us note that if the pattern matching is perfect, then the distance is 0.)

*Pattern parsing (pattern syntax analysis)* is the main recognition technique in the *syntactic approach*. A set of reference patterns in the form of well-formed structures is treated as a formal language.[18] The syntax of this language is defined by a finite set of *generative rules*. (Generative rules have been introduced in Sec. 1.2.) The set of these rules constitutes the *formal (generative) grammar*. Before we continue our considerations concerning the syntactic pattern recognition paradigm, let us analyze the following examples.

We have introduced the example of aldose monosaccharide structures in the previous section. As we have seen, each monosaccharide structure can be constructed with the three *primitives* only, namely $C$ (carbon), $O$ (oxygen) and $H$ (hydrogen).

---

[15]Therefore we have used the general term *structural/syntactic approach* till now.

[16]Sometimes a class is represented by one *template pattern*.

[17]For simplicity, let us assume that we compare strings of the same length.

[18]This set can be finite or infinite.

However, what is more interesting is that all 30 aldose monosaccharide structures can be constructed with four structural subpatterns only, which are shown in Fig. 1.7a.[19] The examples of trioses (three carbon atoms), tetroses (four carbon atoms) and pentoses (five carbon atoms) are shown in Figs. 1.7b, c and d. (The examples of various hexoses (six carbon atoms) have been already shown in Figs. 1.6a, b and c.) Since there are only four *reusable* structural subpatterns for constructing all the aldose monosaccharide structures, we need to define only four generative rules. These rules are shown in Fig. 1.7e.[20] For example, if we want to generate the glyceraldehyde structure (Fig. 1.7b), we should apply rule (1) once, then rule (2) twice and rule (4) at the end, as it is shown in Fig. 1.7f.[21]

In the area of computer vision, the reusability of a small number of simple structural subpatterns is frequent e.g., in shape analysis. The exemplary set of primitives used for constructing shapes of printed capitals is shown in Fig. 1.7g. Firstly, we define the structural pattern for a capital **I** which consists of four straight vertical segment primitives, as is shown in Fig. 1.7h. As we will see, this pattern constitutes a reusable subpattern, let us call it *LSV* (*Long Straight Vertical*), which will be used for constructing other capitals shown in Fig. 1.7h. Secondly, we define the structural pattern for a capital **P**. We can reuse the subpattern *LSV* (this being marked with a dashed line in the figure as a reused subpattern) and we have to define a new substructure representing a "loop", let us call it *LP*, situated at the upper part of the **P** (this being marked with a bold line in the figure as a new subpattern). Then, in defining the structural pattern for a capital **B**, we do not need to define any new subpatterns, since we can (re)use *LSV* and *LP* etc. Of course, equally in this case we are able to use a small number of generative rules because of the small number of reusable structural subpatterns.

Thus, if structures from a set of reference patterns can be composed of a small number of substructures,[22] then this set can be represented by the small number of generative rules that define its syntax. It is an important factor influencing the efficiency of the recognition process, because we use here the *pattern parsing* technique which consists of checking whether an unknown pattern can be constructed with generative rules. Thus, a small number of rules considerably reduces the computation time of the pattern parsing.

Summing up, if a set of reference patterns can be composed of a small number of substructures, then the pattern parsing technique can be less time consuming than the pattern matching technique which consists of the (exhaustive) comparison of an unknown pattern with all the reference patterns. In as far as space efficiency

---

[19]Substructure (4) consists of a single primitive *H*.

[20]We do not define generative grammar here in a formal way. We merely show how generative rules can be used for constructing structural patterns. The issue of defining a formal grammar that generates a language of structural patterns is presented in Sec. 3.1.

[21]The reader can check that in order to generate a galactose structure (Fig. 1.6c), one should apply a sequence of rules: (1), (2), (3), (3), (2), (2), (4).

[22]*A small number of substructures* means here *small in comparison with the number of reference patterns*.

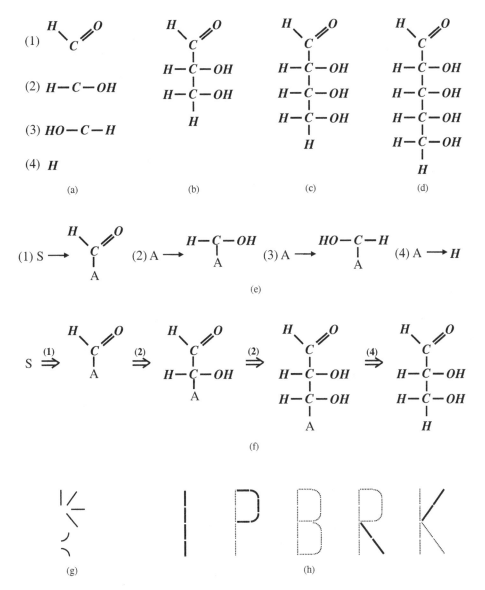

Fig. 1.7 (a) The reusable set of substructures for constructing structures of aldose monosaccharides. (b) Glyceraldehyde. (c) Erythrose. (d) Ribose. (e) The rules for constructing structures of aldose monosaccharides. (f) Generating of the glyceraldehyde pattern with the rules. (g) The set of primitives for constructing shapes (printed capitals). (h) The example of the reusability of substructures for constructing shapes.

is concerned, a small number of generative rules means that a formal grammar is a compact/condensed representation of a (usually huge) set of reference patterns. Therefore, in such a case the syntactic approach should be considered as a competitive approach in relation to the structural one.

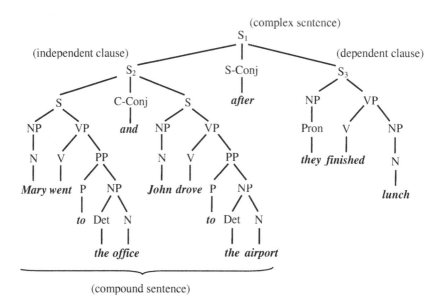

Fig. 1.8   Exemplary hierarchical structure in natural language processing.

### 1.3.3   *Hierarchy-Oriented Multilevel Recognition*

The syntactic approach prevails over the structural one, if the recognition process is multilevel. That is, in order to recognize some complex pattern $P$ one has to recognize (usually simpler) the patterns $P_1, P_2, \ldots, P_n$ which are substructures of $P$.[23] The patterns $P_1, P_2, \ldots, P_n$ can be decomposed into still simpler patterns etc. Let us consider the example from the area of natural language processing. Let us adopt the following rule.

(1) $< S_1 > \rightarrow < S_2 > < S\text{-}Conj> < S_3 >$,

where $< S_1 >$ means a *complex sentence*, $< S_2 >$ means an *independent clause* of $< S_1 >$, $< S\text{-}Conj>$ means a *subordinating conjunction* and $< S_3 >$ means a *dependent clause* of $< S_1 >$.

This rule defines the way of constructing a (well-formed) structure for any complex sentence. However, in order to make it useful in practice we have to define rules for constructing (well-formed) structures of $< S_2 >$ and $< S_3 >$ at the lower level of the syntactic hierarchy. Therefore, let us introduce e.g., the following rules.[24]

(2) $< S_2 > \rightarrow < S > < C\text{-}Conj> < S >$ ,

(3) $< S_3 > \rightarrow < NP > < VP >$ ,

(4) $< S\text{-}Conj> \rightarrow$ **after** ,

---

[23]The patterns $P_1, P_2, \ldots, P_n$ can constitute the goal of the recognition procedure themselves in other cases.

[24]We are not defining here the complete set of rules of syntax for the English language, but only exemplary rules.

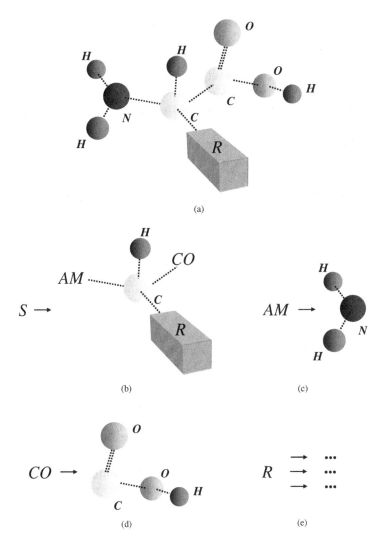

Fig. 1.9  (a) The generic structure of amino acids.  (b) The highest-level rule generating the generic structure of any amino acid.  (c) The second-level rule generating the amine group.  (d) The second-level rule generating the carboxyl group.  (e) The second-level rules generating side chains which are specific to various amino acids.

where $<S>$ means a *simple sentence*, $<C-Conj>$ means a *coordinating conjunction*, $<NP>$ means a *noun phrase* and $<VP>$ means a *verb phrase*.

On the one hand, the rules (2) and (3) define the substructures of a complex sentence. On the other hand, they define two well-formed structures of English syntax - rule (2) describes the structure of a *compound sentence* and rule (3) describes one of the structures of a *simple sentence*.

The use of rules (1)-(4) in the (hierarchical) syntax analysis of the sentence: **Mary went to the office and John drove to the airport after they finished** *lunch.* is shown in Fig. 1.8.[25] The sentence is described as a complex sentence which consists of an independent clause and a dependent clause at the highest level of the structure. At the lower level, one can see that the independent clause is a compound sentence and the dependent clause is a simple sentence and so on. Thus, we can analyze the structure of the pattern (of the form of the language sentence in our example) at various levels of the part-of/generalization hierarchy. This hierarchy is expressed by the hierarchy of generative rules of formal grammar.

Let us consider another example of hierarchical syntax analysis. The generic structure of any amino acid is shown in Fig. 1.9a.[26] The structure can be analyzed hierarchically. As we can see, it contains the following substructures: an amine functional group ($-NH_2$), a carboxyl functional group ($-COOH$) and a side chain ($R$ group) which is specific to each amino acid.[27] The highest-level rule expressing this generic structure is shown in Fig. 1.9b, whereas the second-level rules which generate the amine and carboxyl functional groups are shown in Figs. 1.9 c and d, respectively. Let us note that these rules are used for generating all 500 amino acids.

In the previous section we have shown that identifying structural subpatterns allows us to reuse them, which improves the time and space efficiency of the recognition procedures used. In this section we have shown that hierarchy-oriented recognition allows us to identify *meaningful substructures* which can be used for *describing* patterns in terms of their *(multilevel) syntactical characterization*. If such a syntax-based characterization/description of patterns is required rather than their (simple) classification, then the syntactic approach is to be recommended.

In our chemical examples we identified functional groups (e.g., aldehyde, amine and carboxyl groups) as substructures specific for certain classes of chemical compounds. Let us note that functional groups are responsible for the specific chemical reactions of these compounds. That is, we can, for example, predict the behavior of compounds, if we are able to recognize the functional group substructures. The issue of such a structure-based interpretation of patterns is discussed in the following section.

### 1.3.4  *Requirement of Structure-Based Interpretation*

As we have mentioned above, in some application areas generating a structure-based *characterization* of a *pattern* is the goal of the pattern recognition task. Sometimes, even a more difficult goal is to be achieved, that is *interpreting objects* (systems, processes etc.) represented by structural patterns. *Interpretation* means here providing the meaning, stating the essential qualities, explaining the behavior etc. In

---

[25] The reader can easily identify other rules used in this example.

[26] Since there are ca. 500 naturally occurring amino acids, the effect of the reusability of structural subpatterns, discussed in the previous section, is considerable in the case of the use of the syntactic approach.

[27] The whole structure contains equally a carbon atom and a hydrogen atom.

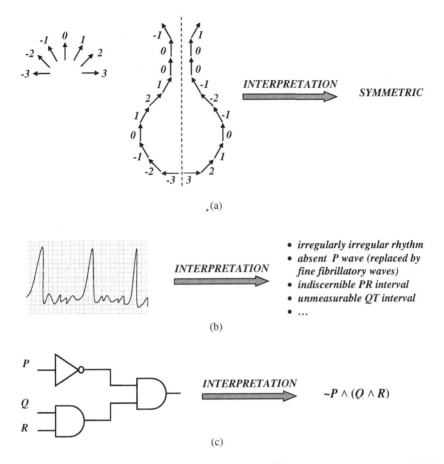

Fig. 1.10 (a) A shape analysis for discovering symmetry. (b) An interpretation of an ECG chart for diagnosing (atrial fibrillation). (c) An interpretation of an electronic circuit for recognizing its function.

the area of computer vision, interpretation typically consists of discovering certain general shape characteristics, like regularities (e.g., shape symmetry, see Fig. 1.10a), irregularities etc. The quantitative knowledge-based interpretation of the specific pattern substructures can be performed in order to:

- identify the behavioral characteristics of objects represented by structural patterns, e.g., predicting the behavior of chemical compounds on the basis of the specific functional groups recognized,
- understand processes represented by structural patterns, e.g., generating interpretations of ECG charts for diagnosing (see Fig. 1.10b),
- predict the functional properties and modes of behaving of systems represented by structural patterns, e.g., interpreting electronic circuits for recognizing their functions (see Fig. 1.10c).

If the objects are so complex that this interpretation can be made only by inferring their global properties from the characteristics of the *substructures* they are composed of, then syntax analysis (parsing) seems to be the most effective technique for such a structural-based interpretation. Therefore, the syntactic approach is to be highly recommended in this case.

# Chapter 2

# Methodology of Syntactic Pattern Recognition

In the previous chapter we have discussed the premises which constitute indications for choosing the syntactic approach for solving a pattern recognition problem. All these premises determine the use of structural patterns and the representation of their syntax with the help of the finite set of generative rules which constitute the formal grammar. We will discuss these two fundamental assumptions of syntactic pattern recognition in a more detailed way in the following sections.

## 2.1 Structural Patterns: Strings, Trees and Graphs

Three types of structural patterns are applied in syntactic pattern recognition: strings, trees and graphs. The adequate pattern type is applied depending on the characteristics of the relationships that are defined among the elements of the structures represented.

A linear structure is the simplest one. Any element of such a structure can be in a relationship with at most two other elements, i.e., with its predecessor and its successor.[1] Moreover, we define one type of the relationship, called the *concatenation*, for linear structures. The patterns used for representing linear structures (of objects/phenomena) are called *strings*. A typical application of strings is representing phenomena charts which have structural characteristics. Strings are used for representing charts of physiological phenomena, e.g., for electrocardiography (ECG), electroencephalography (EEG), pulse wave analysis (PWA), auditory brainstem response (ABR) audiometry, cardiotocography (CTG). They can also represent charts generated by artefactual systems, such as economic systems (technical analysis charts), industrial system process signals etc. From a mathematical point of view (order theory) strings are totally ordered sets.

The part of an ECG signal is shown, for example, in Fig. 2.1a. Let us assume the subset of a set of primitives depicted in Fig. 2.1b. Then, the ECG signal can be represented with the primitives as can be seen in Fig. 2.1c. The linear-structure pattern is defined in Fig. 2.1d as well as the corresponding string. (Let us note that, in fact, a string is a linear graph.)

---

[1] The first and the last elements are in a relationship with the only one element in such a structure.

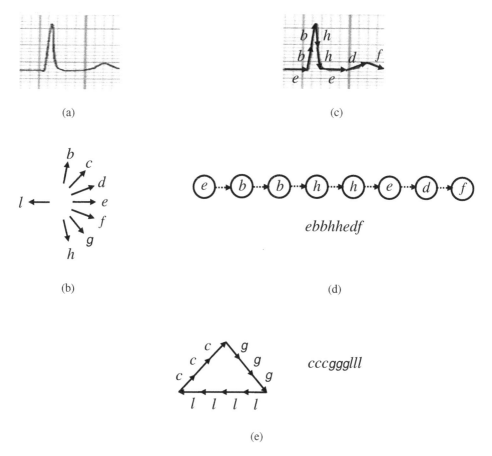

Fig. 2.1   Representing objects/phenomena with strings. (a) The part of an ECG signal. (b) The subset of the exemplary set of primitives. (c) Representing the ECG signal with the primitives. (d) The linear-structure pattern and the corresponding string. (e) Representing the contour with the string.

Representing 2D shapes is another typical application of strings. For example, a contour of a triangle and its representation with the primitives defined is shown in Fig. 2.1e.

*Trees*, which are acyclic (connected) graphs[2] allow us to represent much more complex structural objects/systems than strings. Any element of a tree structure can be in a relationship with many other elements. The typical applications of tree-based models include image analysis and processing, optical character recognition, texture analysis, structure analysis in seismology, natural language processing, speech recognition, analysis of visual events and bioinformatics (representations of macromolecular structures).

For example, the structure of the valine amino acid shown in Fig. 2.2a is depicted

---

[2]The formal definitions concerning trees are presented in Chap. 7.

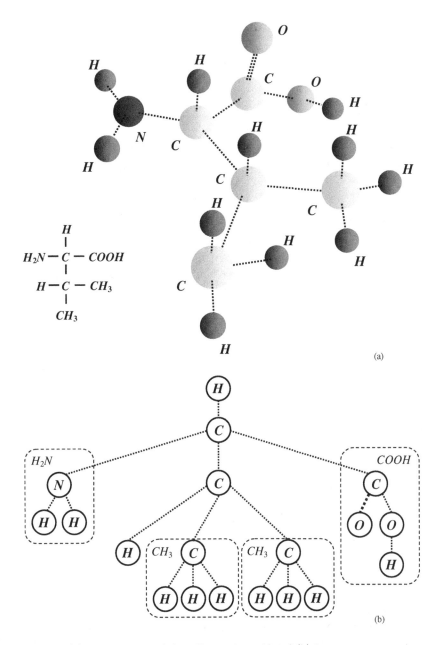

Fig. 2.2 (a) The structure of the valine amino acid and (b) its tree representation.

by the tree shown in Fig. 2.2b. Let us note that from a mathematical point of view trees are partially ordered sets (posets).

If the structures to be represented contain cycles, as in the structure of the phenylalanine amino acid shown in Fig. 2.3, then *graphs* are used. In syntactic pat-

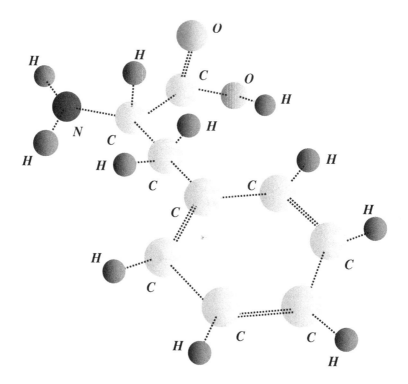

Fig. 2.3   The graph structure of the phenylalanine amino acid.

tern recognition both undirected graphs and directed graphs are applied, depending
on the type of relationships between the pairs of the structure elements considered.
If the relationships are symmetric, like a relation "is bound to" in Figs. 2.2a and
2.3, then the graphs are undirected. If the relationships are asymmetric, like those
considered in scene analysis, then the graphs are directed.

For example, the spatial (3D) and placement relationships are distinguished in
the scene shown in Fig. 2.4a. The scene consists of five objects: the chair ($C$), the
speaker ($S$), the vase ($V$), the pedestal ($P$) and the radiator ($R$). Four relationships
between the pairs of these objects are distinguished: **right, behind-right, behind-
left** and **on**. The structural pattern of the scene in the form of the directed graph
is depicted in Fig. 2.4b. Let us note that, in general, no order is defined for graphs.

The fundamental taxonomy of the syntactic pattern recognition methods is defined just on the basis of the type of the structural patterns applied. Therefore, the
methods in this book are divided into string-, tree-, and graph-based models, which
are presented in Parts: II, III and IV, respectively.

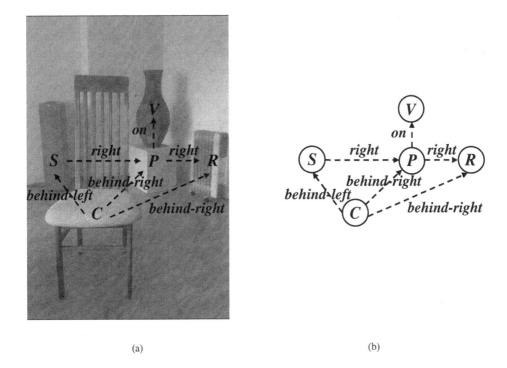

(a)                                       (b)

Fig. 2.4   (a) The scene and (b) its graph representation.

## 2.2   Formal Tools: Grammars - Automata - Induction Algorithms

Three basic formalisms are used in syntactic pattern recognition: a (generative) grammar, a syntax analyzer (automaton) and a language inference (induction) algorithm (cf. Fig. 2.5a). Let us present their roles in syntactic pattern recognition[3]

As we have stated in Sec. 1.3.2, a *(generative) grammar* is a formalism which is used to define the syntax of a formal language treated as a set of structural patterns. The set of *generative rules* is a basic element of the grammar. The grammar is a generative tool, i.e., it can generate any structural pattern of the language considered. Although it plays an auxiliary role, i.e., it is not used for recognition directly, usually it is defined, because its rules allow a human being (i.e., a system designer) to perceive the language syntax in an intuitive way.[4] Later, generative rules will be called *(grammar) productions*. Grammars are introduced with formal definitions in the book and denoted in the following way.

**Definition 2.1** (*<Name of>* **Grammar):** ...

---

[3]Of course, these formalisms are also used in other areas of computer science, e.g., compiler design theory, and then they play different roles from the one presented in this book.

[4]In the case of (the simplest) regular string languages both (regular) grammar rules and (finite-state) automaton transitions are easily perceivable. However, for more complex classes of formal languages, (grammar) rules are a more intuitive way of expressing a language syntax.

A *syntax analyzer* or *parser* means here a formal tool which is defined for a given language (of structural patterns) and constructed on the basis of the grammar generating this language. A parser checks whether a pattern belongs to the language (i.e., it is syntactically correct). Apart from this classification task, a parser can generate an interpretation of the analyzed pattern (cf. Fig. 2.5a). Thus, a parser is a basic formal tool for syntactic pattern recognition. *Parsing schemes* are introduced with formal definitions of corresponding *automata* or with *parser algorithms*[5] in the book and denoted in the following way.

**Parsing Scheme 2.1:** *<Name of Automaton/Parser>*

. . .

Whereas a parsing scheme is specific to the type of the automaton/syntax analyzer, its control table (cf. Fig. 2.5b) is defined on the basis of the productions of a corresponding grammar.[6] Therefore, we need a system which generates the control table on the basis of the set of productions. Such systems, called *parser generators*, are defined for standard syntax analyzers within compiler design theory (see Sec. 3.1).

The last issue concerns constructing a grammar for a given language. In the case of typical applications of the theory of formal languages in computer science (e.g., programming languages and compilers design) formalisms of grammars and automata are sufficient. Grammars are constructed on the basis of the pre-defined syntax of (artefactual) languages.[7] In syntactic pattern recognition, however, a (pattern) language is usually given by a sample of (structural) patterns (a learning set). Therefore, we need a *language inference (induction)* algorithm which generates grammars or automata on the basis of the sample. *Language induction schemes* are introduced as algorithms in the book and denoted in the following way.

**Induction Scheme 2.1:** *<Name of Inference Algorithm>*

. . .

The general scheme of the syntactic pattern recognition system is shown in Fig. 2.5b. The system can work in two modes. In the *learning mode* the system generates the control table of the syntax analyzer, whereas in the *recognition mode* the system classifies an unknown image/object and can provide its interpretation. The *preprocessing* module decomposes an image/object into the primitives. If the syntactic pattern recognition system is constructed in the area of computer vision, this module performs firstly the important operations of *image processing* [Fu and Rosenfeld (1976)] including, e.g.,:

---

[5]Depending on which way is more convenient for the reader.
[6]That is, the control table changes, if the set of structural patterns (i.e., the language) changes.
[7]That is, the syntax of programming languages is given.

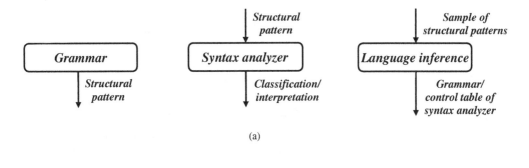

(a)

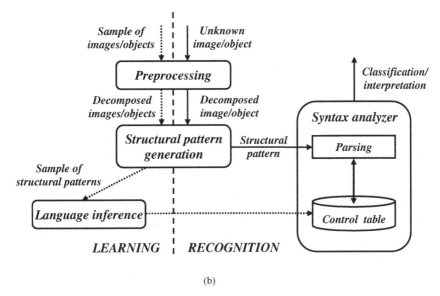

(b)

Fig. 2.5   (a) Formal tools and (b) the general scheme of the syntactic pattern recognition system.

- noise reduction,
- smoothing,
- contrast enhancement,
- image restoration.

For example, the input image shown in Fig. 2.6a during the preprocessing phase is filtered and smoothed, which gives the preprocessed image shown in Fig. 2.6b.

Secondly, the image is decomposed into primitives. For any specific recognition problem the set of primitives has to be pre-defined. The decomposition is usually performed using the computer vision operations of edge/boundary detection and image segmentation.

For our exemplary ECG application the primitives: <PR>, <R>, <ST+> and <T+> from this set are shown in Fig. 2.6c. The sub-image (marked in Fig. 2.6b) decomposed in such a way that these primitives are identified is shown in Fig. 2.6d.

Issues of image processing are not presented in the book. The reader is referred to classic monographs on image processing [Gonzales and Woods (2008); Jain (1989); Pratt (2013); Rosenfeld and Kak (1982); Sonka *et al.* (2015)] and handbooks on computer vision [Chen *et al.* (1993, 1999); Chen and Wang (2005); Chen (2010, 2016)]. The impact of image processing on syntactic pattern recognition is discussed in Chap. 13.

After an image is preprocessed and decomposed into primitives its structural pattern is generated (cf. Fig. 2.5b). In the case of string patterns this phase is usually trivial. For example, for our exemplary ECG sub-image its structural pattern is defined just by concatenating the succeeding primitives, i.e., it is of the form <PR><R><ST+><T+>. However, in the case of tree patterns or graph patterns, especially when various relationships between pairs of primitives can be defined, the issue of a structural pattern generation is more complex.

A definition of classes of grammars which have a strong descriptive power and the corresponding parsing algorithms of the low time complexity is the first main objective of research into syntactic pattern recognition [Flasiński (2016b)]. The (standard) theory of formal languages[8] delivers two classes of grammars, i.e., the regular and context-free ones with the corresponding two types of automata, i.e., the finite-state and pushdown ones, respectively. These two standard formalisms are introduced in the context of syntactic pattern recognition in the first part of Chap. 3 (Sections: 3.1 and 3.2). In the second part of Chap. 3 (Section 3.3) the models of syntactic recognition of vague/distorted patterns, i.e., stochastic languages, fuzzy languages, error-correcting parsers and hidden Markov models, are presented.

For some applications the descriptive/discriminating power of context-free grammars and (standard) pushdown syntax analyzers is too low. In such cases we cannot use context-sensitive grammars since the corresponding linear bounded automata are computationally inefficient. In order to solve this problem, *enhanced* classes of string grammars are defined. The syntactic pattern recognition models based on such enhanced classes are introduced in Chap. 4.

Of course, we increase the descriptive/discriminating power of the syntactic pattern recognition models when we represent images/objects with tree and graph structural patterns. Then, we have to use tree grammars/automata and graph grammars/parsers. The syntactic pattern recognition models based on these advanced formalisms are presented in Chapters 7 and 10, respectively.

A definition of language inference (induction) algorithms is the second main objective of research in syntactic pattern recognition [Flasiński (2016b)]. Inference algorithms of string, tree and graph languages are introduced in Chapters 5, 8 and 11, respectively.

Chapters 6, 9 and 12 contain surveys on the applications of string-, tree- and graph-based models of the syntactic pattern recognition presented in Parts II, III and IV of the book.

---

[8]Notions of the theory of formal languages are included in Appendix A.

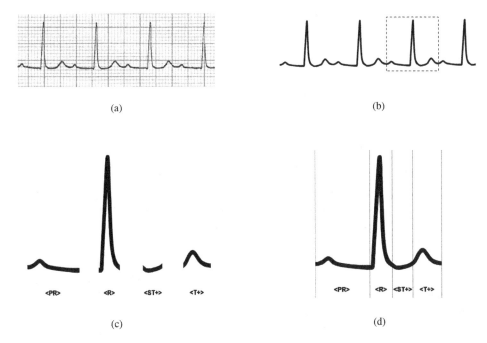

Fig. 2.6   Image processing in the ECG syntactic pattern recognition system: (a) The exemplary input image, (b) the image after preprocessing, (c) the exemplary primitives and (d) the decomposed image.

The last part of the book contains two chapters. A summary of the results and the open problems in syntactic pattern recognition are presented in Chap. 13. The methodological issues which influence future research into syntactic pattern recognition methods are discussed in Chap. 14.

## 2.3   Place of Syntactic Pattern Recognition in Computer Science

To summarize this methodological chapter we discuss the place of syntactic pattern recognition in computer science. This is shown in Fig. 2.7.[9] The relation between *pattern recognition* and *syntactic pattern recognition* has been discussed in the previous chapter.

Syntactic pattern recognition is also closely related to the area of computer vision. In fact, most of the syntactic pattern recognition applications, based on string, tree and graph models, are developed in this area. *Computer vision* is a research field in which the research goal is the development of systems performing tasks as performed by the human visual system. Since we refer here to the *human* visual system, computer vision is sometimes seen as a part of Artificial Intelligence

---

[9]The theory of formal languages and automata is also used in theoretical computer science (computability theory, computational complexity theory), mathematical logic (formal theories, formal systems, model theory etc.) and mathematics (e.g., combinatorics on words).

(AI) [Flasiński (2016a)]. The basic research areas of computer vision include the following issues.

(1) Image acquisition.
(2) Image preprocessing.
(3) Feature[10] extraction.
(4) Image segmentation.
(5) Image representation generation.
(6) Image recognition.

Let us note that all these phases are to be performed in a syntactic pattern recognition system used for *image* recognition. In the scheme of the syntactic pattern recognition system shown in Fig. 2.5b, we have assumed that an image has been obtained in a computer (point 1 in the list above). The operations of points 2-4 are included in the *preprocessing* phase in the scheme, whereas *image representation generation* (point 5) consists of *structural pattern generation* in the syntactic pattern recognition system. *Image recognition* (point 6) is performed with the help of the *syntax analyzer* in the system. Thus, syntactic pattern recognition concerns, in fact, recognizing structural patterns of images.[11]

Other important research areas of computer vision include: color and shading processing, texture processing, 3D vision, tracking, motion and virtual reality. The issues of computer vision which are outside the area of syntactic pattern recognition are not presented in the present book. The reader is referred to monographs on computer vision [Ballard and Brown (1982); Chen *et al.* (1993, 1999); Chen and Wang (2005); Chen (2010, 2011, 2016); Davis (2012); Forsyth and Ponce (2012); Jain *et al.* (1995); Klette (2014); Marr (1982); Shapiro and Stockman (2001); Steger *et al.* (2018); Szeliski (2011)]

Formal languages applied for constructing syntactic pattern recognition models in the computer vision area are called *visual pattern languages* in this book (cf. Fig. 2.7). Their applications include[12]

- shape and picture analysis,
- optical character recognition (OCR),
- analysis of medical images,
- scene analysis
- analysis of visual events and activities (including sign language recognition and anomaly behavior detection),
- analysis of architectural objects,
- texture analysis,
- fingerprint recognition.

---

[10]For example, edges, corners, ellipses, blobs and ridges are image features.
[11]These structural patterns have to be obtained with the help of methods which belong to other subareas of computer vision.
[12]These applications are surveyed in Chaps. 6, 9 and 12.

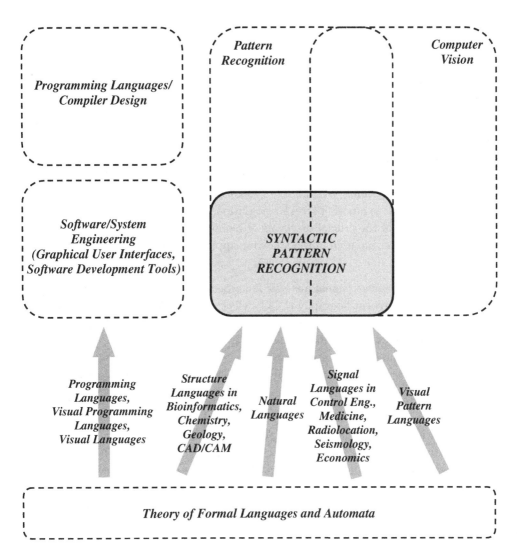

Fig. 2.7 The place of syntactic pattern recognition in computer science.

Syntactic pattern recognition is also applied for recognizing *natural languages* (cf. Fig. 2.7). Stochastic finite-state automata, fuzzy regular grammars, weighted finite-state transducers, hidden Markov models, $k$-testable languages, $LR(k)$ parsers and error-correcting Cocke-Younger-Kasami parsers have been applied for *speech recognition*. Stochastic context-free grammars, stochastic tree grammars, $LR(k)$ parsers and Cocke-Younger-Kasami parsers have been used in the area of *Natural Language Processing (NLP)*.

*Structure languages* in syntactic pattern recognition represent structures of natural objects and artifacts. They are applied for

- structure analysis of RNA/DNA, protein secondary structure prediction, etc., in *bioinformatics*,
- structure analysis in *chemistry*,
- structure analysis in *geology*,
- feature recognition in *computer aided design and manufacturing* (*CAD/CAM*).

Extensive research into syntactic-pattern-recognition-based methods for bioinformatics was launched in the last decade of the 20th century. It has resulted in the development of many efficient analysis models based on the inference of stochastic regular grammars, hidden Markov models, stochastic context-free grammars, stochastic Tree Adjoining Grammars (TAGs) and stochastic tree grammars. Indeed, it seems that syntactic pattern recognition will deliver the basic formal tools for solving many of the crucial problems of bioinformatics in the 21st century.

*Signal languages* are used in the following applications areas of syntactic pattern recognition.

- *Control engineering* (signal analysis for process monitoring and control),
- *medicine* (electrocardiography (ECG), electroencephalography (EEG), etc.),
- *radiolocation* (radar target recognition, radar surveillance and tracking, infrared location of airborne objects, etc.),
- *seismology* (analysis of seismic wavelets, detection of bright spots),
- *finance/economics* (technical analysis, time series analysis in economics).

*Programming languages/compiler design* has been the main application area of the theory of formal languages and automata since the beginning of computer science (cf. Fig. 2.7). It has delivered all the standard syntax analyzers for recognizing string context-free languages, including: $LL(k)$ languages, $LR(k)$ languages, precedence parsing, Earley parsing and Cocke-Younger-Kasami parsing.[13] *Visual (programming) languages* used in *software/system engineering* have been developed since the 1980s. Since some formal models of visual languages are used in syntactic pattern recognition, we present them in a concise way in Chap. 4.

---

[13]These models are presented in Chap. 3.

# PART 2
# STRING-BASED MODELS

## Chapter 3

# Pattern Recognition Based on Regular and CF Grammars

String-based models of syntactic pattern recognition are defined with the help of Chomsky's generative grammars[1] [Chomsky (1956, 1959, 1965)]. According to the Chomsky hierarchy, these grammars can be divided into four types depending on their *generative power*. Since the notion of the generative power of a type of grammar is crucial in syntactic pattern recognition (not only for Chomsky's string grammars), we shall introduce it now.

Let $L(G)$ be a language generated by a grammar $G$. Let $X$ denote a type of grammars. The corresponding class $X$ of languages constitutes the set

$$\mathcal{L}(X) = \{L : \ \exists \ G \ of \ the \ type \ X \ such \ that \ L = L(G)\}.$$

That is, $\mathcal{L}(X)$ is the set of all the languages $L$ which can be generated by any grammar $G$ of the class $X$. We say that grammars of a type $X$ have greater generative power than grammars of a type $Y$ iff $\mathcal{L}(Y) \subsetneq \mathcal{L}(X)$.

Let $UNR$, $CSG$, $CFG$ and $REG$ denote the following types of Chomsky's grammars: unrestricted, context-sensitive, context-free and regular, respectively. The following theorem establishes the Chomsky hierarchy.[2]

**Theorem 3.1 (Chomsky Hierarchy [Chomsky (1959)])**

$$\mathcal{L}(REG) \subsetneq \mathcal{L}(CFG) \subsetneq \mathcal{L}(CSG) \subsetneq \mathcal{L}(UNR)$$

A formal grammar is the generator of a set of pattern structural representations[3] in syntactic pattern recognition, whereas a formal automaton is used for recognizing/accepting these representations. The following four types of formal automata[4] are recognizers of languages generated by Chomsky's grammars: a Turing machine, *TM* [Turing (1937)], a linear-bounded automaton, *LBA* [Myhill (1960);

---

[1] The formal definitions concerning Chomsky's generative grammars are included in Appendix A.1.

[2] Languages generated by unrestricted grammars are sometimes called recursively enumerable (RE) or recognizable.

[3] As we have mentioned, a set of pattern structural representations is treated as a formal language in syntactic pattern recognition.

[4] The definitions of formal automata are included in Appendix A.2.

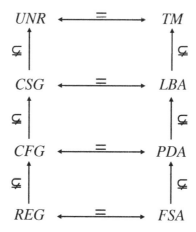

Fig. 3.1   The relations among the classes of string languages.

Kuroda (1964)], a pushdown automaton, *PDA* [Chomsky (1962)] and a finite-state automaton, *FSA* [Shannon (1948); Kleene (1956); Chomsky and Miller (1958); Rabin and Scott (1959)]. Now, let us denote a set of all the languages $L$ which can be accepted/recognized by an automaton $A$ of a class $X$ with $\mathcal{L}(X)$. The following theorem establishes the correspondence between grammars and automata [Chomsky (1959, 1962); Bar-Hillel *et al.* (1961); Schützenberger (1963); Landweber (1963); Davis (1958)].

### Theorem 3.2 (Grammars - Automata Correspondence)

$$\mathcal{L}(REG) = \mathcal{L}(FSA)$$
$$\mathcal{L}(CFG) = \mathcal{L}(PDA)$$
$$\mathcal{L}(CSG) = \mathcal{L}(LBA)$$
$$\mathcal{L}(UNR) = \mathcal{L}(TM)$$

On the basis of both theorems we can define the diagram which presents the relations among the classes of languages generated by Chomsky's grammars and the classes of languages accepted/recognized by corresponding automata as in Fig. 3.1.

Although unrestricted and context-sensitive grammars are of great generative power, they are not used in syntactic pattern recognition because the corresponding automata, i.e. *TM* and *LBA*, are inefficient computationally. Therefore, in Sec. 3.1 and 3.2 ideas of constructing syntactic pattern recognition models which are based on regular and context-free grammars are introduced. The extensions of such models for the recognition of vague/distorted patterns are presented in Sec. 3.3. All the notions and denotations of formal language theory used in this chapter are introduced in Appendix A.

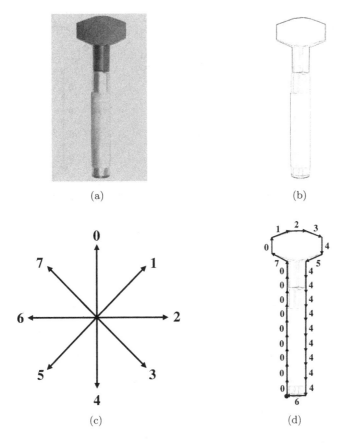

Fig. 3.2 Representation of the object with Freeman chain codes.

## 3.1 Recognition with Finite-State Automata

As we have mentioned in Chap. 2, a syntactic pattern recognition model consists of three basic formalisms: a grammar, a syntax analyzer and a language inference algorithm. Additionally, for generating a parser control table on the basis of a set of grammar productions a parser generator is needed. The issue of a parser control generation is a standard problem of compiler design theory. Therefore, we present the issue *only* for finite-state automata in this section and for $LL(k)$ parsers in the next section, just to show the problem. In the case of the remaining parsing schemes the reader is referred to classic textbooks on compiler design theory [Aho *et al.* (2007); Cooper and Torczon (2011); Grune *et al.* (2012); Mak (2009); Muchnick (1997)]. Language inference schemes will be discussed for string-, tree- and graph-based models in Chapters: 5, 8 and 11, respectively. However, in this section the idea of canonical grammar induction will be introduced.

Let us begin by presenting the basic ideas and formalisms for the recognition

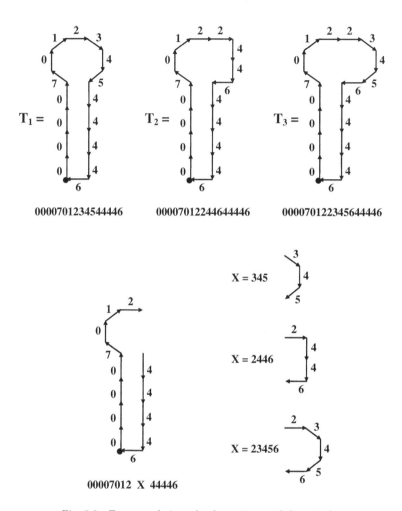

Fig. 3.3   Freeman chain codes for contours of three tools.

of patterns described with regular languages with an example of a contour recognition[5]. Let us assume that for a contour description Freeman chain codes [Freeman (1961); Feder (1968)] are used as structural primitives, as shown in Fig. 3.2. If we determine the starting point as the leftmost and lowermost point of a contour (marked with a dot in Fig. 3.2 d), then a wrench is represented with the word 00000000070123454444444446. We treat this word as belonging to a formal language over a set of (terminal) symbols $\Sigma_T = \{0, 1, 2, 3, 4, 5, 6, 7\}$ which are interpreted as Freeman chain codes.

Now, we shall consider an example of defining a regular grammar[6] for a set of structural patterns treated as a formal language. Patterns $T_1$, $T_2$ and $T_3$ represented with the Freeman chain codes 0000701234544446, 00007012244644446 and

---

[5] A recognition of contours is one of typical applications of string-based methods.

[6] A regular grammar is defined in Appendix A.1.

000070122345644446, respectively, are shown in Fig. 3.3. The grammar is defined in the following way. ($\Sigma_T$ has already been defined above.)

$G = (\Sigma_N, \Sigma_T, P, S)$, where:

$\Sigma_N = \{S, A_1, A_2, \ldots, A_{20}\}$,

$\Sigma_T = \{0, 1, 2, 3, 4, 5, 6, 7\}$,

$P$ consists of the following productions:

Productions generating the representation of the tool $T_1$.

(1) $S \rightarrow 0A_1$　　(5) $A_4 \rightarrow 7A_5$　　(9) $A_8 \rightarrow 3A_9$　　(13) $A_{12} \rightarrow 4A_{13}$

(2) $A_1 \rightarrow 0A_2$　　(6) $A_5 \rightarrow 0A_6$　　(10) $A_9 \rightarrow 4A_{10}$　　(14) $A_{13} \rightarrow 4A_{14}$

(3) $A_2 \rightarrow 0A_3$　　(7) $A_6 \rightarrow 1A_7$　　(11) $A_{10} \rightarrow 5A_{11}$　　(15) $A_{14} \rightarrow 4A_{15}$

(4) $A_3 \rightarrow 0A_4$　　(8) $A_7 \rightarrow 2A_8$　　(12) $A_{11} \rightarrow 4A_{12}$　　(16) $A_{15} \rightarrow 6$

Productions generating the representation of the tool $T_2$: (1), (2), (3), (4), (5), (6), (7), (8), (12), (13), (14), (15), (16) and the following ones.

(17) $A_8 \rightarrow 2A_{16}$　　(18) $A_{16} \rightarrow 4A_{17}$　　(19) $A_{17} \rightarrow 4A_{18}$　　(20) $A_{18} \rightarrow 6A_{11}$

Productions generating the representation of the tool $T_3$: (1), (2), (3), (4), (5), (6), (7), (8), (12), (13), (14), (15), (16), (17), (20) and the following ones.

(21) $A_{16} \rightarrow 3A_{19}$　　(22) $A_{19} \rightarrow 4A_{20}$　　(23) $A_{20} \rightarrow 5A_{18}$

For example, let us derive the chain code representation of the tool $T_2$. (The following sequence of productions is applied: 1, 2, 3, 4, 5, 6, 7, 8, 17, 18, 19, 20, 12, 13, 14, 15, 16.)

$S \Rightarrow 0A_1 \Rightarrow 00A_2 \Rightarrow 000A_3 \Rightarrow 0000A_4 \Rightarrow 00007A_5 \Rightarrow 000070A_6 \Rightarrow 0000701A_7 \Rightarrow$
$\Rightarrow 00007012A_8 \Rightarrow 000070122A_{16} \Rightarrow 0000701224A_{17} \Rightarrow 00007012244A_{18} \Rightarrow$
$\Rightarrow 000070122446A_{11} \Rightarrow 0000701224464A_{12} \Rightarrow 00007012244644A_{13} \Rightarrow$
$\Rightarrow 000070122446444A_{14} \Rightarrow 0000701224464444A_{15} \Rightarrow 00007012244644446 .$

This example has been presented also in order to show the essential idea of syntactic pattern recognition, as discussed in Chap. 1. Let us notice that each pattern $T_i$ consists of two subpatterns (substructures) as shown in Fig. 3.3. The first subpattern, denoted by $00007012X44446$ in Fig. 3.3, is common to all the patterns. The patterns differ from each other in the second subpattern, denoted by $X$ in Fig. 3.3. Therefore, after defining all the productions for the pattern $T_1$, for the patterns $T_2$ and $T_3$ we have defined those productions generating the second subpattern ($X$) only. (For generating their first subpattern we can use productions which have already been defined for $T_1$.) This advantageous effect enhances as the number of patterns increases and the patterns are decomposable into various combinations of simpler subpatterns hierarchically. (Primitives are the simplest subpatterns at the bottom of such a hierarchy.)

Now, before constructing a finite-state automaton for the grammar $G$, we introduce the general rules of constructing finite-state automata on the basis of regular grammars.[7]

Let $G = (\Sigma_N, \Sigma_T, P, S)$ be a (right-) regular grammar.[8] A finite-state automaton[9] $A = (Q, \Sigma_T, \delta, q_0, F)$ such that $L(A) = L(G)$ is constructed in the following way.

(1) $Q := \Sigma_N$.
(2) $q_0 := S$.
(3) $F := \{T\}$.
(4) For every $A \rightarrow aB \in P$, $A, B \in \Sigma_N, a \in \Sigma_T$ add a transition $\delta(A, a) = B$. (If a production is in the recursive form $A \rightarrow aA$, then add a transition $\delta(A, a) = A$.)
(5) For every $A \rightarrow a \in P$, $A \in \Sigma_N, a \in \Sigma_T$ add a transition $\delta(A, a) = T$.

Let us define the automaton $A$ for the grammar $G$ according to the rules introduced.

$A = (Q, \Sigma_T, \delta, q_0, F)$, where:
$Q = \{S, A_1, A_2, \ldots, A_{20}, T\}$,
$\Sigma_T = \{0, 1, 2, 3, 4, 5, 6, 7\}$,
$q_0 = S$,
$F = \{T\}$,
$\delta : Q \times \Sigma_T \longrightarrow Q$ is defined as follows (the productions are presented for each transition as well):

| | | | | |
|---|---|---|---|---|
| (1) $S \rightarrow 0A_1$, | $\delta(S, 0) = A_1$ | | (13) $A_{12} \rightarrow 4A_{13}$, | $\delta(A_{12}, 4) = A_{13}$ |
| (2) $A_1 \rightarrow 0A_2$, | $\delta(A_1, 0) = A_2$ | | (14) $A_{13} \rightarrow 4A_{14}$, | $\delta(A_{13}, 4) = A_{14}$ |
| (3) $A_2 \rightarrow 0A_3$, | $\delta(A_2, 0) = A_3$ | | (15) $A_{14} \rightarrow 4A_{15}$, | $\delta(A_{14}, 4) = A_{15}$ |
| (4) $A_3 \rightarrow 0A_4$, | $\delta(A_3, 0) = A_4$ | | (16) $A_{15} \rightarrow 6$, | $\delta(A_{15}, 6) = T$ |
| (5) $A_4 \rightarrow 7A_5$, | $\delta(A_4, 7) = A_5$ | | (17) $A_8 \rightarrow 2A_{16}$, | $\delta(A_8, 2) = A_{16}$ |
| (6) $A_5 \rightarrow 0A_6$, | $\delta(A_5, 0) = A_6$ | | (18) $A_{16} \rightarrow 4A_{17}$, | $\delta(A_{16}, 4) = A_{17}$ |
| (7) $A_6 \rightarrow 1A_7$, | $\delta(A_6, 1) = A_7$ | | (19) $A_{17} \rightarrow 4A_{18}$, | $\delta(A_{17}, 4) = A_{18}$ |
| (8) $A_7 \rightarrow 2A_8$, | $\delta(A_7, 2) = A_8$ | | (20) $A_{18} \rightarrow 6A_{11}$, | $\delta(A_{18}, 6) = A_{11}$ |
| (9) $A_8 \rightarrow 3A_9$, | $\delta(A_8, 3) = A_9$ | | (21) $A_{16} \rightarrow 3A_{19}$, | $\delta(A_{16}, 3) = A_{19}$ |
| (10) $A_9 \rightarrow 4A_{10}$, | $\delta(A_9, 4) = A_{10}$ | | (22) $A_{19} \rightarrow 4A_{20}$, | $\delta(A_{19}, 4) = A_{20}$ |
| (11) $A_{10} \rightarrow 5A_{11}$, | $\delta(A_{10}, 5) = A_{11}$ | | (23) $A_{20} \rightarrow 5A_{18}$, | $\delta(A_{20}, 5) = A_{18}$ |
| (12) $A_{11} \rightarrow 4A_{12}$, | $\delta(A_{11}, 4) = A_{12}$ | | | |

---

[7] One can construct a parser (control) generator according to these rules.
[8] We assume that $G$ is a $\lambda$-free grammar, cf. Definition A.6 in Appendix A.1.
[9] A finite-state automaton is defined in Appendix A.2.

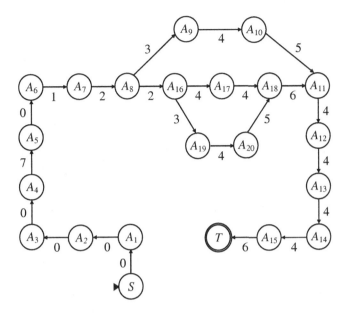

Fig. 3.4   The finite state automaton $A$ which recognizes the contours of three tools.

The diagram of the automaton $A$ is shown in Fig. 3.4.

For example, parsing of the chain code representation of the tool $T_2$ is performed by the automaton $A$ in the following way:

$(S, 00007012244644446) \vdash (A_1, 0007012244644446) \vdash (A_2, 007012244644446) \vdash$
$\vdash (A_3, 07012244644446) \vdash (A_4, 7012244644446) \vdash (A_5, 012244644446) \vdash$
$\vdash (A_6, 12244644446) \vdash (A_7, 2244644446) \vdash (A_8, 244644446) \vdash (A_{16}, 44644446) \vdash$
$\vdash (A_{17}, 4644446) \vdash (A_{18}, 644446) \vdash (A_{11}, 44446) \vdash (A_{12}, 4446) \vdash (A_{13}, 446) \vdash$
$\vdash (A_{14}, 46) \vdash (A_{15}, 6) \vdash (T, )$ .

Thus, the automaton $A$ has accepted the representation of $T_2$, i.e. it has recognized this representation as belonging to $L(A) = L(G)$. One can easily notice that testing whether $w \in L(A)$ is efficient. It takes $\mathcal{O}(n)$ time, where $n$ is the length of $w$.

Let us introduce the following denotation. Let $\Sigma$ be a set of symbols, $\mathbb{N}$ be a set of natural numbers (with 0). If $a \in \Sigma$, $n \in \mathbb{N}$, then

$$a^n = \underbrace{aa \dots a}_{n \ times} .$$

$a^0 = \lambda$, where $\lambda$ is the empty word. For example, the representation of the tool $T_2$: $00007012244644446 = 0^4 7012^2 4^2 64^4 6$. This denotation can be extended for groups of symbols, i.e., $(abc)^3 = (abc)(abc)(abc) = abcabcabc$, $a, b, c \in \Sigma$.

As we have discussed in Chap. 2, there are two main scenarios of defining a grammar in syntactic pattern recognition. Firstly, a grammar $G$ can be generated with a grammatical inference (induction) algorithm, if a set of sample patterns

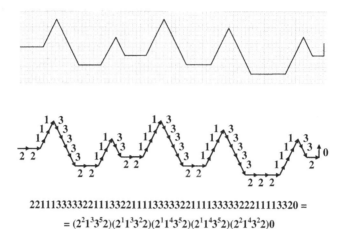

$$2211133333322111332211111333333221111333333222111113320 =$$
$$= (2^2 1^3 3^5 2)(2^1 1^3 3^2 2)(2^1 1^4 3^5 2)(2^1 1^4 3^5 2)(2^2 1^4 3^2 2)0$$

Fig. 3.5　An exemplary waveform of the regular language $L$.

is available.[10] Secondly, a grammar $G$ can be defined by hand, if the formalized characteristics of a language $L$ which represents the patterns considered are given. In the second case after defining $G$ we have to prove that $L = L(G)$, i.e., that we can generate $L$ and only $L$ with grammar productions. Thus, we should prove that $L \subseteq L(G)$ and $L \supseteq L(G)$. We consider this issue with the following example:

Let there be given the set of waveforms[11] of the form shown in Fig. 3.5. They are described with the subset of Freeman chain codes $\Sigma_T = \{0, 1, 2, 3\}$. The language that represents the waveforms is defined as $L = \{\alpha \in \Sigma_T^+ : \alpha = (2^{k_1} 1^{m_1} 3^{n_1} 2)(2^{k_2} 1^{m_2} 3^{n_2} 2) \ldots (2^{k_j} 1^{m_j} 3^{n_j} 2)0, \ k_i \geq 1, \ m_i \geq 1, \ n_i \geq 1, \ i = 1, \ldots, j\} \cup \{ \ 0 \ \}$. That is, each pattern consists of $j$ waves, $j \geq 0$, and there is one symbol 0 at the end of the whole pattern. Each wave consists of: the sequence of 2s $(2^{k_i}, k_i \geq 1)$, then the sequence of 1s $(1^{m_i}, m_i \geq 1)$, then the sequence of 3s $(3^{n_i}, n_i \geq 1)$, and it ends with 2.

Let us define the grammar $G$ such that $L = L(G)$.
$G = (\Sigma_N, \Sigma_T, P, S)$, where:
$\Sigma_N = \{S, A, B, C\}$,
$P$ consists of the following productions.

(1) $S \rightarrow 2A$　(3) $A \rightarrow 1B$　(5) $B \rightarrow 3C$　(7) $C \rightarrow 2S$

(2) $A \rightarrow 2A$　(4) $B \rightarrow 1B$　(6) $C \rightarrow 3C$　(8) $S \rightarrow 0$

Now, let us prove that $L = L(G)$. Firstly, we should show that $L \subseteq L(G)$, which means that for any $\alpha$ if $\alpha \in L$, then $\alpha \in L(G)$. That is, we should show that if we take any $\alpha$ which is of the form described by the definition of $L$, then we can generate it with productions of the grammar $G$.

---

[10]A set of sample patterns is represented as the set of the sample words of a formal language.
[11]A recognition of waveforms is one of the typical applications of string-based methods.

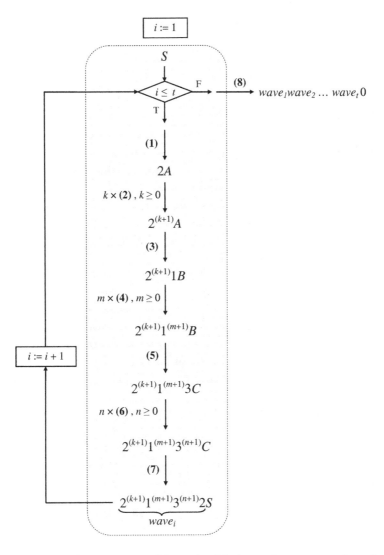

Fig. 3.6    Scheme of generating possible words with the regular grammar of waveforms.

Firstly, let us take $\alpha = 0$, i.e., $j = 0$. To generate it we should apply production 8 once.

Let us take any

$$\alpha = \underbrace{(2^{p_1}1^{r_1}3^{s_1}2)}_{wave_1}\underbrace{(2^{p_2}1^{r_2}3^{s_2}2)}_{wave_2}\ldots\underbrace{(2^{p_t}1^{r_t}3^{s_t}2)}_{wave_t}0 \; , p_i \geq 1, \; r_i \geq 1, \; s_i \geq 1, \; i = 1,\ldots,t \; .$$

One can easily notice that in order to generate $wave_1$ the following derivation sequence should be performed.

(1) Production 1 should be applied once.

(2) Production 2 should be applied ($p_1 - 1$) times.
(3) Production 3 should be applied once.
(4) Production 4 should be applied ($r_1 - 1$) times.
(5) Production 5 should be applied once.
(6) Production 6 should be applied ($s_1 - 1$) times.
(7) Production 7 should be applied once.

After this derivation sequence we obtain the string $2^{p_1} 1^{r_1} 3^{s_1} 2S$. If $t > 1$, then we should continue the derivation according to the scheme defined above, otherwise we should apply production 8. After generating all the waves we should apply production 8. In this way we have proved that $L \subseteq L(G)$.

Now, we should prove that $L \supseteq L(G)$, which means that for any $\alpha$ if $\alpha \in L(G)$, then $\alpha \in L$. That is, we should show that if we take any $\alpha \in \Sigma_T^+$ which is derived from $S$, then $\alpha$ is of the form described by the definition of $L$. A scheme of possible sequences of productions in $G$ is shown in Fig. 3.6.

Firstly, we can apply production 8 and finish a derivation generating the word $\alpha = 0 \in L$. If we apply for $S$ production 1 we have to perform a derivation sequence included in the grey area in Fig. 3.6. This sequence generates a string consisting of a wave belonging to $L$ and concatenated with $S$. Then, we are again at the starting point. So we can apply production 8 and finish the derivation which generates the word $\alpha \in L$ or we can begin the generation of the next wave. Anyway, one can easily see that if we perform a sequence of productions of $G$ which finishes with $\alpha \in \Sigma_T^+$, then $\alpha \in L$.[12]

At the end of this section we introduce a simple algorithm of inference for regular grammars. Let us assume that $S_+ = \{\alpha_i \in \Sigma_T^+ \mid \alpha_i = a_{i_1} a_{i_2} \ldots a_{i_{k(i)}}, \ i = 1, \ldots, s\}$ is a set of words representing a language $L$, called a *positive sample*. A *canonical grammar* [Fu and Booth (1975a)][13] $G = (\Sigma_N, \Sigma_T, P, S)$ generating $S_+$ is inferred with the following scheme.

---

**Induction Scheme 3.1: Canonical Grammar Inference**

$\Sigma_N := \{S\}; \ \Sigma_T := \emptyset; \ P := \emptyset;$
**for** $i := 1$ **to** $s$ **do**
   **if** $\alpha_i = a_{i_1} a_{i_2} \ldots a_{i_{k(i)}}$ **then**
      **begin**
         $P := P \cup \{S \to a_{i_1} X_{i_1}, \ X_{i_1} \to a_{i_2} X_{i_2}, \ \ldots, \ X_{i_{(k(i)-1)}} \to a_{i_{k(i)}}\};$
         $\Sigma_T := \Sigma_T \cup \{a_{i_1}, a_{i_2}, \ldots, a_{i_{k(i)}}\};$
         $\Sigma_N := \Sigma_N \cup \{X_{i_1}, X_{i_2}, \ldots, X_{i_{(k(i)-1)}}\};$
      **end;**

---

[12]Let us notice that the condition $L \supseteq L(G)$ is really essential from a practical point of view. If it did not hold, an automaton $A$ constructed for a grammar $G$ would accept words which do not belong to $L$.

[13]Induction of a canonical grammar is the first phase of various inference methods.

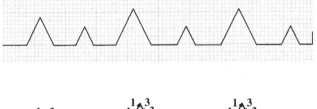

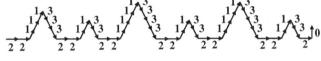

$$(2^21^33^32)(2^11^23^22)(2^11^43^42)(2^11^23^22)(2^11^43^42)(2^11^23^22)0$$

Fig. 3.7   An exemplary symmetric waveform of the context-free language $L$.

For example, if $S^+ = \{0, 212, 5434\}$, then the algorithm infers a grammar $G$ containing the following productions.

(1) $S \rightarrow 0$     (3) $X_1 \rightarrow 1X_2$   (5) $S \rightarrow 5X_3$     (7) $X_4 \rightarrow 3X_5$

(2) $S \rightarrow 2X_1$   (4) $X_2 \rightarrow 2$     (6) $X_3 \rightarrow 4X_4$   (8) $X_5 \rightarrow 4$

## 3.2   Recognition of CF Languages

Context-free (*CF*) languages are widely used for constructing string-based pattern recognition models. This results from the fact that their basic formal characteristics, i.e., generative power and computational efficiency are well-balanced. Let us come back to our example of waveforms considered in a previous section. We modify the example by requiring waveforms to be of the regular form shown in Fig. 3.7.

Each wave is now symmetric, which means that its descending part consists of the same number of primitives as its ascending part. Formally, this new language representing the *symmetric* waveforms is defined as $L = \{\alpha \in \Sigma_T^+ : \alpha = (2^{k_1}1^{m_1}3^{m_1}2)(2^{k_2}1^{m_2}3^{m_2}2)\ldots(2^{k_j}1^{m_j}3^{m_j}2)0, \ k_i \geq 1, \ m_i \geq 2, \ i = 1, \ldots, j\} \cup \{0\}$. Its formula differs from the one defined in a previous section in requiring the same number of 1s as 3s (i.e., $1^{m_i}3^{m_i}$ instead of $1^{m_i}3^{n_i}$).[14] Of course, we cannot generate this new language with a regular grammar, since the form of a regular grammar production makes obtaining such a symmetry impossible.[15]
For the *symmetric wave language* $L$ we define the *CF* grammar $G$ such that $L = L(G)$ in the following way.
$G = (\Sigma_N, \Sigma_T, P, S)$, where:
$\Sigma_N = \{S, A, B\},$

---

[14]Additionally, for simplicity of a grammar, we require a wave consists of at least four primitives.
[15]We can generate waveforms belonging to the *symmetric wave language* $L$ with the help of a grammar $G$ defined in a previous section, i.e. $L \subseteq L(G)$. However, the condition $L \supseteq L(G)$ obviously does not hold.

$P$ consists of the following productions.

$$(1)\ S\ \rightarrow\ 2A \quad (3)\ A\ \rightarrow\ 1B32S \quad (5)\ B\ \rightarrow\ 13$$

$$(2)\ A\ \rightarrow\ 2A \quad (4)\ B\ \rightarrow\ 1B3 \quad\ (6)\ S\ \rightarrow\ 0$$

As we have mentioned above context-free (*CF*) languages are useful for syntactic pattern recognition because their generative power and computational efficiency are well-balanced. Although, in general, pushdown automata recognizing these languages are not as efficient as finite-state automata, we can define polynomial syntax analysis algorithms for *CF* languages and even linear-time algorithms for certain subclasses of *CF* languages. Before we define such algorithms and *CF* subclasses, let us consider the following issues.

Firstly, let us note that, in the case of context-free grammars, one can derive a word in a number of ways[16]. For example, we can generate the word 2113320 with the symmetric wave grammar $G$ defined above applying a production to the left-most nonterminal in any sentential form as follows (replaced nonterminals are underlined, derivation step denotations (arrows) are marked with indices of the productions applied):

$$S \xrightarrow{(1)} 2\underline{A} \xrightarrow{(3)} 21\underline{B}32S \xrightarrow{(5)} 211332\underline{S} \xrightarrow{(6)} 2113320 \ .$$

Such derivations are called *leftmost*.

We can also generate the word applying productions to the right-most nonterminals as follows:

$$S \xrightarrow{(1)} 2\underline{A} \xrightarrow{(3)} 21B32\underline{S} \xrightarrow{(6)} 21\underline{B}320 \xrightarrow{(5)} 2113320 \ .$$

Such derivations are called *rightmost* (or *canonical*).

In order to reduce parsing time complexity we can require a grammar to be not ambiguous (i.e., to be unambiguous). A grammar is *ambiguous* if we can define more than one leftmost or more than one rightmost derivation for the same word.

Secondly, we define a *derivation tree* which can be used for representing a derivation process. A single derivation tree shows how a word (or a sentential form) is derived from the start symbol disregarding the order of applying productions. For example, the derivation of the word 2113320 from our example above is represented by the last derivation tree in Fig. 3.8a. The leaves of the tree read from left to right represent the word. At the same time, as we can see in Fig. 3.8a, the sequence of derivation trees of sentential forms generated during the derivation is a convenient way of representing the derivation. One can easily notice that the leftmost derivation of 2113320 is shown in this figure.

There are two general parsing strategies. The main idea of *top-down parsing* consists in analyzing successive symbols of a word in order to find its leftmost derivation. This strategy for our exemplary word 2113320 is shown in Fig. 3.8b. We

---

[16]If we derive words of a regular language, as in a previous section, we can do this in only one way, because there is only one nonterminal symbol in any sentential form (at the end of the form).

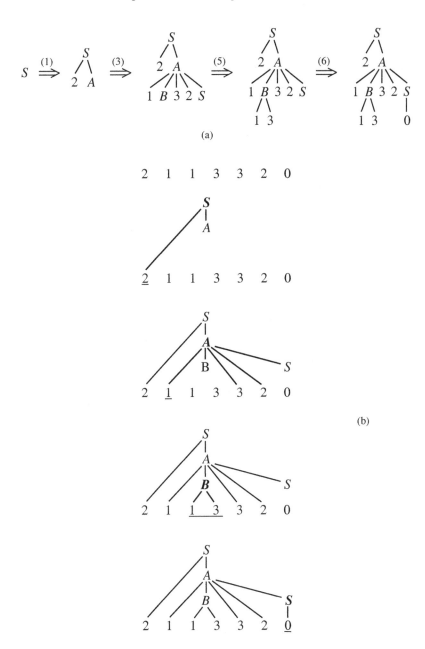

Fig. 3.8   Example of leftmost derivation (a) and top-down parsing (b).

begin with the start symbol and we try to construct the derivation tree expanding it in a top-down manner. Given the nonterminal to be expanded and the prefix of the word (underlined in Fig. 3.8b), we try to predict the production to be applied.[17]

---

[17]In the case of *backtracking parsing* more than one production can match.

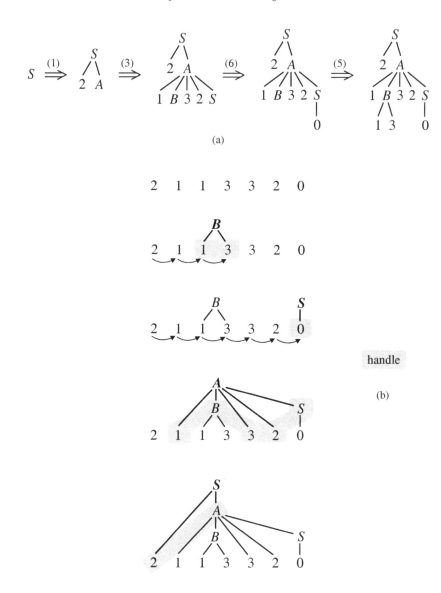

Fig. 3.9   Example of rightmost derivation (a) and bottom-up parsing (b).

The *bottom-up parsing* strategy is based on the rightmost derivation. The rightmost derivation for our exemplary word 2113320 is shown in Fig. 3.9a and its bottom-up parsing is depicted in Fig. 3.9b. This time, as one can see, we construct the derivation tree beginning with its bottom, i.e., beginning at the leaves in order to reach its root. Now, in reading the word we look for those substrings that are right-hand sides of productions. Such substrings are called *handles* and are marked with a grey color in Fig. 3.9b. Once a handle is identified it is replaced (reduced) by the corresponding left-hand side, which is called a *reduction*.

In the following subsections we introduce the basic models of *CF* languages parsing: $LL(k)$, $LR(k)$, precedence-based, Earley parser and CYK.

### 3.2.1 *LL(k) Languages*

The $LL(k)$ parser[18] [Lewis II and Stearns (1968); Rosenkrantz and Stearns (1970)] performs a top-down parsing. It makes predictions according to the Polish prefix (pre-order) traversal of a derivation tree. The parser works deterministically (i.e., without backtracking) if it looks ahead to the $k$-length substrings of an input word. It is defined for an $LL(k)$ subclass of context-free grammars. Firstly, let us introduce this subclass.

Let $G = (\Sigma_N, \Sigma_T, P, S)$ be a context-free grammar, $\eta \in \Sigma^*$, and $| x |$ denote the length of a string $x \in \Sigma^*$.

$FIRST_k(\eta)$ denotes a set of all the terminal prefixes of the strings of the length $k$ (or of a length less than $k$, if a terminal string shorter than $k$ is derived from $\alpha$) that can be derived from $\eta$ in the grammar $G$, i.e.

$$FIRST_k(\eta) = \{x \in \Sigma_T^* : (\eta \overset{*}{\Rightarrow} x\beta \wedge | x |= k) \vee (\eta \overset{*}{\Rightarrow} x \wedge | x |< k) , \ \beta \in \Sigma^*\}.$$

**Definition 3.1 ($LL(k)$ Grammar):** Let $G = (\Sigma_N, \Sigma_T, P, S)$ be a context-free grammar, the leftmost derivation in $G$ be denoted with $\overset{*}{\underset{l(G)}{\Rightarrow}}$ . $G$ is called an $LL(k)$ grammar iff for every two leftmost derivations

$$S \overset{*}{\underset{l(G)}{\Rightarrow}} \alpha A\theta \underset{l(G)}{\Rightarrow} \alpha\beta\theta \overset{*}{\underset{l(G)}{\Rightarrow}} \alpha x$$

$$S \overset{*}{\underset{l(G)}{\Rightarrow}} \alpha A\theta \underset{l(G)}{\Rightarrow} \alpha\gamma\theta \overset{*}{\underset{l(G)}{\Rightarrow}} \alpha y,$$

where $\alpha, x, y \in \Sigma_T^*$, $\beta, \gamma, \theta \in \Sigma^*$, $A \in \Sigma_N$, the following condition holds.

If $FIRST_k(x) = FIRST_k(y)$, then $\beta = \gamma$.

Thus, for every derivation step of a word $w$ in $G$, we are able to choose a production in an unambiguous way by analyzing a part of $w$ that is of length $k$. We say that $G$ has the *property of an unambiguous choice of a production given the $k$-length prefix*[19] *in a leftmost derivation*. We will see in Chap. 10 that a similar property will be defined for parsable $ETPL(k)$ graph grammars which are analogous to (string) $LL(k)$ grammars.

For simplicity reasons, we assume $k = 1$ in our considerations. Let us notice that our previous grammar generating the symmetric wave language is not $LL(1)$. Let us look at Fig. 3.8b once more. One can easily see that if we want to choose a proper production for a nonterminal $B$ we have to analyze a prefix of the length $k = 2$ (underlined in the figure). If it is equal to the substring 13 (as in the figure),

---

[18]**LL** means that it scans a word from **L**eft to right generating it according to a **L**eftmost derivation.

[19]The $k$-length prefix means here the prefix of a part of $w$ that has not been parsed till now. In the definition this part is denoted by $x$.

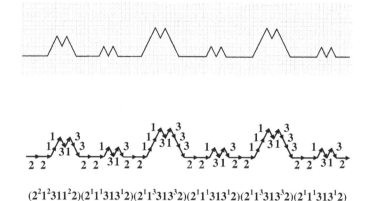

$$(2^21^2311^22)(2^11^1313^12)(2^11^3313^32)(2^11^1313^12)(2^11^3313^32)(2^11^1313^12)$$

Fig. 3.10   Exemplary symmetric waves with "craters" of the $LL(1)$ language $L$.

then we should choose production 5. However, if it is equal to the substring 11, then we should choose production 4. (The grammar is $LL(2)$, in fact.) In order to consider an $LL(1)$ grammar, let us modify our language a little bit. We assume that there is a "crater" instead of a "peak" at the top of each wave, as it is shown in Fig. 3.10. Additionally, we assume that there is no symbol 0 at the end of the whole pattern.[20]

Formally, the *symmetric waves with craters language* is defined as $L = \{\alpha \in \Sigma_T^+ : \alpha = (2^{k_1}1^{m_1}313^{m_1}2)(2^{k_2}1^{m_2}313^{m_2}2)\ldots(2^{k_j}1^{m_j}313^{m_j}2),\ k_i \geq 1,\ m_i \geq 1,\ i = 1,\ldots,j\} \cup \{\lambda\}$. Let us define the $LL(1)$ grammar $G$ which generates $L$. $G = (\Sigma_N, \Sigma_T, P, S)$, where:
$\Sigma_N = \{S, A, B\}$,
$P$ consists of the following productions.

$(1)\ S \;\to\; 2A$   $(3)\ A \;\to\; 1B32S$   $(5)\ B \;\to\; 31$

$(2)\ A \;\to\; 2A$   $(4)\ B \;\to\; 1B3$   $(6)\ S \;\to\; \lambda$

The last production replaces $S$ with the empty word ($\lambda$).

Now, we can introduce the idea of $LL(1)$ parsing.[21] A configuration of an $LL(1)$ parser is of the form (*input* , *stack* , *output*), where *stack* is used as working memory, indices of the productions identified are written to *output*. The parser works according to its *control table* which defines a proper action on the basis of a symbol read from *input* and the top of *stack*.[22] For our grammar $G$ the

---

[20]For our further considerations we want to define a lambda production. Hence, the lack of 0 at the end.

[21]We do not present here "technical" issues which concern defining an $LL(k)$ grammar for an LL($k$) language (eliminating ambiguity, removing left recursion, left factoring). The reader is referred to the classic textbooks on compiler design theory mentioned at the beginning of Sec. 3.1.

[22]Let us note that a control table corresponds to a transition function in a formal definition of an automaton.

Table 3.1   $LL(1)$ control table $M$.

| | | INPUT | | | |
|---|---|---|---|---|---|
| | | 1 | 2 | 3 | $\perp$ |
| | $S$ | $err$ | 1 | $err$ | 6 |
| S | $A$ | 3 | 2 | $err$ | $err$ |
| T | $B$ | 4 | $err$ | 5 | $err$ |
| A | 1 | $rem$ | $err$ | $err$ | $err$ |
| C | 2 | $err$ | $rem$ | $err$ | $err$ |
| K | 3 | $err$ | $err$ | $rem$ | $err$ |
| | $\perp$ | $err$ | $err$ | $err$ | $acc$ |

parser control $M$ is defined in Table 3.1. (Indices inside the table are indices of the productions.)

If a production is identified, the parser pops its left-hand side from *stack*, pushes its right-hand side onto *stack* and writes the production index to *output*. If a symbol read from *input* is equal to a symbol at the top of *stack*, then the symbol is *removed* (*rem*) from *stack* and the next symbol is read.[23] *Acc* means the acceptance of the word, *err* means an error. The initial configuration is of the form $(a_1a_2\ldots a_n\perp,\ S\perp,\ \lambda)$, where $a_1a_2\ldots a_n$ is a word to be parsed, $\perp$ is used as the end-marker of the word and the bottom-marker of the stack.

Let us consider the following example. Parsing of the symmetric waveform with craters 211313322213132 is performed according to Table 3.1 as follows:

$(211313322213132\perp,\ S\perp,\ ) \vdash (211313322213132\perp,\ 2A\perp,\ 1) \vdash$
$\vdash (11313322213132\perp,\ A\perp,\ 1) \vdash (11313322213132\perp,\ 1B32S\perp,13) \vdash$
$\vdash (1313322213132\perp,\ B32S\perp,\ 13) \vdash (1313322213132\perp,\ 1B332S\perp,\ 134) \vdash$
$\vdash (313322213132\perp,\ B332S\perp,\ 134) \vdash (313322213132\perp,\ 31332S\perp,\ 1345) \vdash$
$\vdash (13322213132\perp,\ 1332S\perp,\ 1345) \vdash (3322213132\perp,\ 332S\perp,\ 1345) \vdash$
$\vdash (322213132\perp,\ 32S\perp,\ 1345) \vdash (22213132\perp,\ 2S\perp,\ 1345) \vdash$
$\vdash (2213132\perp,\ S\perp,\ 1345) \vdash (2213132\perp,\ 2A\perp,\ 13451) \vdash$
$\vdash (213132\perp,\ A\perp,\ 13451) \vdash (213132\perp,\ 2A\perp,\ 134512) \vdash$
$\vdash (13132\perp,\ A\perp,\ 134512) \vdash (13132\perp,\ 1B32S\perp,\ 1345123) \vdash$
$\vdash (3132\perp,\ B32S\perp,\ 1345123) \vdash (3132\perp,\ 3132S\perp,\ 13451235) \vdash$
$\vdash (132\perp,\ 132S\perp,\ 13451235) \vdash (32\perp,\ 32S\perp,\ 13451235) \vdash$
$\vdash (2\perp,\ 2S\perp,\ 13451235) \vdash (\perp,\ S\perp,\ 13451235) \vdash (\perp,\ \perp,\ 134512356) \vdash acc.$

Before we present the $LL(1)$ parsing algorithm, we introduce its data structures and functions.

---

[23]We assume that every symbol read from *input* is valid, i.e. either it belongs to $\Sigma_T$ or it is equal to the end-marker.

- $M$ - the parser control table,[24]
- *read_input*() - the function reads one symbol from *input*,
- *move_head*() - the function moves the reading head one position to the right,
- *stack_top*() - the function gives the top element of *stack* (without removing it),
- *push_onto_stack*($\beta$) - the function pushes $\beta$ onto *stack*,
- *pop_from_stack*() - the function removes an element from *stack*,
- *write_output*($k$) - the function writes $k$ to *output*,
- *is_terminal*($A$) - the Boolean function which checks whether $A$ is terminal.

---

**Parsing Scheme 3.1: $LL(1)$ Parser**

```
/* Initial configuration: (a₁a₂...aₙ⊥ , S⊥ , λ) */
error := 0;
x := read_input();
repeat
    A := stack_top();
    if is_terminal(A) or A = ⊥ then
        if A = x then
            begin
                pop_from_stack();
                move_head();
                x := read_input();
            end;
        else error := 1;
    else
        if M[A, x] = (k) A → β then
            begin
                pop_from_stack();
                push_onto_stack(β);
                write_output(k);
            end;
        else error := 1;
until A = ⊥ or error = 1;
```

$LL(k)$ parsing is efficient. Let us present the following theorem.

**Theorem 3.3 ($LL(k)$ Parsing Complexity [Lewis and Stearns (1968)] )**

*The running time of the parsing algorithm for $LL(k)$ grammars is $\mathcal{O}(n)$, where $n$ is the input length.*

---

[24] For clarity reasons the algorithm has been constructed so that it uses only the part of a control table which is defined for stack *nonterminals* (e.g. only the first three rows of Table 3.1).

At the end of this section we define the rules of constructing an $LL(1)$ parsing control table on the basis of productions of an $LL(1)$ grammar [Aho *et al.* (2007)]. Firstly, however, let us introduce the following notion.

$FOLLOW_k(A)$, $A \in \Sigma_N$ denotes a set of all the terminal strings of the length $k$ (or of the length less than $k$)[25] that can occur immediately to the right of $A$ in some sentential form of a derivation in $G^{26}$, i.e.:

$$FOLLOW_k(A) = \{x \in \Sigma_T^* : S \xRightarrow{*} \alpha A \theta \land x \in FIRST_k(\theta) , \alpha, \theta \in \Sigma^*\}.$$

Let $G = (\Sigma_N, \Sigma_T, P, S)$ be an $LL(1)$ grammar. A parsing control table $M$ for $G$ is constructed in the following way.

(1) For every $(i)$ $X \to \alpha \in P$, $X \in \Sigma_N$, $\alpha \in \Sigma^*$ such that $x \in FIRST_1(\alpha)$, $x \neq \lambda$, add $(i)$ to $M[X, x]$.
(2) For every $(j)$ $Y \to \beta \in P$, $Y \in \Sigma_N$, $\beta \in \Sigma^*$ such that $\lambda \in FIRST_1(\beta)$, add $(j)$ to $M[Y, y]$ for every $y \in FOLLOW_1(Y)$. (If $\bot \in FOLLOW_1(Y)$, add $(j)$ to $M[Y, \bot]$.)
(3) Add *acc* to $M[\bot, \bot]$.
(4) Add *err* for every remaining entry of $M$.

Let us note that Table 3.1 has been constructed according to the rules (1)–(4). For example,

- $M[S, 2] = 1$, since (1) $S \to 2A \in P$ and $2 \in FIRST_1(2A)$,
- $M[A, 2] = 2$, since (2) $A \to 2A \in P$ and $2 \in FIRST_1(2A)$,
- $M[A, 1] = 3$, since (3) $A \to 1B32S \in P$ and $1 \in FIRST_1(1B32S)$,
- $M[B, 1] = 4$, since (4) $B \to 1B3 \in P$ and $1 \in FIRST_1(1B3)$,
- $M[B, 3] = 5$, since (5) $B \to 31 \in P$ and $3 \in FIRST_1(31)$,
- $M[S, \bot] = 6$, since (6) $S \to \lambda \in P$ and $\bot \in FOLLOW_1(S)$.

### 3.2.2  *LR(k) Languages*

The $LR(k)$ parser[27] [Knuth (1965)] performs a bottom-up parsing. It performs reductions according to the Reverse Polish (post-order) traversal of a derivation tree. The parser works deterministically if it looks ahead to the $k$-length strings beyond handles. Let us define $LR(k)$ grammars as follows.

---

[25] See $FIRST_k$ at the beginning of this section.
[26] If $A$ is the rightmost symbol of some sentential form, then $\bot \in FOLLOW_k(A)$.
[27] **LR** means that it scans a word from **L**eft to right generating it according to a **R**ightmost derivation.

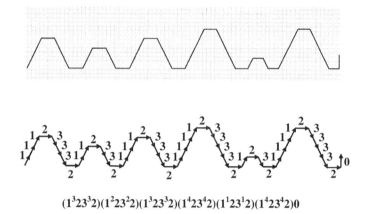

$$(1^3 23^3 2)(1^2 23^2 2)(1^3 23^3 2)(1^4 23^4 2)(1^1 23^1 2)(1^4 23^4 2)0$$

Fig. 3.11  Exemplary symmetric waves with "flat tops" of the $LR(1)$ language $L$.

**Definition 3.2 ($LR(k)$ Grammar):** Let $G = (\Sigma_N, \Sigma_T, P, S)$ be a context-free grammar, the rightmost derivation in $G$ be denoted with $\underset{r(G)}{\overset{*}{\Longrightarrow}}$ . $G$ is called an $LR(k)$ grammar iff for every two rightmost derivations

$$S \underset{r(G)}{\overset{*}{\Longrightarrow}} \alpha A w \underset{r(G)}{\Longrightarrow} \alpha \beta w$$

$$S \underset{r(G)}{\overset{*}{\Longrightarrow}} \gamma B y \underset{r(G)}{\Longrightarrow} \alpha \beta x,$$

where $w, x, y \in \Sigma_T^*$, $\alpha, \beta, \gamma \in \Sigma^*$, $A, B \in \Sigma_N$, the following condition holds.

If $FIRST_k(w) = FIRST_k(x)$ then $\alpha = \gamma$ , $A = B$ , $x = y$.

Thus, for every right-sentential form we can identify a handle and we can choose a production in an unambiguous way by looking at most $k$ symbols beyond the handle. We say that $G$ has the *property of an identification of a handle and an unambiguous choice of a production given $k$ symbols beyond the handle in a right-sentential form*. We will see in Chap. 10 that a similar property will be defined for parsable $ETPR(k)$ graph grammars which are analogous to (string) $LR(k)$ grammars.

Now, we introduce the succeeding version of the language of waveforms that is useful for considering bottom-up schemes of parsing. The *symmetric waves with flat tops language* is defined as $L = \{\alpha \in \Sigma_T^+ : \alpha = (1^{m_1} 23^{m_1} 2)(1^{m_2} 23^{m_2} 2) \ldots (1^{m_j} 23^{m_j} 2), m_i \geq 1, i = 1, \ldots, j\}$. The exemplary waveform belonging to $L$ is shown in Fig. 3.11. Let us define the $LR(1)$ grammar $G$ which generates $L$.

$G = (\Sigma_N, \Sigma_T, P, S)$, where:

$\Sigma_N = \{S, B\}$,

$P$ consists of the following productions:

Table 3.2   $LR(1)$ control table $M$.

| | | ACTION | | | | | GOTO | |
|---|---|---|---|---|---|---|---|---|
| | | **0** | **1** | **2** | **3** | **⊥** | **S** | **B** |
| | $I_0$ | $I_3$ | $I_2$ | | | | $I_1$ | |
| | $I_1$ | | | | | *acc* | | |
| | $I_2$ | | $I_5$ | $I_6$ | | | | $I_4$ |
| S | $I_3$ | | | | | 4 | | |
| T | $I_4$ | | | | $I_7$ | | | |
| A | $I_5$ | | $I_5$ | $I_6$ | | | | $I_8$ |
| T | $I_6$ | | | | 3 | | | |
| E | $I_7$ | | | $I_9$ | | | | |
| | $I_8$ | | | | $I_{10}$ | | | |
| | $I_9$ | $I_3$ | $I_2$ | | | | $I_{11}$ | |
| | $I_{10}$ | | | | 2 | | | |
| | $I_{11}$ | | | | | 1 | | |

$$(1)\ S\ \rightarrow\ 1B32S \qquad (3)\ B\ \rightarrow\ 2$$

$$(2)\ B\ \rightarrow\ 1B3 \qquad (4)\ S\ \rightarrow\ 0$$

Let us present the idea of $LR(k)$ parsing.[28] A configuration of an $LR(1)$ parser is defined as (*stack* , *input* , *output*), where *stack*, *input*, *output* play the same role as for $LL(1)$.[29] The parser works according to the control table $M$ which is defined in Table 3.2 for our grammar $G$. The table is divided into two parts **ACTION** and **GOTO** and it contains production indices and *states* $(I_0, I_1, \ldots)$.[30] The parser reads one symbol $x$ from *input* and chooses a proper action according to **ACTION**$[I_{top}, x]$, where $I_{top}$ is the state on top of the stack. If the action is defined as the state $I'$, then both $x$ (firstly) and $I'$ are pushed onto *stack*. If the action is defined as a production, then the parser pops the handle (with associated states) from *stack*, pushes its left-hand side $A$ onto *stack* and writes the production index to *output*. In order to push a proper state onto the top of *stack*, i.e., after the left-hand side nonterminal $A$, the parser chooses this state according to **GOTO**$[I_{prec}, A]$, where $I_{prec}$ is the state preceding $A$. The initial configuration is of the form $(I_0$ , $\underline{a_1 a_2 \ldots a_n} \perp$ , $\lambda)$, where $a_1 a_2 \ldots a_n$ is a word to be parsed, $\perp$ is its end-marker, $I_0$ is the start state.

We shall consider the following example. Parsing of the symmetric waveform

---

[28] We do not present here issues which relate to defining various $LR$-type parsers for $LR$-type grammars ($SLR$, $LALR$, etc.). The reader is referred to the classic textbooks on compiler design theory mentioned at the beginning of Sec. 3.1.

[29] Let us notice that in this instance *stack* is the first element.

[30] Additionally, the acceptance state is denoted with *acc*, error states are denoted with spaces.

with flat tops pattern 11233212320 is performed according to Table 3.2 as follows.

| | | | | |
|---|---|---|---|---|
| $(I_0$ | $, 11233212320\perp$ | , | $)$ | $\vdash$ |
| $(I_0 1 I_2$ | $, 1233212320\perp$ | , | $)$ | $\vdash$ |
| $(I_0 1 I_2 1 I_5$ | $, 233212320\perp$ | , | $)$ | $\vdash$ |
| $(I_0 1 I_2 1 I_5 \underline{2 I_6}$ | $, 33212320\perp$ | , | $)$ | $\vdash$ |
| $(I_0 1 I_2 1 I_5 B I_8$ | $, 33212320\perp$ | , | $3)$ | $\vdash$ |
| $(I_0 1 I_2 \underline{1 I_5 B I_8 3 I_{10}}$ | $, 3212320\perp$ | , | $3)$ | $\vdash$ |
| $(I_0 1 I_2 B I_4$ | $, 3212320\perp$ | , | $32)$ | $\vdash$ |
| $(I_0 1 I_2 B I_4 3 I_7$ | $, 212320\perp$ | , | $32)$ | $\vdash$ |
| $(I_0 1 I_2 B I_4 3 I_7 2 I_9$ | $, 12320\perp$ | , | $32)$ | $\vdash$ |
| $(I_0 1 I_2 B I_4 3 I_7 2 I_9 1 I_2$ | $, 2320\perp$ | , | $32)$ | $\vdash$ |
| $(I_0 1 I_2 B I_4 3 I_7 2 I_9 1 I_2 \underline{2 I_6}$ | $, 320\perp$ | , | $32)$ | $\vdash$ |
| $(I_0 1 I_2 B I_4 3 I_7 2 I_9 1 I_2 B I_4$ | $, 320\perp$ | , | $323)$ | $\vdash$ |
| $(I_0 1 I_2 B I_4 3 I_7 2 I_9 1 I_2 B I_4 3 I_7$ | $, 20\perp$ | , | $323)$ | $\vdash$ |
| $(I_0 1 I_2 B I_4 3 I_7 2 I_9 1 I_2 B I_4 3 I_7 2 I_9$ | $, 0\perp$ | , | $323)$ | $\vdash$ |
| $(I_0 1 I_2 B I_4 3 I_7 2 I_9 1 I_2 B I_4 3 I_7 2 I_9 \underline{0 I_3}$ | $, \perp$ | , | $323)$ | $\vdash$ |
| $(I_0 1 I_2 B I_4 3 I_7 2 I_9 \underline{1 I_2 B I_4 3 I_7 2 I_9 S I_{11}}$ | $, \perp$ | , | $3234)$ | $\vdash$ |
| $(I_0 \underline{1 I_2 B I_4 3 I_7 2 I_9 S I_{11}}$ | $, \perp$ | , | $32341)$ | $\vdash$ |
| $(I_0 S I_1$ | $, \perp$ | , | $323411)$ | $\vdash$ *acc* |

At the end of this section we will present the $LR(1)$ parsing algorithm. Its functions are defined in the same way as for the $LL(1)$ parsing algorithm (Parsing Scheme 3.1) except for one thing - the function *pop_from_stack*$(m)$ removes $m$ symbols from *stack*.

Although $LR$-type grammars have greater generative power than the $LL$-type ones[31], their parsing is as efficient as for $LL$, which is stated by the following theorem.

**Theorem 3.4 ($LR(k)$ Parsing Complexity [Knuth (1965)])**

*The running time of the parsing algorithm for $LR(k)$ grammars is $\mathcal{O}(n)$, where $n$ is the input length.*

---

[31] We shall discuss this issue in Section 3.2.6.

And here is the algorithm.

---

**Parsing Scheme 3.2: *LR*(1) Parser**

```
/* Initial configuration: (I₀ , a₁a₂...aₙ⊥ , λ) */
```
$/*$ Initial configuration: $(I_0 , \underline{a_1}a_2 \ldots a_n \perp , \lambda)$ $*/$
$error := 0;$
$accept := 0;$
$x := read\_input();$
**repeat**
  $I := stack\_top();$
  **if ACTION**$[I, x] =$ "shift $I_m$" **then**
    **begin**
      $push\_onto\_stack(x);$
      $push\_onto\_stack(I_m);$
      $move\_head();$
      $x := read\_input();$
    **end;**
  **else if ACTION**$[I, x] =$ "reduce $(k)$ $A \rightarrow \beta$" **then**
    **begin**
      $number\_of\_symbols := 2 * length(\beta);$
      $pop\_from\_stack(number\_of\_symbols);$
      $I := stack\_top();$
      $push\_onto\_stack(A);$
      $state := \mathbf{GOTO}[I, A];$
      $push\_onto\_stack(state);$
      $write\_output(k);$
    **end;**
  **else if ACTION**$[I, x] =$ "accept" **then** $accept := 1;$
  **else** $error := 1;$
**until** $accept = 1$ **or** $error = 1;$

---

### 3.2.3 *Precedence Parsing*

The idea of precedence parsing was introduced in [Floyd (1963)] for operator-precedence grammars and was developed for simple precedence grammars in [Wirth and Weber (1966)]. It is based on *precedence relations* which allow a deterministic bottom-up parser to identify handles on a stack. Let us begin by defining these relations.[32]

Let $G = (\Sigma_N, \Sigma_T, P, S)$ be a context-free grammar, $X, Y \in \Sigma \cup \{ \perp \}$. The precedence relations $\doteq$, $\lessdot$, $\gtrdot$ are defined as follows.
$X \doteq Y \iff \exists A \rightarrow \alpha X Y \beta \subset P$, $\alpha, \beta \in \Sigma^*$ (Fig. 3.12a).

---

[32]We are considering here the Wirth-Weber model.

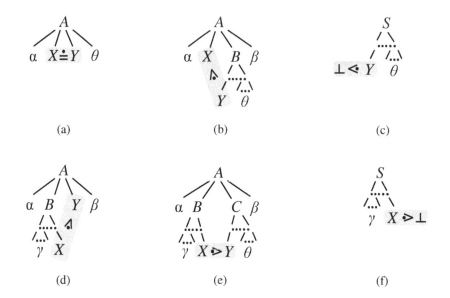

Fig. 3.12 Precedence relations.

$X \lessdot Y \iff \exists\, A \to \alpha X B \beta \in P \;\wedge\; \exists\, B \xRightarrow[G]{+} Y\theta,\; \alpha,\beta,\theta \in \Sigma^*,\; B \in \Sigma_N$
(Fig. 3.12b) or
$\qquad X = \bot \;\wedge\; \exists\, S \xRightarrow[G]{+} Y\theta,\; \theta \in \Sigma^*$ (Fig. 3.12c).

$X \gtrdot Y \iff \exists\, A \to \alpha B Y \beta \in P \;\wedge\; \exists\, B \xRightarrow[G]{+} \gamma X,\; Y \in \Sigma_T,\; \alpha,\beta,\gamma \in \Sigma^*,\; B \in \Sigma_N$
(Fig. 3.12d) or
$\qquad \exists\, A \to \alpha B C \beta \in P \;\wedge\; \exists\, B \xRightarrow[G]{+} \gamma X \;\wedge\; \exists\, C \xRightarrow[G]{+} Y\theta,\; Y \in \Sigma_T,$
$\qquad \alpha,\beta,\gamma,\theta \in \Sigma^*,\; B,C \in \Sigma_N$ (Fig. 3.12e) or
$\qquad Y = \bot \;\wedge\; \exists\, S \xRightarrow[G]{+} \gamma X,\; \gamma \in \Sigma^*$ (Fig. 3.12f).

Now, we can introduce the following definition.[33]

> **Definition 3.3 (Simple Precedence Grammar):** Let $G$ be a context-free grammar. $G$ is called a simple precedence grammar iff
> - it is $\lambda$-free,
> - it is uniquely invertible,
> - all its symbols are useful and
> - for each pair of symbols there is only one precedence relation.

We present the idea of precedence parsing with the use of the grammar $G$ introduced in a previous section.[34] Table 3.3 is the precedence table **REL** for $G$. An example of precedence parsing is given below the table.

---

[33]The notions used in the definition are introduced in Appendix A.1.
[34]The grammar G is both $LR(k)$ and (simple) precedence.

Table 3.3  Precedence control table **REL**.

|   | S | B | 0 | 1 | 2 | 3 | ⊥ |
|---|---|---|---|---|---|---|---|
| S |   |   |   |   |   |   | > |
| B |   |   |   |   |   | ≐ |   |
| 0 |   |   |   |   |   |   | > |
| 1 |   | ≐ |   |   | < | < |   |
| 2 | ≐ |   |   | < | < |   | > |
| 3 |   |   |   |   |   | ≐ | > |
| ⊥ | < |   |   |   | < |   |   |

| | | | |
|---|---|---|---|
| (⊥ | ,11233212320⊥ , | ) | ⊥ < 1 |
| (⊥ < 1 | ,1233212320⊥ , | ) | 1 < 1 |
| (⊥ < 1 < 1 | ,233212320⊥ , | ) | 1 < 2 |
| (⊥ < 1 < 1 <u>< 2 ></u> | ,33212320⊥ , | ) | 2 > 3 |
| (⊥ < 1 < 1 ≐ B | ,33212320⊥ , | 3) | 1 ≐ B |
| (⊥ < 1 < 1 ≐ B ≐ 3 | ,3212320⊥ , | 3) | B ≐ 3 |
| (⊥ < 1 <u>< 1 ≐ B ≐ 3 ></u> | ,3212320⊥ , | 3) | 3 > 3 |
| (⊥ < 1 ≐ B | ,3212320⊥ , | 32) | B ≐ 3 |
| (⊥ < 1 ≐ B ≐ 3 | ,212320⊥ , | 32) | 3 ≐ 2 |
| (⊥ < 1 ≐ B ≐ 3 ≐ 2 | ,12320⊥ , | 32) | 2 < 1 |
| (⊥ < 1 ≐ B ≐ 3 ≐ 2 < 1 | ,2320⊥ , | 32) | 1 < 2 |
| (⊥ < 1 ≐ B ≐ 3 ≐ 2 < 1 <u>< 2 ></u> | ,320⊥ , | 32) | 2 > 3 |
| (⊥ < 1 ≐ B ≐ 3 ≐ 2 < 1 ≐ B | ,320⊥ , | 323) | 1 ≐ B |
| (⊥ < 1 ≐ B ≐ 3 ≐ 2 < 1 ≐ B ≐ 3 | ,20⊥ , | 323) | B ≐ 3 |
| (⊥ < 1 ≐ B ≐ 3 ≐ 2 < 1 ≐ B ≐ 3 ≐ 2 | ,0⊥ , | 323) | 3 ≐ 2 |
| (⊥ < 1 ≐ B ≐ 3 ≐ 2 < 1 ≐ B ≐ 3 ≐ 2 ≐ 0 | ,⊥ , | 323) | 2 ≐ 0 |
| (⊥ < 1 ≐ B ≐ 3 ≐ 2 <u>< 1 ≐ B ≐ 3 ≐ 2 ≐ 0 ></u> | ,⊥ , | 323) | 0 > ⊥ |
| (⊥ < 1 ≐ B ≐ 3 ≐ 2 ≐ S | ,⊥ , | 3231) | 2 ≐ S |
| (⊥ <u>< 1 ≐ B ≐ 3 ≐ 2 ≐ S ></u> | ,⊥ , | 3231) | S > ⊥ |
| (⊥ < S | ,⊥ , | 32311) |  |

Let us analyze this example. A configuration of a precedence parser is defined as (*stack* , *input* , *output*), where *stack*, *input*, *output* play the same role as for $LR(1)$. The initial configuration is of the form $(\perp,\ \underline{a_1}a_2\ldots a_n\perp,\ \lambda)$, where $a_1 a_2 \ldots a_n$ is a word to be parsed, $\perp$ is used as the end-marker of the word and the bottom-marker of the stack.

Let $Z$ be a symbol on top of the stack. The parser reads one symbol $x$ from *input* and finds a precedence relation between $Z$ and $x$ in the precedence table **REL**. (Comparing $Z$ and $x$ with the help of the relation found is shown in the second column of our example.) If the relation is $<$ or $\doteq$, then both the relation (firstly) and $x$ are pushed onto *stack*. If the relation is $>$, then the parser identifies the handle. The handle, called here the *pivot*[35], is limited with the identified relation $>$ at the top of *stack* and the nearest $<$ (i.e., the pivot is of the form $<\ldots \doteq \ldots \doteq \ldots\ldots \doteq \ldots \doteq \ldots >$ ). The parser pops the pivot from *stack*. Then, it identifies the production due to the unique invertibility of the grammar. Finally, it finds a precedence relation between the new $Z$ (top of *stack*) and the left-hand side of the production *lhs* and pushes this relation (firstly) and *lhs* onto *stack*. (That is, in the fourth line the pivot $\underline{<\mathbf{2}>}$ is found. It is reduced with the production: (3) $B \to 2$ of the grammar $G$ to $lhs = B$. After popping the pivot from *stack*, there is **1** at the top. We push $\doteq \mathbf{B}$ onto *stack*, since **REL**$[\mathbf{1}, \mathbf{B}] = $ " $\doteq$ " .) The production index is written to *output*.

Although simple precedence grammars are less powerful than $LR$ grammars, they are used in practical applications because of their simplicity as well as their efficiency. Let us present the following theorem.

**Theorem 3.5 ([Wirth and Weber (1966)] Parser Complexity)**

*The running time of the parsing algorithm for simple precedence grammars is $\mathcal{O}(n)$, where $n$ is the input length.*

At the end of this section we will present the precedence parsing algorithm. It uses functions which have been defined for $LL(1)$ and $LR(1)$ parsing algorithms (Parsing Schemes 3.1 and 3.2) in previous sections. Additionally, let us introduce the following functions.

- *identify_pivot_on_stack*() - the function identifies and extracts the pivot which ends at the top of *stack*,
- *identify_production*(*pivot*) - the functions finds a proper production on the basis of *pivot* and gives its index,
- *pop_from_stack*(*pivot*) - the function removes *pivot* from *stack*,
- *left_hand_side*(*prod_index*) - the function gives the left-hand side *lhs* of the production *prod_index*.

---

[35]Pivots are underlined in the example.

**Parsing Scheme 3.3: Precedence Parser**

/* Initial configuration: $(\perp, \underline{a_1}a_2 \dots a_n\perp, \lambda)$ */
$error := 0;$
$accept := 0;$
$x := read\_input();$
**repeat**
  $Z := stack\_top();$
  $rel := \mathbf{REL}[Z, x];$
  **if** $rel = $ " $<$ " **or** $rel = $ " $\doteq$ " **then**
    **begin**
      $push\_onto\_stack(rel);$
      $push\_onto\_stack(x);$
      $move\_head();$
      $x := read\_input();$
    **end;**
  **else if** $rel = $ " $>$ " **then**
    **begin**
      $pivot := identify\_pivot\_on\_stack();$
      $prod\_index := identify\_production(pivot);$
      **if** $prod\_index \neq 0$ **then**
        **begin**
          $pop\_from\_stack(pivot);$
          $Z := stack\_top();$
          $A := left\_hand\_side(prod\_index);$
          $rel := \mathbf{REL}[Z, A];$
          $push\_onto\_stack(rel);$
          $push\_onto\_stack(A);$
          $write\_output(prod\_index);$
        **end;**
      **else** $error := 1;$
    **end;**
  **else** $error := 1;$
**until** $configuration = (\perp < S, \perp, \pi)$ **or** $error = 1;$

### 3.2.4 *Earley Parser*

The Earley parser [Earley (1970)] does not require the imposing any additional conditions on the form of a context-free grammar. Therefore, it is frequently used in practical applications and especially in syntactic pattern recognition. Let us present the basic notions and functions of this model.

Let us introduce the Earley dot notation. Let $G = (\Sigma_N, \Sigma_T, P, S)$ be a context-free grammar. If $A \to \alpha\beta \in P$, then $A \to \alpha_\bullet\beta$ denotes a situation during parsing in which $\alpha$ has already been analyzed.

For a word to be parsed $w = a_1 a_2 \ldots a_n$ the parser generates a sequence of state sets $I(0), I(1), \ldots, I(n)$. A state set $I(i)$ consists of state items of the form $[A \to \alpha_\bullet\beta, \; j]$, where $j$ denotes a position in the word $w$ at which the parser began matching the production $A \to \alpha\beta$. Firstly, the parser *initializes* the state set $I(0) = \{ \; [S \to _\bullet\gamma, \; 0] \; \}$, where $S$ is the start symbol of $G$. Then, it repeatedly performs the following three operations for each state set $I(k)$, $k = 0, 1, \ldots, n$.

- *predict* - for each $[A \to \alpha_\bullet B\beta, \; i] \in I(k)$ for each $B \to \theta \in P$ add $[B \to _\bullet\theta, \; k]$ to $I(k)$. Let us note that $B \in \Sigma_N$.
- *scan* - for each $[A \to \alpha_\bullet x\beta, \; i] \in I(k)$ such that $x = a_{k+1}$ add $[A \to \alpha x_\bullet\beta, \; i]$ to $I(k+1)$. Let us note that $x \in \Sigma_T$.
- *complete* - for each $[A \to \omega_\bullet, \; i] \in I(k)$ for each $I(i)$ if $[C \to \alpha_\bullet A\beta, \; j] \in I(i)$, then add $[C \to \alpha A_\bullet\beta, \; j]$ to $I(k)$. The item $[A \to \omega_\bullet, \; i]$ is called a *final state*.

The word $w = a_1 a_2 \ldots a_n$ is accepted if a state item of the form $[S \to \phi_\bullet, \; 0]$ belongs to $I(n)$.

Let us present the idea of Earley parsing with the use of the grammar $G$ introduced in Sec. 3.2.2. We will analyze the waveform $a_1 a_2 a_3 a_4 a_5 = 12320$. Each item is characterized additionally with a type of operation used for its generation.

| Input | State set | State items | Operation |
|---|---|---|---|
| | $I(0)$ | $[S \to _\bullet 1B32S, \; 0]$ | *initialize* |
| | | $[S \to _\bullet 0, \; 0]$ | *initialize* |
| $a_1 = 1$ | $I(1)$ | $[S \to 1_\bullet B32S, \; 0]$ | *scan* |
| | | $[B \to _\bullet 1B3, \; 1]$ | *predict* |
| | | $[B \to _\bullet 2, \; 1]$ | *predict* |
| $a_2 = 2$ | $I(2)$ | $[B \to 2_\bullet, \; 1]$ | *scan* |
| | | $[S \to 1B_\bullet 32S, \; 0]$ | *complete* |
| $a_3 = 3$ | $I(3)$ | $[S \to 1B3_\bullet 2S, \; 0]$ | *scan* |
| $a_4 = 2$ | $I(4)$ | $[S \to 1B32_\bullet S, \; 0]$ | *scan* |
| | | $[S \to _\bullet 1B32S, \; 4]$ | *predict* |
| | | $[S \to _\bullet 0, \; 4]$ | *predict* |
| $a_5 = 0$ | $I(5)$ | $[S \to 0_\bullet, \; 4]$ | *scan* |
| | | $[S \to 1B32S_\bullet, \; 0]$ | *complete* |

The word 12320 is accepted since the item $[S \to 1B32S_\bullet,\ 0]$ belongs to $I(5)$.

Before we present the Earley parsing algorithm, we introduce its functions.

- *predictor*($k$) - the function performs the *predict* operation for the state set $I(k)$,
- *scanner*($k$) - the function performs the *scan* operation for the state set $I(k)$,
- *completer*($k$) - the function performs the *complete* operation for the state $I(k)$,
- *initialize_I*(0)*_state_set*() - the function initializes the state set $I(0)$,
- *final_state*(*state*) - the function which checks whether *state* is a final set,
- *after_dot_symbol*(*state*) - the function gives the symbol which is after the dot in *state*,
- *is_empty*($W$) - the function which checks whether the set $W$ is empty,
- *final_state_from_S*($I(n)$) - the function which checks whether there is the final state with $S$ in the left-hand side in the state set $I(n)$.

---

**Parsing Scheme 3.4: Earley Parser**

*error* := 0;
*accept* := 0;
*initialize_I*(0)*_state_set*();
$k$ := 0;
**repeat**
    **for each** *state* **in** $I(k)$ **do**
      **if** *final_state*(*state*) **then** *completer*($k$)
      **else**
        **begin**
          $X$ := *after_dot_symbol*(*state*);
          **if** *is_terminal*($X$) **then** *scanner*($k$)
          **else** *predictor*($k$);
        **end**;
    **if** $k < n$ **and** *is_empty*($I(k+1)$) **then** *error* := 1;
    **if** $k = n$ **then if** *final_state_from_S*($I(n)$) **then** *accept* := 1 **else** *error* := 1;
    $k$ := $k + 1$;
**until** *accept* = 1 **or** *error* = 1;

---

Derivation sequences can be easily reconstructed on the basis of state sets.

At the end of this section let us present the following theorem.

**Theorem 3.6 ([Earley (1970)] Parser Complexity)**

*The running time of the Earley parsing algorithm for context-free grammars is $\mathcal{O}(n^3)$, where $n$ is the input length. If the grammar is unambiguous then the running time is $\mathcal{O}(n^2)$.*

### 3.2.5   *Cocke-Younger-Kasami Parser*

The idea of a parsing algorithm presented in this section was developed indepen-
dently in [Kasami (1965)], [Younger (1967)] and [Cocke and Schwartz (1970)]. The
CYK algorithm is defined for context-free grammars in Chomsky Normal Form
(CNF) [Chomsky (1959)]. Let is introduce this form.[36]

> **Definition 3.4 (Chomsky Normal Form (CNF)):** Let $G = (\Sigma_N, \Sigma_T, P, S)$
> be a context-free grammar. $G$ is in Chomsky Normal Form (CNF) iff
> • all its productions are in one of the following forms:
>
> $$A \to BC, \ A, B, C \in \Sigma_N \text{ or}$$
> $$A \to a, \ A \in \Sigma_N, \ a \in \Sigma_T \ ,$$
>
> • all its symbols are useful.

This requirement is not restrictive because every context-free grammar can be
transformed to CNF.

In order to present the idea of the CYK algorithm we introduce, firstly, an exemplary grammar in Chomsky Normal Form. Let us consider the following example.
Sometimes we analyze visual objects in order to test whether they are symmetric.
For example, such an object (a vase) is shown in Fig. 3.13a. In order to make
such an analysis we can scan rows of pixels (row by row). If an object is symmetric
then each row should be in the form of palindrome. For simplicity reasons, let us
assume that (only) three grey levels occur in considered images: white ($w$), grey
($g$) and black ($b$). For example, a row of pixels shown in Fig. 3.13b can be coded
with $gwwgggwbwgggwwg$. Let us formalize the *language of palindromic forms* as
$L = \{\alpha \in \Sigma_T^+ : \alpha = \gamma b\theta, \ \gamma, \theta \in \{w, g\}^+, \ \theta = \gamma^R, \ R$ is the reversal operation $\}$. The
grammar $G$ which generates $L$ is defined as follows.
$G = (\Sigma_N, \Sigma_T, P, S)$, where:
$\Sigma_N = \{S, X, Y, W_1, W_2, G_1, G_2\}$,
$\Sigma_T = \{w, g, b\}$,
$P$ consists of the following productions.

$$\begin{array}{lll}
(1) \ S \to W_1 X & (4) \ Y \to SG_2 & (7) \ W_2 \to w \\
(2) \ X \to SW_2 & (5) \ S \to b & (8) \ G_1 \to g \\
(3) \ S \to G_1 Y & (6) \ W_1 \to w & (9) \ G_2 \to g
\end{array}$$

Now, we introduce the idea of the CYK parsing algorithm. For a word to be
parsed $w = a_1 a_2 \ldots a_n$, the parser generates the table $T$. The scheme of such a
table for a word $a_1 a_2 \ldots a_5$ (of the length 5) is shown in Fig. 3.13c. A CYK parsing
table has the following property. If a nonterminal $X$ is in the table entry $T_{i,m}$ then

---

[36]For applications in syntactic pattern recognition we can consider grammars which are $\lambda$-free, cf.
Definition A.5 in Appendix A.1.

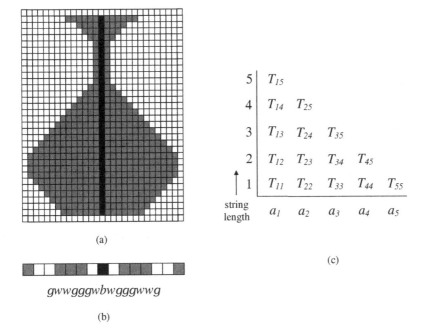

(a)

| 5 | $T_{15}$ | | | | |
|---|---|---|---|---|---|
| 4 | $T_{14}$ | $T_{25}$ | | | |
| 3 | $T_{13}$ | $T_{24}$ | $T_{35}$ | | |
| 2 | $T_{12}$ | $T_{23}$ | $T_{34}$ | $T_{45}$ | |
| 1 | $T_{11}$ | $T_{22}$ | $T_{33}$ | $T_{44}$ | $T_{55}$ |
| string length | $a_1$ | $a_2$ | $a_3$ | $a_4$ | $a_5$ |

(c)

*gwwgggwbwgggwwg*

(b)

Fig. 3.13 (a),(b) A symmetric object as a sequence of palindromic words. (c) The scheme of the CYK parsing table.

$X \xRightarrow[G]{+} a_i \dots a_m$. Let us note that $i$ is the index of the first symbol of $v = a_i \dots a_m$, $(m - i + 1)$ is the length of $v$ (cf. Fig. 3.13c).

Firstly, the algorithm computes the first (lowest) row ($l = 1$, i.e., the parser analyzes the substrings of $w$ of the length 1). For each $a_i, i = 1, 2, \dots, n$ for each production of the form $A \to a_i$, the nonterminal $A$ is added to the table entry $T_{i,i}$.

Then, the algorithm iterates with $l = 2, \dots, n$, i.e., it analyzes the substrings of $w$ of the length $l = 2$, then it analyzes the substrings of $w$ of the length $l = 3$, etc. For each substring $v$ of length 2 and greater the parser analyzes the possible partitions of $v$ into two parts $v_1$ and $v_2$ (i.e. $v = v_1v_2$) and checks whether there is a production of the form $A \to BC$ such that $B \xRightarrow[G]{+} v_1$ and $C \xRightarrow[G]{+} v_2$. If so, it means obviously that $A \xRightarrow[G]{+} v$.

Let us notice that the CYK parser is constructed with *dynamic programming technique*. If it checks whether $A \in T_{i,m}$, it has $T_{i,k}$ and $T_{(k+1),m}$ already computed ($k$ is the place of dividing $v$ into $v_1$ and $v_2$). Of course, $w \in L(G)$, if $S \in T_{1,n}$ (i.e., $S \xRightarrow[G]{+} a_1a_2 \dots a_n = w$).

Now, let us consider the parsing of the palindrome $w = a_1a_2a_3a_4a_5 = wgbgw$. Table 3.4 is the parsing table generated for the grammar $G$ and the word $w$. Productions in brackets are used to show why nonterminals have been added to entries. For example, analyzing substrings of the length $l = 2$ the parser adds $Y$ to the entry $T_{3,4}$ (for the substring $a_3a_4 = bg$) because:

Table 3.4    Parsing table $T$ generated with the CYK parser.

| $l$ | $i=1$ | $i=2$ | $i=3$ | $i=4$ | $i=5$ |
|---|---|---|---|---|---|
| 5 | $S$ <br> $(S \longrightarrow W_1 X)$ | | | | |
| 4 | — | $X$ <br> $(X \longrightarrow SW_2)$ | | | |
| 3 | — | $S$ <br> $(S \longrightarrow G_1 Y)$ | — | | |
| 2 | — | — | $Y$ <br> $(Y \longrightarrow SG_2)$ | — | |
| 1 | $W_1, W_2$ <br> $(W_1 \longrightarrow w)$ <br> $(W_2 \longrightarrow w)$ | $G_1, G_2$ <br> $(G_1 \longrightarrow g)$ <br> $(G_2 \longrightarrow g)$ | $S$ <br> $(S \longrightarrow b)$ | $G_1, G_2$ <br> $(G_1 \longrightarrow g)$ <br> $(G_2 \longrightarrow g)$ | $W_1, W_2$ <br> $(W_1 \longrightarrow w)$ <br> $(W_2 \longrightarrow w)$ |
| | $a_1 = w$ | $a_2 = g$ | $a_3 = b$ | $a_4 = g$ | $a_5 = w$ |

$i \rightarrow$

- there is the production $Y \rightarrow SG_2 \in P$ and
- $S \xRightarrow[G]{+} b$ (i.e., $S \in T_{3,3}$) and $G_2 \xRightarrow[G]{+} g$ (i.e., $G_2 \in T_{4,4}$).

Now, we can present the CYK parsing algorithm. The function $add(X, T_{j,m})$ adds nonterminal $X$ to the parsing table entry $T_{j,m}$.

## Parsing Scheme 3.5: CYK Parser

```
/* Input word: a₁a₂...aₙ */
error := 0;
accept := 0;
initialize_first_row();
for l := 2 to n do
   for i := 1 to n − l + 1 do
      for k := i to i + l − 2 do
         for each B in T_{i,k} do
            for each C in T_{(k+1),(i+l−1)} do
               if A → BC in P then add(A, T_{i,(i+l−1)});
if S in T_{1,n} then accept := 1 else error := 1;
```

At the end of this section we present the following theorem.

## Theorem 3.7 (CYK Parser Complexity [Hopcroft *et al.* (2006)])

*The running time of the CYK parsing algorithm for context-free grammars in CNF is $\mathcal{O}(n^3)$, where $n$ is the input length.*

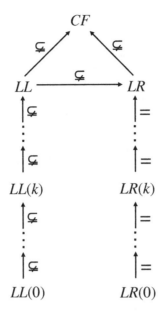

Fig. 3.14   The relations among $LL$ and $LR$ languages.

### 3.2.6   *Summary of Parsers for CF Languages*

Five classic parsing algorithms for context-free languages: $LL(k)$, $LR(k)$, precedence-based, Earley and CYK have been introduced. The $LL(k)$ and $LR(k)$ parsers are basic algorithms in compiler design theory [Hopcroft *et al.* (2006)] because they are fast (cf. Theorems 3.3 and 3.4) and easy-to-design.[37] The $LR$ parser was generalized ($GLR$ parser) in [Tomita (1985, 1987)]. Moreover, a variety of parser generators for $LL$-type and $LR$-type parsers have been developed. At the same time, research into their power properties has resulted in their complete characteristics (see [Rosenkrantz and Stearns (1970)] for $LL(k)$, [Knuth (1965); Mickunas *et al.* (1976)] for $LR(k)$), which can be summarized as in Fig. 3.14.

On the other hand, we can use $LL$-type, $LR$-type and precedence-based parsing techniques only if the corresponding subclasses of context-free grammars are strong enough to generate languages of the structural patterns considered. Otherwise, we have to employ the Earley or CYK parsing techniques. The use of enhanced context-free grammars, which will be presented in Chap. 4, can be another way to handle the problem. In this case syntax analysis algorithms are to be modified.

The comparison of the context-free grammar parsing algorithms introduced in this chapter is presented in Table 3.5.

---

[37] In fact, precedence-based parsers have the same advantages.

Table 3.5   The comparison of *CF* parsing methods.

| Method | Constraints imposed on grammar | Running time |
|---|---|---|
| $LL(k)$ | an unambiguous choice of a production given the $k$-length prefix in a leftmost-derivation (cf. Definition 3.1) | $\mathcal{O}(n)$ |
| $LR(k)$ | an identification of a handle and an unambiguous choice of a production, given $k$ symbols beyond the handle in a right-sentential form (cf. Definition 3.2) | $\mathcal{O}(n)$ |
| (simple) precedence | $\lambda$-freeness, unique invertibility, usefulness of symbols, only one precedence relation for each pair of symbols (cf. Definition 3.3) | $\mathcal{O}(n)$ |
| Earley | none/unambiguity | $\mathcal{O}(n^3)/\mathcal{O}(n^2)$ |
| CYK | none (CNF) | $\mathcal{O}(n^3)$ |

## 3.3   Recognition of Vague/Distorted Patterns

In practical applications structural patterns are often vague/distorted. In order to deal with this problem we construct syntactic pattern recognition models introducing some measures of uncertainty/ambiguity to grammars. The models can be based on probability theory (a probability-based measure), fuzzy set theory (a membership function-based measure), the theory of metric spaces (a metric/distance-based measure). The choice of a convenient approach depends on the characteristics of the pattern recognition problem to be solved. Let us consider this issue, assuming that $C$ is a class of vague/distorted patterns.

Generally, we use the *probabilistic/stochastic approach*, if some patterns in the class $C$ occur more often than others. If $C$ is characterized by the language $L$, we can assign the probability $p(x)$ to every string $x \in L$. Let us note that the following conditions must hold: $0 < p(x) \leq 1$, $\sum_{x \in L} p(x) = 1$ and the assignment of $p(x)$ to $x$ conforms to the principles of probability theory, especially statistical information for estimating a probability distribution is available. Once we have probabilities assigned to strings of $L$ and the grammar $G$ such that $L = L(G)$, we can define the stochastic grammar $G_s$ which corresponds to $G$ by calculating/estimating the productions probabilities. $G_s$ generates strings with (approximately) the same probabilities as those estimated originally.

Sometimes, we are not able to use a probability measure for the following reasons. Statistical information may be unavailable. Information on patterns may be based on subjective experience, expert opinions, etc. A measure we are able to define may not conforms to the conditions of a probability measure. In this case we can use the *fuzzy set approach*, defining the fuzzy grammar $G_f$ for $G$ by assigning membership grades to the productions according to a membership function defined for the set $L$ (treated here as a fuzzy set).

In probabilistic and fuzzy approaches vague patterns are treated as better or worse (more or less frequent) examples of the class $C$. In the *error-correcting ap-*

*proach* we consider distorted/deformed versions of structural representations of reference (template) patterns for the language $L$.[38] Sometimes we assume that structural representations can be corrupted because of errors which occur at an image preprocessing stage [Fu (1982)]. In this approach we define error-transformations for strings and the expanded grammar $G_e$ including *error productions* based on these transformations which generates also erroneous strings. Then, the distance of a vague pattern to the template can be calculated on the basis of the number of error productions used in the derivation of the pattern.

If vague patterns are generated by stochastic processes, the *hidden Markov model* (*HMM*) is often used. We shall introduce this model in the last section.

The extended models for vague/distorted patterns can be constructed for various types of grammars of the Chomsky hierarchy. We introduce them for regular grammars and corresponding finite-state automata. (The extensions for context-free grammars and various parsers are defined analogously (see also [Fu (1982)]).)

### 3.3.1 *Stochastic Languages*

Let us introduce the notion of stochastic regular grammar [Grenander (1967); Fu and Li (1969); Salomaa (1969); Fu (1971); Booth and Thompson (1973)].

**Definition 3.5 (Stochastic Regular Grammar):** A ($\lambda$-free) stochastic regular (right-regular) grammar is a quadruple

$$G = (\Sigma_N, \Sigma_T, P, S), \text{ where}$$

$\Sigma_N$ is a set of nonterminal symbols,
$\Sigma_T$ is a set of terminal symbols,
$P$ is a set of stochastic productions of the form:

$$A_i \xrightarrow{p_{ij}} \gamma_{ij}, \quad i = 1, \ldots, n, \ j = 1, \ldots, m_i,$$

in which $A_i \in \Sigma_N$ , $\gamma_{ij} \in \Sigma_T \cup \Sigma_T \Sigma_N$, $p_{ij}$ is the probability related to the application of the production such that

$$0 < p_{ij} \leq 1 \ , \ \sum_{j=1}^{m_i} p_{ij} = 1 \ ,$$

$S$ is the start symbol (axiom), $S \in \Sigma_N$.

For stochastic grammars we extend the notion of a derivation (cf. Definition A.2 in Appendix A.1) in the following way. Let the string $\theta$ be derived directly from the string $\beta$ as the result of applying the production $A_i \xrightarrow{p_{ij}} \gamma_{ij}$, i.e.

$$\beta \xrightarrow{p_{ij}} \theta \ .$$

We say that $\beta$ derives directly $\theta$ with the probability $p_{ij}$.

---

[38]Let us notice the analogy to template matching method in decision-theoretic pattern recognition.

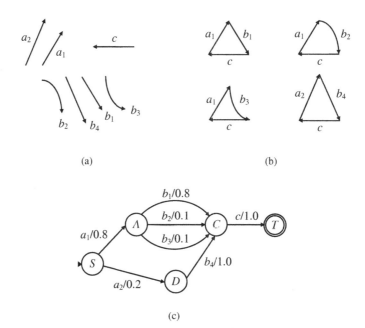

(a)                                              (b)

(c)

Fig. 3.15   (a) Primitives for describing vague triangles. (b) Sample triangles. (c) A stochastic *FSA* which recognizes sample triangles.

If there exists the following sequence of derivational steps

$$\alpha_k \xrightarrow{p_k} \alpha_{k+1} \ , \ k = 1, \ldots, r - 1$$

then we say that $\alpha_1$ derives $\alpha_r$ with the probability $p = \prod_{k=1}^{r} p_k$, denoted $\alpha_1 \xrightarrow{p}{}_{*} \alpha_r$.

Now, we can define the stochastic (regular) language generated by the grammar.

**Definition 3.6 (Stochastic Regular Language Generated):** The language generated by the stochastic regular grammar $G = (\Sigma_N, \Sigma_T, P, S)$ is the set

$$L(G) = \{(\phi, p(\phi)) : \phi \in \Sigma_T^*, \ S \xrightarrow{p_v}{}_{*} \phi, \ v = 1, \ldots, s, \ p(\phi) = \sum_{v=1}^{s} p_v\},$$

where $s$ is the number of all the different derivations of $\phi$ from $S$ and $p_v$ is the probability of the $v$th derivation of $\phi$.

Let the primitives used for representing vague triangle patterns be defined as in Fig. 3.15a. Let there be 64 patterns $a_1 b_1 c$, 8 patterns $a_1 b_2 c$, 8 patterns $a_1 b_3 c$ and 20 patterns $a_2 b_4 c$ in the sample $S$ (cf. Fig. 3.15b). We can estimate probabilities from the relative frequencies of pattern occurrences as follows: $p(a_1 b_1 c) = 0.64$, $p(a_1 b_2 c) = 0.08$, $p(a_1 b_3 c) = 0.08$ and $p(a_2 b_4 c) = 0.2$. One can easily check that the

following stochastic regular grammar $G$ generates the sample $S$. (Probabilities of productions are defined as $p(i)$, where $i$ is a production index.)
$G = (\Sigma_N, \Sigma_T, P, S)$, where:
$\Sigma_N = \{S, A, C, D\}$,
$\Sigma_T = \{a_1, a_2, b_1, b_2, b_3, c\}$,
$P$ consists of the following productions.

$$(1)\ S \to a_1 A, \ p(1) = 0.8 \qquad (5)\ C \to c, \ p(5) = 1.0$$

$$(2)\ A \to b_1 C, \ p(2) = 0.8 \qquad (6)\ S \to a_2 D, \ p(6) = 0.2$$

$$(3)\ A \to b_2 C, \ p(3) = 0.1 \qquad (7)\ D \to b_4 C, \ p(7) = 1.0$$

$$(4)\ A \to b_3 C, \ p(4) = 0.1$$

For example, productions 1, 2, 5 are applied to derive the pattern $a_1 b_1 c$ and the corresponding probability is[39]

$$p(a_1 b_1 c) = p(1) \cdot p(2) \cdot p(5) = 0.64 \ .$$

Let us introduce the notion of stochastic finite-state automaton [Rabin (1963); Turakainen (1968); Fu and Li (1969)].

---

**Parsing Scheme 3.6: Stochastic Finite-State Automaton**

A stochastic finite-state automaton is a quintuple

$$A = (Q, \Sigma_T, \Pi, \pi_0, \pi_F), \text{ where}$$

$Q$ is a set of $n$ states,
$\Sigma_T$ is a finite set of input symbols,
$\Pi$ is a mapping of $\Sigma_T$ into the set of $n \times n$ stochastic state-transition matrices such that

$$\Pi(a) = [\pi_{ij}(a)]_{n \times n} \ , \ \pi_{ij} \geq 0 \ , \ \sum_{j=1}^{n} \pi_{ij} = 1 \ , \ i = 1, \ldots, n \ ,$$

where $\pi_{ij}(a)$ is the probability of the transition from state $q_i$ to state $q_j$ when the symbol $a$ has been read,
$\pi_0$ is an $n$-dimensional row vector representing the initial state distribution such that its first component is equal to 1 and the remaining components are equal to 0,
$\pi_F$ is an $n$-dimensional column vector such that its $k$th component is equal to 1 if $q_k$ is the final state and 0 otherwise.

---

The mapping $\Pi$ can be extended for the domain $\Sigma_T^+$ in the following way.

---

[39]Let us note that each pattern from the sample $S$ has only one derivation. If some pattern had more derivations in the grammar, the probabilities of these derivations would be added together.

$$\Pi(a_1...a_k) = \Pi(a_1) \cdot .... \cdot \Pi(a_k), \ a_i \in \Sigma_T, i = 1, \ldots, k.$$

Now, we can define the stochastic (regular) language accepted by the automaton [Fu and Li (1969)].

> **Definition 3.7 ($\Lambda$-Stochastic Regular Language Accepted):** The $\Lambda$-stochastic regular language accepted with a threshold $\Lambda$, $0 \leq \Lambda < 1$ by the stochastic finite-state automaton $A = (Q, \Sigma_T, \Pi, \pi_0, \pi_F)$ is the set
>
> $$L(A, \Lambda) = \{\phi \in \Sigma_T^* : \ \pi_0 \cdot \Pi(\phi) \cdot \pi_F > \Lambda\}.$$

Before constructing the stochastic finite-state automaton for our exemplary stochastic grammar $G$, we shall introduce the general rules of constructing stochastic *FSAs* on the basis of stochastic regular grammars.
Let $G = (\Sigma_N, \Sigma_T, P, S)$ be a stochastic regular grammar.[40] A stochastic finite-state automaton $A = (Q, \Sigma_T, \Pi, \pi_0, \pi_F)$ such that $L(A) = L(G)$ is constructed in the following way.

(1) Let $\Sigma_N = \{A_1 = S, A_2, \ldots, A_n\}$.
    $Q := \Sigma_N \cup \{A_{n+1} = T, A_{n+2} = R\}$, where $A_{n+1} = T$ is the termination state, $A_{n+2} = R$ is the rejection state[41]. Further, we assume that the states are ordered, i.e. $(A_1 = S, A_2, \ldots A_n, A_{n+1}, A_{n+2})$.

(2) $\pi_0 := \begin{bmatrix} 1 \ 0 \ 0 \ \ldots \ 0 \end{bmatrix}$, an $(n+2)$-dimensional row vector.

(3) $\pi_F := \begin{bmatrix} 0 \ 0 \ \ldots \ 1 \ 0 \end{bmatrix}^T$, an $(n+2)$-dimensional column vector.

(4) Let $\Sigma_T = \{a^1, a^2, \ldots, a^l\}$.
    Every state transition matrix $\Pi(a^k) = [\pi_{ij}(a^k)]_{(n+2) \times (n+2)}$, $k = 1, 2, \ldots, l$ is defined in the following way.
    For every $(A_i \rightarrow a^k B_j, \ p_{ij}^k) \in P$, where $p_{ij}^k$ is the probability of the production: $\pi_{ij}(a^k) := p_{ij}^k$.
    For every $(A_i \rightarrow a^k, \ p_{i0}^k) \in P$, where $p_{i0}^k$ is the probability of the production: $\pi_{i(n+1)}(a^k) := p_{i0}^k$.
    The remaining entries of $\Pi(a^k)$, except for the $(n+2)$th column, set to 0.
    The entries in the $(n+2)$th column set to such values that $\Pi(a^k)$ is a right stochastic matrix.

According to these rules, we are able to construct the stochastic finite-state automaton $A$ for our exemplary stochastic regular grammar $G$ (see Fig. 3.15c). We define the rows and columns of the six-dimensional stochastic state-transition matrices assuming the following ordering of the states $(S, A, C, D, T, R)$.

---

[40]We assume that $G$ is a $\lambda$-free grammar, cf. Definition A.6 in Appendix A.1.
[41]State-transition matrices of a stochastic *FSA* are right stochastic matrices. A right stochastic matrix is a square matrix of nonnegative real numbers, with each row summing to 1. The rejection state $A_{n+2} = R$ is introduced for normalization purposes, i.e., matrix entries belonging to "its" column $(n+2)$ contain values such that each row is summing to 1.

$$\Pi(a_1) = \begin{bmatrix} 0 & 0.8 & 0 & 0 & 0 & 0.2 \\ 0 & 0 & 0 & 0 & 0 & 1 \\ 0 & 0 & 0 & 0 & 0 & 1 \\ 0 & 0 & 0 & 0 & 0 & 1 \\ 0 & 0 & 0 & 0 & 0 & 1 \\ 0 & 0 & 0 & 0 & 0 & 1 \end{bmatrix} \quad \Pi(a_2) = \begin{bmatrix} 0 & 0 & 0 & 0.2 & 0 & 0.8 \\ 0 & 0 & 0 & 0 & 0 & 1 \\ 0 & 0 & 0 & 0 & 0 & 1 \\ 0 & 0 & 0 & 0 & 0 & 1 \\ 0 & 0 & 0 & 0 & 0 & 1 \\ 0 & 0 & 0 & 0 & 0 & 1 \end{bmatrix} \quad \Pi(b_1) = \begin{bmatrix} 0 & 0 & 0 & 0 & 0 & 1 \\ 0 & 0 & 0.8 & 0 & 0 & 0.2 \\ 0 & 0 & 0 & 0 & 0 & 1 \\ 0 & 0 & 0 & 0 & 0 & 1 \\ 0 & 0 & 0 & 0 & 0 & 1 \\ 0 & 0 & 0 & 0 & 0 & 1 \end{bmatrix}$$

$$\Pi(b_2) = \Pi(b_3) = \begin{bmatrix} 0 & 0 & 0 & 0 & 0 & 1 \\ 0 & 0 & 0.1 & 0 & 0 & 0.9 \\ 0 & 0 & 0 & 0 & 0 & 1 \\ 0 & 0 & 0 & 0 & 0 & 1 \\ 0 & 0 & 0 & 0 & 0 & 1 \\ 0 & 0 & 0 & 0 & 0 & 1 \end{bmatrix} \quad \Pi(b_4) = \begin{bmatrix} 0 & 0 & 0 & 0 & 0 & 1 \\ 0 & 0 & 0 & 0 & 0 & 1 \\ 0 & 0 & 0 & 0 & 0 & 1 \\ 0 & 0 & 1 & 0 & 0 & 0 \\ 0 & 0 & 0 & 0 & 0 & 1 \\ 0 & 0 & 0 & 0 & 0 & 1 \end{bmatrix} \quad \Pi(c) = \begin{bmatrix} 0 & 0 & 0 & 0 & 0 & 1 \\ 0 & 0 & 0 & 0 & 0 & 1 \\ 0 & 0 & 0 & 0 & 1 & 0 \\ 0 & 0 & 0 & 0 & 0 & 1 \\ 0 & 0 & 0 & 0 & 0 & 1 \\ 0 & 0 & 0 & 0 & 0 & 1 \end{bmatrix}$$

Let us analyze the pattern $a_1 b_1 c$ with the automaton $A$. One can easily check that

$$\pi_0 \cdot \Pi(a_1 b_1 c) \cdot \pi_F = \pi_0 \cdot \Pi(a_1) \cdot \Pi(b_1) \cdot \Pi(c) \cdot \pi_F = 0.64 \ .$$

According to Definition 3.7, the pattern $a_1 b_1 c$ will belong to the $\Lambda$-stochastic regular language accepted by the automaton $A$, if the threshold $\Lambda$ is set to a value which is less than 0.64.

If the pattern classes $\omega_1, \omega_2, \ldots, \omega_C$ are represented by the stochastic grammars $G_1, G_2, \ldots, G_C$, respectively, then a *maximum-likelihood classifier* assigns a string pattern $\phi$ to class $\omega_k$ if

$$p(\phi \mid G_k) = \max_{i=1,\ldots,C} \{p(\phi \mid G_i)\},$$

where $p(\phi \mid G_i)$ is the probability of generating $\phi$ by $G$.

Stochastic context-free languages are defined in an analogous way to stochastic regular languages [Huang and Fu (1971); Persoon and Fu (1975); Tsai and Fu (1979); Thomason (1990a)]. Probabilities are assigned to grammar productions as well as to parser operations. The issue of estimating probability measures associated with grammars and automata is discussed in [Fu (1982)] as well.

Using stochastic regular grammars and stochastic finite-state automata we treat patterns as being generated by stochastic processes [Vidal *et al.* (2005a,b)]. We have also assumed implicitly that a stochastic process is somehow observable, i.e., any transition between two states is related to one symbol. In presenting hidden Markov models in Section 3.3.4 we abandon this restriction.

### 3.3.2   *Fuzzy Languages*

As we have mentioned at the beginning of Sec. 3.3, if we are not able to use a probability measure, we can treat a language of vague patterns as a fuzzy set. Let us begin with the classic definition of a fuzzy set [Zadeh (1965)].

Let $U$ be a nonempty space. A set $A$, $A \subseteq U$, is called a fuzzy set iff $A = \{(x, \mu(x)) : x \in U\}$, where $\mu : U \longrightarrow [0, 1]$ is a membership function, which is defined as follows

$$\mu(x) = \begin{cases} 0, & x \notin A, \\ 1, & x \in A, \\ m, \ m \in (0,1), & x \text{ belongs to } A \text{ with a grade of membership } m. \end{cases}$$

Now, we can define fuzzy regular grammar [Zadeh (1969); Mizumoto *et al.* (1972)].

**Definition 3.8 (Fuzzy Regular Grammar):** A fuzzy regular (right-regular) grammar is a quadruple

$$G = (\Sigma_N, \Sigma_T, P, S), \text{ where}$$

$\Sigma_N$ is a set of nonterminal symbols,
$\Sigma_T$ is a set of terminal symbols,
$P$ is a set of fuzzy productions of the form:

$$A_i \xrightarrow{\mu_{ij}} \gamma_{ij}, \quad i = 1, \ldots, n, \ j = 1, \ldots, m_i,$$

in which $A_i \in \Sigma_N$ , $\gamma_{ij} \in \Sigma_T \cup \Sigma_T \Sigma_N$, $\mu_{ij}$ is the grade of membership related to the application of the production such that $0 \leq \mu_{ij} \leq 1$
$S$ is the start symbol (axiom), $S \in \Sigma_N$.

A derivation for fuzzy grammars is extended in the following way (cf. Definition A.2 in Appendix A.1). Let the string $\theta$ be derived directly from the string $\beta$ as the result of applying the production $A_i \xrightarrow{\mu_{ij}} \gamma_{ij}$, i.e.

$$\beta \xrightarrow{\mu_{ij}} \theta \ .$$

We say that $\beta$ derives directly $\theta$ with the membership grade $\mu_{ij}$.
If there exists the following sequence of derivational steps

$$\alpha_k \xrightarrow{\mu_{k}} \alpha_{k+1} \ , \ k = 1, \ldots, (r-1)$$

then we say that $\alpha_1$ derives $\alpha_r$ with the membership grade

$$\mu = \min_{k=1,\ldots,(r-1)} \{\mu_k\},$$

denoted $\alpha_1 \overset{\mu}{\underset{*}{\Longrightarrow}} \alpha_r$.

Let us define the fuzzy (regular) language generated by the grammar [Lee and Zadeh (1969)].

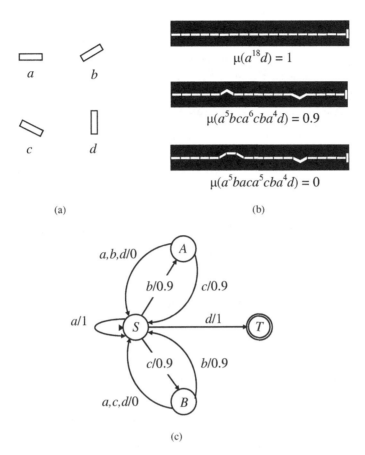

$$\mu(a^{18}d) = 1$$

$$\mu(a^5bca^6cba^4d) = 0.9$$

$$\mu(a^5baca^5cba^4d) = 0$$

(a)          (b)

(c)

Fig. 3.16   (a) Primitives for describing vague path patterns. (b) Exemplary paths. (c) A fuzzy *FSA* which recognizes the language of vague paths.

**Definition 3.9 (Fuzzy Regular Language Generated):** The language generated by the fuzzy regular grammar $G = (\Sigma_N, \Sigma_T, P, S)$ is the set

$$L(G) = \{(\phi, \mu(\phi)) : \phi \in \Sigma_T^*, \ S \xrightarrow{\mu_v}_{*} \phi, \ v = 1, \ldots, s, \ \mu(\phi) = \max_{v=1,\ldots,s} \{\mu_v\}\},$$

where $s$ is the number of all the different derivations of $\phi$ from $S$ and $\mu_v$ is the membership grade of the $v$th derivation of $\phi$. We say that $\phi$ belongs to $L(G)$ with the membership grade $\mu(\phi)$.

Let us consider the following example of an industrial visual inspection system. A recognition of paths which consist of straight segments is one of the system tasks. We assume that segments may be not ideally straight as shown in Fig. 3.16b. Assuming the structural primitives shown in Fig. 3.16a, we tolerate small distortions represented by the substrings *bc* and *cb*.[12] If a segment is ideally straight

---

[12] Each segment is finished with the end-marker *d*.

(e.g., the first segment $a^{18}d$ in Fig. 3.16b) then it belongs to the (fuzzy) set of straight segments with the membership grade 1. If it contains distortions of the form $bc$ or $cb$ (e.g. the second segment $a^5bca^6cba^4d$) then it belongs to the set of straight segments with the membership grade 0.9. Otherwise, the segment is rejected (e.g. the third segment $a^5baca^5cba^4d$ with the membership grade 0). The fuzzy regular grammar $G$ which generates the fuzzy language of vague segments is defined as follows.

$G = (\Sigma_N, \Sigma_T, P, S)$, where:

$\Sigma_N = \{S, A, B\}$,

$\Sigma_T = \{a, b, c, d\}$,

$P$ consists of the following productions.

|  |  |
|---|---|
| (1) $S \rightarrow aS$, $\mu(1) = 1$ | (6) $S \rightarrow cB$, $\mu(6) = 0.9$ |
| (2) $S \rightarrow bA$, $\mu(2) = 0.9$ | (7) $B \rightarrow bS$, $\mu(7) = 0.9$ |
| (3) $A \rightarrow cS$, $\mu(3) = 0.9$ | (8) $B \rightarrow aS$, $\mu(8) = 0$ |
| (4) $A \rightarrow aS$, $\mu(4) = 0$ | (9) $B \rightarrow cS$, $\mu(9) = 0$ |
| (5) $A \rightarrow bS$, $\mu(5) = 0$ | (10) $S \rightarrow d$, $\mu(10) = 1$ |

For example, in order to generate the pattern $aabcad$ the following sequence of productions should be applied: (1), (1), (2), (3), (1), (10) and the corresponding membership grade is

$$\mu(aabcad) = \min\{\mu(1), \mu(1), \mu(2), \mu(3), \mu(1), \mu(10)\} = 0.9.$$

Let us define a fuzzy finite-state automaton [Santos (1968, 1976); Wee and Fu (1969); Mizumoto *et al.* (1969); Thomason (1973); Thomason and Marinos (1974)].

---

**Parsing Scheme 3.7: Fuzzy Finite-State Automaton**

A fuzzy finite-state automaton is a quintuple

$$A = (Q, \Sigma_T, M, \mu_0, \mu_F), \text{ where}$$

$Q$ is a set of $n$ states,

$\Sigma_T$ is a finite set of input symbols,

M is a mapping of $\Sigma_T$ into the set of $n \times n$ fuzzy state-transition matrices such that

$$M(a) = [\mu_{ij}(a)]_{n \times n}, \ 0 \leq \mu_{ij}(a) \leq 1, \ i = 1, \ldots, n, \ j = 1, \ldots, n,$$

where $\mu_{ij}(a)$ is the grade of the transition from state $q_i$ to state $q_j$ when the symbol $a$ has been read,

$\mu_0$ is an $n$-dimensional row vector representing the initial state,

$\mu_F$ is an $n$-dimensional column vector representing the final states.

In order to define a language accepted by a (max-min) fuzzy automaton [Malik and Mordeson (1996)] we introduce firstly notions of: the (minimum-based) fuzzy (binary) relation and the max-min composition of fuzzy relations.

Let $\mu_X$ and $\mu_Y$ be the membership functions of the fuzzy sets $X$ and $Y$, respectively. The fuzzy relation $X \times Y$ is defined by its membership function $\mu_{X \times Y}(x, y) = min\{\mu_X(x), \mu_Y(y)\}$.

Let $R_1 \subseteq X \times Z$, $R_2 \subseteq Z \times Y$ be fuzzy relations. The max-min composition of $R_1$ and $R_2$, denoted by $R_1 \circ R_2$ or $maxmin(R_1, R_2)$, is defined as follows:

$$R_1 \circ R_2(x, y) = \max_{z \in Z}\{min\{R_1(x, z), R_2(z, y)\}\}.$$

Now, we can extend the mapping $M$ for the domain $\Sigma_T^*$ in the following way.[43]

$$M(a_1...a_k) = M(a_1) \circ \ldots \circ M(a_k), \ a_i \in \Sigma_T, i = 1, \ldots, k.$$

Finally, let us define a fuzzy (regular) language accepted by the automaton [Wee and Fu (1969); Mizumoto *et al.* (1975)].

**Definition 3.10 (Fuzzy Regular Language Accepted):** The fuzzy regular language accepted with a threshold $\Lambda$, $0 \leq \Lambda < 1$ by the fuzzy max-min finite-state automaton $A = (Q, \Sigma_T, M, \mu_0, \mu_F)$ is the set

$$L(A, \Lambda) = \{\phi \in \Sigma_T^* : \ \mu(\phi) = \mu_0 \circ M(\phi) \circ \mu_F > \Lambda\}.$$

The rules of constructing fuzzy finite-state automata on the basis of fuzzy regular grammars are analogous to those defined for stochastic automata/grammars introduced in a previous section.[44] Therefore, we do not present them here.

The fuzzy state-transition matrices and vectors of the fuzzy automaton $A$ constructed for our exemplary fuzzy grammar $G$ (see Fig. 3.16c) are defined in the following way. (Rows and columns of the fuzzy state-transition matrices are defined assuming the following ordering of the states $(S, A, B, T)$.) $\mu_0 = \begin{bmatrix} 1 & 0 & 0 & 0 \end{bmatrix}$,

$\mu_F := \begin{bmatrix} 0 & 0 & 0 & 1 \end{bmatrix}^T$.

$$M(a) = \begin{bmatrix} 1 & 0 & 0 & 0 \\ 0 & 0 & 0 & 0 \\ 0 & 0 & 0 & 0 \\ 0 & 0 & 0 & 0 \end{bmatrix} \quad M(b) = \begin{bmatrix} 0 & 0.9 & 0 & 0 \\ 0 & 0 & 0 & 0 \\ 0.9 & 0 & 0 & 0 \\ 0 & 0 & 0 & 0 \end{bmatrix} \quad M(c) = \begin{bmatrix} 0 & 0 & 0.9 & 0 \\ 0.9 & 0 & 0 & 0 \\ 0 & 0 & 0 & 0 \\ 0 & 0 & 0 & 0 \end{bmatrix} \quad M(d) = \begin{bmatrix} 0 & 0 & 0 & 1 \\ 0 & 0 & 0 & 0 \\ 0 & 0 & 0 & 0 \\ 0 & 0 & 0 & 0 \end{bmatrix}$$

Let us analyze the pattern *aabcad* with the automaton $A$. It can be easily checked that[45]

---

[43] For the empty string $\lambda$ the matrix $M(\lambda)$ can be defined as the identity matrix.

[44] Of course, we do not introduce the rejection state $R$ in case of fuzzy automata.

[45] Let us notice that the max-min composition $\circ$ of matrices is analogous to a multiplication of matrices. Instead of multiplying entries we apply the *minimum* operation. Instead of summing the multiplication results we apply the *maximum* operation.

$$\mu(aabcad) = \mu_0 \circ M(aabcad) \circ \mu_F =$$
$$\mu_0 \circ M(a) \circ M(a) \circ M(b) \circ M(c) \circ M(a) \circ M(d) \circ \mu_F = 0.9 \; .$$

According to Definition 3.10, the pattern *aabcad* will belong to the fuzzy regular language accepted by the automaton $A$, if the threshold $\Lambda$ is set to a value which is less than 0.9.

Fuzzy *CF* languages [Santos (1974); Bucurescu and Pascu (1981); Asveld (2005a,b)] are defined in an analogous way to fuzzy regular languages. Membership grades assigned to productions and transitions. Fuzzy automata are presented in [Mordeson and Malik (2002)] and fuzzy transducers in [Thomason (1974b)].

### 3.3.3    *Error-Correcting Parsing*

As we have mentioned at the beginning of Sec. 3.3, structural representations are sometimes distorted because of errors occurring at an image preprocessing stage [Fu (1982)]. Three types of errors are considered for string representations in the error-correcting model: substitution, deletion and insertion.

A substitution error consists in replacing a symbol by another symbol. Let us return to our example of the fuzzy language of vague segments defined in a previous section. We have decided to tolerate small distortions of the form *bc* and *cb*. A distortion of the form *bc* is shown in Fig. 3.17a. Now, let us look at Fig. 3.17b. Although a pattern shown in this figure is less distorted than the pattern in Fig. 3.17a, the second primitive of the distortion has been classified as *a* because of the small inclination angle, which results in rejecting this pattern (represented with $a^k(ba)a^n$). The substitution error consists in replacing *c* by *a*.

Whereas substitution errors are often caused by primitive recognition errors, deletion and insertion errors occur frequently due to segmentation errors. Let us consider an example of a deletion error. It consists in removing a symbol from a string representing a reference pattern. Let us look at Fig. 3.17c. Due to a segmentation error, the boundary of an object has been located incorrectly, resulting in generating the chain code string 1177 instead of the (correct) chain code string 11077.

The third type of errors, insertion, consists in including incorrectly a symbol to a string.

Let us present the idea of error-correcting parsing before introducing its formal definitions. Firstly, we define error transformations which allow us to model three types of errors introduced above. (Using these transformations various distances between strings can be defined.) Secondly, on the basis of a reference grammar $G$ generating representations of patterns considered, the so-called *expanded grammar* $G_e$ which contains additionally *error productions* is constructed. For every production of $G$, error-productions are introduced with the help of the error transformations and the costs of these errors are defined.[46] Finally, an automaton/parser is

---

[46]That is, error productions model errors which can occur in strings of $L(G)$.

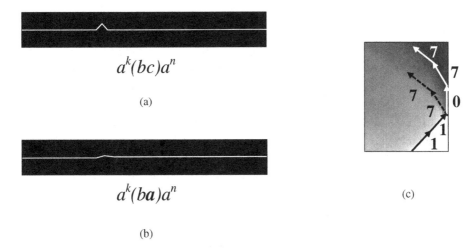

(a)

(b)

(c)

Fig. 3.17 (a) A pattern which belongs to the fuzzy language of vague segments. (b) A pattern which does not belong to the fuzzy language of vague segments. (c) A segmentation error and its consequence.

constructed. Error-correcting automata/parsers are (simple) modifications of their standard counterparts. The costs of errors[47] corresponding to transitions (reduction operations) are added up during parsing, giving, finally, a distance between an analyzed string and a (reference) string of $L(G)$.

Now, we can formalize our considerations. Firstly, let us introduce error transformations [Levenshtein (1966); Thomason (1974a); Fu (1982)]

Let there be given two strings $x, y \in \Sigma_T^*$. A transformation $\mathcal{F} : \Sigma_T^* \longmapsto \Sigma_T^*$ such that $y \in \mathcal{F}(x)$ is called a *string transformation*. We define the following string error transformations.

- Substitution error transformation $\mathcal{F}_S : \eta_1 a \eta_2 \xmapsto{\mathcal{F}_S} \eta_1 b \eta_2$ , $a, b \in \Sigma_T$, $a \neq b$, $\eta_1, \eta_2 \in \Sigma_T^*$.
- Insertion error transformation $\mathcal{F}_I : \eta_1 \eta_2 \xmapsto{\mathcal{F}_I} \eta_1 a \eta_2$ , $a \in \Sigma_T$, $\eta_1, \eta_2 \in \Sigma_T^*$.
- Deletion error transformation $\mathcal{F}_D : \eta_1 a \eta_2 \xmapsto{\mathcal{F}_D} \eta_1 \eta_2$ , $a \in \Sigma_T$, $\eta_1, \eta_2 \in \Sigma_T^*$.

The *distance* $\rho_L(x, y)$ between strings $x$ and $y$ in the sense of the simple Levenshtein metric is defined as the smallest number of string transformations $\mathcal{F}_S, \mathcal{F}_I, \mathcal{F}_D$ required to obtain the string $y$ from the string $x$.

For example, if $x = abcbdbb, y = abcbedba$ then

$$x = abcbdbb \xmapsto{\mathcal{F}_S} abcbdba \xmapsto{\mathcal{F}_I} abcbedba = y \ .$$

The smallest number of string transformations required to obtain $y$ from $x$ is two. Thus, $\rho_L(x, y) = 2$.

Let us ascribe the weights $\sigma, \omega, \gamma$ to the transformations $\mathcal{F}_S, \mathcal{F}_I, \mathcal{F}_D$, respectively. Let $M$ be a sequence of the string transformations applied to obtain the string $y$

---

[47]The cost of a non-error production is equal to 0.

from the string $x$ such that we have used $s_M$ substitution error transformations, $i_M$ insertion error transformations and $d_M$ deletion error transformations. The distance $\rho_{LWTE}(x, y)$ between the strings $x$ and $y$ in the sense of the Levenshtein metric weighted according to the type of error is given by the following formula.

$$\rho_{LWTE}(x, y) = \min_M \{\sigma \cdot s_M + \omega \cdot i_M + \gamma \cdot d_M\}$$

Finally we can define the transformations with various costs depending on various terminal symbols.

Let $S(a, b)$ denote the cost of substituting $a$ by $b$ ($S(a, a) = 0$), $D(a)$ denote the cost of deleting $a$, $I(a, b)$ denote the cost of inserting $b$ before $a$, i.e.,

$$\eta_1 a \eta_2 \overset{\mathcal{F}_I}{\longmapsto} \eta_1 b a \eta_2 \quad a, b \in \Sigma_T, \ \eta_1, \eta_2 \in \Sigma_T^* \ ,$$

and, additionally, let $I_e(b)$ denote the cost of inserting $b$ at the end of a word.
Let $M$ be a sequence of the string transformations applied to obtain the string $y$ from the string $x$ and $c(M)$ denotes the sum of costs $S, I, I_e, D$ of all the transformations of the sequence $M$.
The distance $\rho_{LWE}(x, y)$ between the strings $x$ and $y$ in the sense of the Levenshtein metric weighted with errors is given by the following formula.

$$\rho_{LWE}(x, y) = \min_M \{c(M)\}$$

Now, we shall introduce expanded grammars [Rulot and Vidal (1988)].

**Definition 3.11 (Expanded Grammar):** Let $G = (\Sigma_N, \Sigma_T, P, S)$ be a (reference) regular grammar. $G_e = (\Sigma_N, \Sigma_T', P', S)$ is called an expanded grammar for $G$ iff

$\Sigma_T \subseteq \Sigma_T'$,
$P' = P \cup P_S \cup P_D \cup P_I \cup P_{Ie}$, where
$\qquad P_S = \{(X \to bY, \ S(a, b)) : X \to aY \in P, \ a \in \Sigma_T, \ b \in \Sigma_T', \ a \neq b\} \ \cup$
$\qquad \cup \ \{(X \to b, \ S(a, b)) : X \to a \in P, \ a \in \Sigma_T, \ b \in \Sigma_T', \ a \neq b\}$,
$\qquad P_D = \{(X \to Y, \ D(a)) : X \to aY \in P, \ a \in \Sigma_T\} \ \cup$
$\qquad \cup \ \{(X \to \lambda, \ D(a)) : X \to a \in P, \ a \in \Sigma_T\}$,
$\qquad P_I = \{(X \to bX, \ I(a, b)) : X \to aY \in P, \ a \in \Sigma_T, \ b \in \Sigma_T'\} \ \cup$
$\qquad \cup \ \{(X \to ba, \ I(a, b)) : X \to a \in P, \ a \in \Sigma_T, \ b \in \Sigma_T'\}$,
$\qquad P_{Ie} = \{(X \to ab, \ I_e(b)) : X \to a \in P, \ a \in \Sigma_T, \ b \in \Sigma_T'\}$.
Every non-error production of $P'$ is of the form $(X \to \alpha, \ 0)$, where $X \to \alpha \in P$.

We assume that $\Sigma_T \subseteq \Sigma_T'$, because sometimes we want to add symbols representing additional distortions of terminals of the reference grammar $G$.

Expanded grammars for (reference) context-free grammars are defined in an analogous way.[48] For regular grammars corresponding error-correcting automata

---

[48] Let us notice that an expanded grammar for a regular grammar is not regular because of unit

were presented in [Rulot and Vidal (1988); Huang (2002)]. Error-correcting models for context-free grammars were presented in [Tanaka and Fu (1978)] and error-correcting Earley-based parsers in [Aho and Peterson (1972); Fu (1982)]. The main idea of these models can be formulated as follows:

Let $G$ be a reference grammar, $G_e$ be an expanded grammar for $G$, $A$ be an error-correcting parser (automaton) constructed for $G_e$ and $\rho$ be a metric used in a model. Let $y$ be a string to be recognized. The *minimum-distance error-correcting parser (MDECP)* finds a string $x \in L(G)$ such that
$$\rho(x, y) = \min_z \{\rho(z, y) : z \in L(G)\} \ .$$

At the end of this section we introduce the extensions to the Earley parser which allow one to define its error-correcting version according to the model presented in [Aho and Peterson (1972)].

Let $w = a_1 a_2 \ldots a_n$ be a word to be parsed. The error-correcting Earley parser generates a sequence of state sets $I(0), I(1), \ldots, I(n)$ and computes the minimum distance in the following way.[49] A state set $I(i)$ consists of state items of the form $[A \rightarrow \alpha_\bullet\beta, \ j, \ d]$, where $j, A, \alpha, \beta$ are defined as in Sec. 3.2.4 and $d$ is the minimum number of error transformations required to perform the derivation $\alpha \overset{*}{\Rightarrow} a_{(j+1)} a_{(j+2)} \ldots a_i$. The initialization is made in an analogous way as in Sec. 3.2.4. However, the parser adds a new state item of the form $[A \rightarrow \alpha_\bullet\beta, \ j, \ d]$ in a different way. If there is no state item $[A \rightarrow \alpha_\bullet\beta, \ j, \ d']$ in state set $I(i)$, then the new state is simply added. Otherwise, $[A \rightarrow \alpha_\bullet\beta, \ j, \ d']$ is *replaced* by $[A \rightarrow \alpha_\bullet\beta, \ j, \ d]$ only if $d' > d$.[50]

Three basic operations of the parser, defined for each state $I(k)$, $k = 0, 1, \ldots, n$, are modified with respect to the version presented in Sec. 3.2.4 as follows. Let $G_e = (\Sigma_N, \Sigma_T', P', S)$ be an expanded context-free grammar for $G$.

- *predict* - for each $[A \rightarrow \alpha_\bullet B\beta, \ i, \ d] \in I(k)$ for each $B \rightarrow \theta \in P'$
  add $[B \rightarrow {}_\bullet\theta, \ k, \ 0]$ to $I(k)$.
- *scan* - for each $[A \rightarrow \alpha_\bullet x\beta, \ i, \ 0] \in I(k)$ such that $x = a_{k+1}$
  add $[A \rightarrow \alpha x_\bullet\beta, \ i, \ d]$ to $I(k+1)$.
- *complete* - for each $[A \rightarrow \omega_\bullet, \ i, \ d] \in I(k)$ for each $I(i)$ if $[C \rightarrow \alpha_\bullet A\beta, \ j, \ d'] \in I(i)$, then
  add $[C \rightarrow \alpha A_\bullet\beta, \ j, \ d'']$ to $I(k)$, where $d'' := d + d' + 1$, if $A \rightarrow \omega$ is an error production; and $d'' := d + d'$, otherwise.

The error-correcting Earley parsing algorithm is the same as the Parsing Scheme 3.4 in Sec. 3.2.4.

*Maximum-likelihood error-correcting parsers (MLECPs)*, in which the error-correction model is incorporated into stochastic grammars, were studied in [Fung and Fu (1975); Thomason (1975, 1981); Lu and Fu (1977)]. An error-correcting parser for context-sensitive languages was proposed in [Kobayashi *et al.* (1986)].

---

productions $(X \rightarrow Y)$. An expanded grammar for a context free grammar is context-free.

[49] For simplicity reasons we assume that the simple Levenshtein metric is used.

[50] This way the minimum distance is computed during parsing.

### 3.3.4   *Hidden Markov Model (HMM) and Viterbi Algorithm*

By introducing stochastic systems such as stochastic regular grammars and stochastic *FSAs* in Section 3.3.1 we have, in fact, treated patterns as being generated by stochastic processes. Moreover, we have assumed that a stochastic process is somehow observable, i.e., any transition between two states of the process is related to one "observable" symbol. (A pattern to be analyzed is a sequence of observations in this interpretation.) Of course, the state of a stochastic process does not have to be related one-to-one to the primitive observed. In the hidden Markov model [Markov (1913); Baum and Petrie (1966)] the probability distribution for a set of terminal symbols (primitives) is defined for each state independently. (In the case of *HMMs* we say that a terminal symbol is *emitted* instead of saying that it is *generated/read*).[51] Let us introduce the concept of a hidden Markov model which is analogous to a stochastic finite-state automaton (cf. Parsing Scheme 3.6).

---

**Parsing Scheme 3.8: Hidden Markov Model**

A hidden Markov model is a quintuple

$$HMM = (Q, \Sigma_T, \Pi, E, \pi_0), \text{ where}$$

$Q = \{q_1, q_2, \ldots, q_N\}$ is a set of $N$ states,
$\Sigma_T = \{a_1, a_2, \ldots, a_M\}$ is a finite set of $M$ symbols,
$\Pi : Q \times Q \to \mathbb{R}_{\geq 0}$ is the state-transition probability distribution,
$E : Q \times \Sigma_T \to \mathbb{R}_{\geq 0}$ is the state-based symbol emission probability distribution,
$\pi_0 = [\pi(1), \pi(2), \ldots, \pi(N)]$ is the initial state distribution vector,
and the following conditions hold:

$$\forall q' \in Q \quad \sum_{q'' \in Q} \Pi(q', q'') = 1 \ , \quad \sum_{a \in \Sigma_T} E(q', a) = 1 \ , \quad \sum_{i=1}^{N} \pi(i) = 1 \ .$$

---

$\Pi(q_i, q_j) = \pi_{ij}, i, j = 1, \ldots, N$ is the probability of the transition from state $q_i$ to state $q_j$. $E(q_j, a_m) = e_j(a_m), j = 1, \ldots, N, m = 1, \ldots, M$ is the probability of emitting $a_m$ in state $q_j$. $\pi(i), i = 1, \ldots, N$ is the probability the Markov chain starts in state $q_i$.

Let us consider the following example: let a diagnostic system monitor a parameter of a (stochastic) process. The parameter is monitored in order to find out whether the process is stable and to detect accelerations/decelerations. The behavior of the parameter is tracked with the chart as shown in Fig. 3.18a. The set of primitives used for representing the process patterns is shown in Fig. 3.18b and the pattern shown in Fig. 3.18a is represented as in Fig. 3.18c. Let us define *HMM* for our example in the following way.

---

[51] For some types of *HMMs* symbols are emitted at the transitions (not at the states).

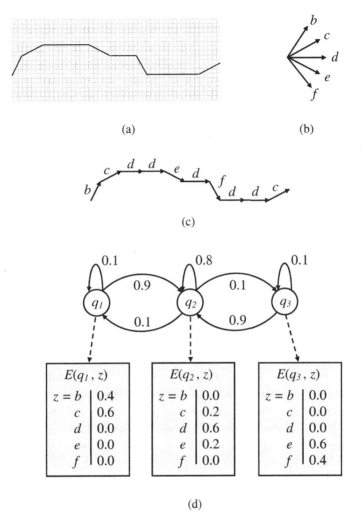

(a)             (b)

(c)

(d)

Fig. 3.18 (a) A pattern corresponding to a process parameter. (b) Primitives for describing the process patterns. (c) The representation of the pattern. (d) *HMM* for the process.

$HMM = (Q, \Sigma_T, \Pi, E, \pi_0)$, where
$Q = \{q_1, q_2, q_3\}$, $q_1$ is the acceleration state, $q_2$ is the in-control state, $q_3$ is the deceleration state,
$\Sigma_T = \{b, c, d, e, f\}$ is shown in Fig. 3.18b,
$\Pi$ and $E$ are defined as follows (the ordering of the symbols $(b, c, d, e, f)$ is assumed)

$$\Pi = \begin{bmatrix} 0.1 \ 0.9 \ 0.0 \\ 0.1 \ 0.8 \ 0.1 \\ 0.0 \ 0.9 \ 0.1 \end{bmatrix} \quad E = \begin{bmatrix} 0.4 \ 0.6 \ 0.0 \ 0.0 \ 0.0 \\ 0.0 \ 0.2 \ 0.6 \ 0.2 \ 0.0 \\ 0.0 \ 0.0 \ 0.0 \ 0.6 \ 0.4 \end{bmatrix}$$

$\pi_0 := \begin{bmatrix} 1.0 \ 0.0 \ 0.0 \end{bmatrix}$, i.e. the process has to start in state $q_1$.

The *HMM* for our example is shown in Fig. 3.18d.

For formal syntactic-stochastic systems like grammars and automata we define what we mean by generating/accepting strings with some probabilities. In the case of hidden Markov models we should also define what we mean when we say that *HMM* emits a string $x \in \Sigma_T^+$ with probability $p(x)$. Let $x = x_1 x_2 \ldots x_T$ be an emitted (observed) string and $z = (z_1, z_2, \ldots, z_T)$ be a valid sequence of states. The probability of $z$ is given by the following formula.

$$p(z) = \pi(z_1) \cdot \Pi(z_1, z_2) \cdot \Pi(z_2, z_3) \cdot \ldots \cdot \Pi(z_{(T-1)}, z_T)$$

The probability of emitting $x$ through $z$ is

$$p(x \mid z) = E(z_1, x_1) \cdot E(z_2, x_2) \cdot \ldots \cdot E(z_T, x_T) \ .$$

Thus, in order to calculate the probability of emitting $x$, we have to take into account all the valid state sequences $Z(x)$ for $x$, which gives the following formula.

$$p(x) = \sum_{z \in Z(x)} p(x \mid z) \cdot p(z)$$

For example, let $x = bcdd$. Then, the probability $p(x)$ is computed as follows.

$$p(bcdd) = p(bcdd \mid q_1 q_1 q_1 q_1) \cdot p(q_1 q_1 q_1 q_1) + p(bcdd \mid q_1 q_1 q_1 q_2) \cdot p(q_1 q_1 q_1 q_2) + \ldots$$

One can notice that computing $p(x)$ according to this formula is inefficient. In general, there are $N^T$ state sequences, where $N$ is the number of states of *HMM*, $T$ is the input length. Therefore, for computing $p(x)$ the forward probability algorithm [Baum *et al.* (1970)] constructed with *dynamic programming technique* is used. In order to make use of this technique we define the probability of being in state $z_t = q_i$ after observing the part $x_1 x_2 \ldots x_t$ of the string $x$, called a partial forward probability, i.e.,

$$f_t(i) = p(x_1 x_2 \ldots x_t, z_t = q_i) \ .$$

Now, the *forward probability algorithm* [Baum *et al.* (1970); Rabiner (1989)] can compute the probabilities $f_t(i)$ and finally $p(x)$ in the following inductive way.

(1) Initialize forward probability:

$$f_1(i) := \pi(i) \cdot e_i(x_1), \ i = 1, \ldots, N \ .$$

(2) Compute partial forward probabilities:

$$f_t(j) := \sum_{i=1}^{N} f_{(t-1)}(i) \pi_{ij} \cdot e_j(x_t), \ t = 2, \ldots, T \ , \ j = 1, \ldots, N \ .$$

(3) Compute probability:

$$p(x) := \sum_{i=1}^{N} f_T(i) \ .$$

The running time of the algorithm is $\mathcal{O}(N^2 \cdot T)$. The forward probability algorithm will be used in Section 5.4 for learning of *HMMs* with the Baum-Welch method.

The forward probability algorithm allows one to compute the probability of generating a pattern $x = x_1 x_2 \ldots x_T$ with *HMM*. However, it does not give us its parse, i.e., the sequence of states associated with its observation. Let us notice that usually there are many such sequences and we would like to find the optimal (the most probable) one. This problem is solved with the Viterbi algorithm [Viterbi (1967)]. The algorithm identifies the most probable sequence of states $(\hat{z}_1, \hat{z}_2, \ldots, \hat{z}_T)$ and computes its probability $\hat{p}$.

In order to use a *dynamic programming technique* we define the (partial) probability $v_t(i)$ of being in state $z_t = q_i$ after observing the part $x_1 x_2 \ldots x_t$ of the string $x$ and assuming that we have passed through the most probable sequence of states

$$v_t(i) = \max_{z_1, z_2, \ldots, z_{(t-1)}} \{ \, p((z_1, z_2, \ldots, z_t = q_i), x_1 x_2 \ldots x_t) \, \} \, .$$

One can easily check that the partial probability $v_t(i)$ can be defined inductively as follows.

$$v_t(j) = \max_{i=1,\ldots,N} \{ \, v_{(t-1)}(i) \pi_{ij} \, \} \cdot e_j(x_t)$$

In order to be able to retrace the complete optimal sequence of states, at each step we store the argument which maximizes the formula above, i.e., the index of the state $q_i$ from which comes the most probable sequence leading to the state $q_j$. We store this index in $best\_predecessor_t(j)$, i.e.,:

$$best\_predecessor_t(j) = \arg\max_{i=1,\ldots,N} \{ \, v_{(t-1)}(i) \pi_{ij} \, \} \, .$$

Now, we can present the Viterbi algorithm.

---

**Parsing Scheme 3.9: Viterbi Algorithm**

**for** $i := 1$ **to** $N$ **do**
  **begin**
    $v_1(i) := \pi(i) \cdot e_i(x_1)$;
    $best\_predecessor_t(j) := 0$;
  **end**;
**for** $t := 2$ **to** $T$ **do**
  **for** $j := 1$ **to** $N$ **do**
    **begin**
      $v_t(j) := \max_{i=1,\ldots,N} \{ v_{(t-1)}(i) \pi_{ij} \} \cdot e_j(x_t)$;
      $best\_predecessor_t(j) := \arg\max_{i=1,\ldots,N} \{ v_{(t-1)}(i) \pi_{ij} \}$;
    **end**;
$\hat{p} := \max_{i=1,\ldots,N} \{ v_{(T)}(i) \}$;
$\hat{z}_T := \arg\max_{i=1,\ldots,N} \{ v_{(T)}(i) \}$;
**for** $t := T - 1$ **downto** $1$ **do**
  $\hat{z}_t := best\_predecessor_{(t+1)}(\hat{z}_{(t+1)})$;

Let us present the following theorem.

**Theorem 3.8 (Viterbi Algorithm Complexity [Viterbi (1967)])**

*The running time of the Viterbi algorithm is $\mathcal{O}(N^2 \cdot T)$, where $N$ is the number of states of HMM, $T$ is the input length.*

As we will see in Chapter 6, *HMM* is used in various applications of syntactic pattern recognition like e.g. gesture recognition, radar tracking, shape recognition, handwritten text recognition, medical image analysis, biological sequence analysis, urban architecture objects analysis [Bunke and Caelli (2001)]. The theory of *HMMs* is presented in [Rabiner (1989); Rabiner and Juang (1993); Jelinek (1997); Manning and Schütze (2003); Jurafsky and Martin (2008)].

In this section we have shown how to enhance grammatical formalisms in order to recognize vague/distorted patterns. Sometimes, however, we have to enhance grammars which generate standard patterns, because the sets of these patterns cannot be represented as context-free languages. We shall consider this problem in the next chapter.

# Chapter 4

# Enhanced String Grammars for Pattern Recognition

In the case of some application areas, the structural patterns are too complex to be modelled by context-free (*CF*) grammars. On the other hand, the class of context-sensitive (*CS*) grammars cannot also be used for the describing of such patterns because the corresponding linear-bounded automata are inefficient computationally. This problem is solved in the following two ways in syntactic pattern recognition:[1]

- the increasing of the *generative power* of *CF* grammars,
- the increasing of the *descriptive power* of string grammars.[2]

The increasing of the *generative power* means here the conceptual modification of the formal definition of a *CF*-type grammar so it can generate certain *CS* languages. Fortunately, the constructing of the (sub)classes of grammars in between *CF* and *CS* grammars is possible. (This issue relates to Parikh's theorem [Parikh (1966)].) Within this methodology, we shall present two main groups of enhanced *CF* grammars: grammars with operator controlled derivations (indexed and linear indexed grammars, head grammars, combinatory categorial grammars, conjunctive grammars and Boolean grammars) in Sec. 4.1 and grammars with programmed derivations (programmed grammars and dynamically programmed grammars) in Sec. 4.2. We introduce here also the model based on *Augmented Regular Expressions* (*AREs*) in Sec. 4.3.

The increasing of the *descriptive power*[3] is achieved in syntactic pattern recognition by the enhancement of the representation scheme (representation mapping). In such a methodological strategy, the structural components of objects (and their relationships) are described in a more adequate way by the representation language, usually by referring to the specific structural and semantic properties of these objects. Firstly, attributed grammars are introduced in Sec. 4.4. Then, various picture language models (*Picture Description Languages*, *PDLs*, two-dimensional automata, matrix/array grammars, shape grammars and *Shape Feature Languages*,

---

[1]The third way consists in the use of the tree or graph grammars which are presented in Parts III and IV of the book.

[2]Sometimes both ways to solve this problem are used at the same time.

[3]Of course, the increasing of the generative power increases the descriptive power as well. However, in some cases it can be insufficient for the solving of a pattern recognition problem.

*SFLs*), which belong to this approach, are presented in Sec. 4.5.
Timed automata are presented in the last section.

## 4.1  Grammars with Operator Controlled Derivations

The increasing of the generative power of *CF* grammars is achieved by the controlling of the derivation process. In this book we present a taxonomy of grammars with controlled derivations from the perspective of syntactic pattern recognition.[4] In the first approach to derivation controlling, certain control operators (conditions, mechanisms) are included within grammar productions. The grammars which belong to this approach are presented in this section. The parsing methods for the enhanced classes of context-free grammars are presented in [Kallmeyer (2010)].

### 4.1.1  *Indexed and Linear Indexed Grammars*

Indexed grammars were presented in [Aho (1968)]. Let us introduce the following definition.

> **Definition 4.1 (Indexed Grammar):** An indexed grammar, *IG*, is a quintuple
>
> $$G = (\Sigma_N, \Sigma_T, I, P, S), \text{ where}$$
>
> $\Sigma_N$ is a set of nonterminal symbols,
> $\Sigma_T$ is a set of terminal symbols,
> $I$ is a set of indices,
> $P$ is a finite set of productions of one of the following three types:
>
> $$1.\ A \longrightarrow \alpha \quad \text{or} \quad 2.\ A[..] \longrightarrow B[i..] \quad \text{or} \quad 3.\ A[i..] \longrightarrow \alpha[..]\ ,$$
>
> where $A$ and $B \in \Sigma_N$, $i \in I$, $[..]$ represents a stack of indices, a string in $I^*$, $\alpha \in \Sigma^*$,
> $S$ is the start symbol (axiom), $S \in \Sigma_N$.

Indices are used in productions to define the context during a derivation. The left-most index is treated as the top element of the stack.

A derivation in indexed grammars is defined in the following way [Aho (1968)]: Let $A, B \in \Sigma_N$, $X_j \in \Sigma$, $\beta \in \Sigma^*$, $\gamma \in \Sigma^*$, $i \in I$, $\theta \in I^*$.

(1) If $A \longrightarrow X_1...X_k$ is a production of type 1, then $\beta A[\theta]\gamma \Rightarrow \beta X_1\theta_1...X_k\theta_k\gamma$, where $\theta_j = [\theta]$ if $X_j \in \Sigma_N$ and $\theta_j = \lambda$ if $X_j \in \Sigma_T$, $j = 1,...k$.
(2) If $A[..] \longrightarrow B[i..]$ is a production of type 2, then $\beta A[\theta]\gamma \Rightarrow \beta B[i\theta]\gamma$.
(3) If $A[i..] \longrightarrow X_1...X_k[..]$ is a production of type 3, then $\beta A[i\theta]\gamma \Rightarrow \beta X_1\theta_1...X_k\theta_k\gamma$, where $\theta_j = [\theta]$ if $X_j \in \Sigma_N$ and $\theta_j = \lambda$ if $X_j \in \Sigma_T$, $j = 1,...k$.

---

[4]A taxonomy defined from the perspective of theoretical computer science can be found, e.g., in [Dassow and Păun (1990); Dassow *et al.* (1997); Dassow (2004)].

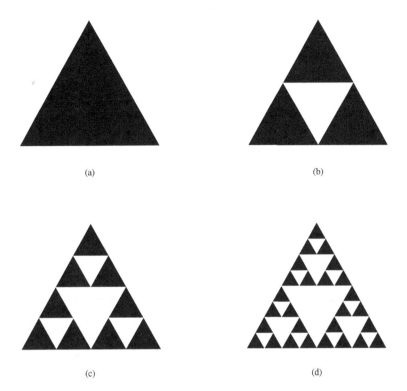

Fig. 4.1   The generation of the Sierpiński Triangle.

For example, let us define the indexed grammar $G$ which generates the Sierpiński Triangle (see Fig. 4.1). Its structure is coded by the string over the set of terminal symbols $\Sigma = \{0, 1, (, )\}$[5] with the help of brackets according to the scheme depicted in Fig. 4.2a in the following way:[6]

- Fig. 4.1b: (1110).
- Fig. 4.1c: ((1110)(1110)(1110)0), etc.

The set of productions $P$ is defined as follows.

---

[5]0 denotes a white triangle and 1 denotes a black triangle.

[6]Let us note that the two above mentioned strategies for the increasing of the generating power of $CF$ grammars are used in this example. The increasing of the *generative power* is obtained by the use of the indexed grammar. The increasing of the *descriptive power* is achieved by the constructing of the following representation scheme: the brackets define the levels of the recursion. The string notation $(ABCD)$ is interpreted as: the left triangle $A$, the upper triangle $B$, the right triangle $C$ and the middle triangle $D$.

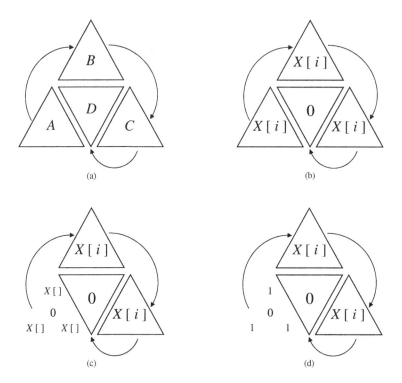

Fig. 4.2   The generation of the Sierpiński Triangle by the indexed grammar.

(1) $S[..] \to S[i..]$                        (the production of type 2)

(2) $S \to (XXX0)$                        (the production of type 1)

(3) $X[i..] \to (XXX0)[..]$    (the production of type 3)

(4) $X \to 1$                              (the production of type 1)

Let us generate, e.g., the Sierpiński Triangle shown in Fig. 4.1c.

$$S[] \xRightarrow{(1)} S[i] \xRightarrow{(2)} (X[i]X[i]X[i]0) \xRightarrow{(3)} ((X[]X[]X[]0)X[i]X[i]0)$$
$$\xRightarrow{2x(3)} ((X[]X[]X[]0)(X[]X[]X[]0)(X[]X[]X[]0)0)$$
$$\xRightarrow{(4)} ((1X[]X[]0)(X[]X[]X[]0)(X[]X[]X[]0)0)$$
$$\xRightarrow{2x(4)} ((1110)(X[]X[]X[]0)(X[]X[]X[]0)0)$$
$$\xRightarrow{6x(4)} ((1110)(1110)(1110)0)$$

The symbol $\xRightarrow{(k)}$ denotes the application of the k-th production and the symbol $\xRightarrow{n\ x(k)}$ denotes the application of the k-th production n times. The number of indices $i$ corresponds to the number of iterations during the generation of the Sierpiński Triangle. The graphical interpretation of the main phases of this derivation is shown in Figs. 4.2b-c.

Let us note that indexed grammars are of a strong generated power. However, a polynomial parsing algorithm has not been defined for them. Therefore, certain subtypes of indexed grammars with better computational properties have been defined. Linear indexed grammars were proposed in [Gazdar (1988)]. Let us introduce the following definition:[7]

**Definition 4.2 (Linear Indexed Grammar):** A linear indexed grammar, *LIG*, is a quintuple

$$G = (\Sigma_N, \Sigma_T, I, P, S), \text{ where}$$

$\Sigma_N$ is a set of nonterminal symbols,
$\Sigma_T$ is a set of terminal symbols,
$I$ is a set of indices,
$P$ is a finite set of productions of one of the following four types:

$$1. \ A[..] \longrightarrow \alpha B[..]\gamma \quad \text{or} \quad 2. \ A[..] \longrightarrow \alpha B[i..]\gamma \quad \text{or}$$
$$3. \ A[i..] \longrightarrow \alpha B[..]\gamma \quad \text{or} \quad 4. \ A[] \longrightarrow \beta \ ,$$

where $A$ and $B \in \Sigma_N$, $i \in I$, $[..]$ represents a stack of indices, a string in $I^*$, $\alpha, \gamma \in \Sigma^*$, $\beta \in \Sigma_T^*$,
$S$ is the start symbol (axiom), $S \in \Sigma_N$.

A derivation for linear indexed grammars differs from that of indexed grammars. At most one right-hand side nonterminal is indicated to receive the copy of the stack.[8]

For example, let us define the linear indexed grammar $G$ which generates the language of squares coded with Freeman chain codes $L = \{0^n 2^n 4^n 6^n, \ n > 0\}$ (see Fig. 4.3a-b).
$G = (\Sigma_N, \Sigma_T, P, S)$, where:
$\Sigma_N = \{S, X\}$,
$P$ consists of the following productions.

(1) $S[..] \to 0S[i..]6$     (the production of type 2)

(2) $S[..] \to X[..]$       (the production of type 1)

(3) $X[i..] \to 2X[..]4$    (the production of type 3)

(4) $X[] \to \lambda$           (the production of type 4)

Let us generate the square $0^2 2^2 4^2 6^2$ shown in Fig. 4.3b.

$$S[] \xrightarrow{(1)} 0S[i]6 \xrightarrow{(1)} 00S[ii]66 \xrightarrow{(2)} 00X[ii]66 \xrightarrow{(3)} 002X[i]466$$
$$\xrightarrow{(3)} 0022X[]4466 \xrightarrow{(4)} 00224466$$

---

[7]We add the fourth type of productions to the definition of linear indexed grammar. Such productions contain no nonterminals on the right-hand side and can generate the empty word.

[8]As we have seen above, in indexed grammars all the right-hand side nonterminals receive copies of the stack.

Linear indexed languages are parsable in polynomial time [Vijay-Shanker and Weir (1994b)]. Other subtypes of indexed grammars, which are parsable in polynomial time include: distributed index grammars [Staudacher (1993)], global index grammars [Castaño (2004)] and sequentially indexed grammars [Eijck van (2008)].

### 4.1.2 *Head Grammars*

Head grammars were presented in [Pollard (1984)]. Let us introduce the following definition.

**Definition 4.3 (Head Grammar):** A head grammar, $HG$, is a quadruple

$$G = (\Sigma_N, \Sigma_T, P, S), \text{ where}$$

$\Sigma_N$ is a set of nonterminal symbols,
$\Sigma_T$ is a set of terminal symbols,
$P$ is a finite set of productions of the form:

$$A \to f(\alpha_1, \ldots, \alpha_n) \text{ or } A \to \alpha_1,$$

where $A \in \Sigma_N$, $\alpha_i$, $i = 1, \ldots, n$, is either a nonterminal symbol or a headed string, $f$ is either a concatenation or a head wrapping operation,
$S$ is the start symbol (axiom), $S \in \Sigma_N$.

The special symbol $\uparrow$ which represents *the head* of the string is defined for head grammars. The grammars generate headed strings or pairs of strings which are denoted by $(u \uparrow v)$ or $(u, v)$. Two types of operations can be performed using the head. The *concatenation* $C_{i,n}$ consists in the joining of $n$ head-divided strings and the inserting of the new head in the string according to the following formula:

$$C_{i,n}(u_1 \uparrow v_1, \ldots, u_i \uparrow v_i, \ldots, u_n \uparrow v_n) = u_1 v_1 \ldots u_i \uparrow v_i \ldots u_n v_n.$$

The *wrapping* $W$ consists in inserting one word into another based on the head position, i.e.,

$$W(u_1 \uparrow v_1, u_2 \uparrow v_2) = u_1 u_2 \uparrow v_2 v_1.$$

For example, let us define the head grammar $G$ which generates our exemplary language of squares $L$ (see Fig. 4.3a-b).
$G = (\Sigma_N, \Sigma_T, P, S)$, where:
$\Sigma_N = \{S, X\}$,
$P$ consists of the following productions.

$$(1) \ S \to C_{1,1}(\lambda \uparrow \lambda) \quad (2) \ S \to C_{2,3}(0 \uparrow \lambda, X, 6 \uparrow \lambda) \quad (3) \ X \to W(S, 2 \uparrow 4)$$

The derivation of the square $0^2 2^2 4^2 6^2$ shown in Fig. 4.3b is performed in the following way.

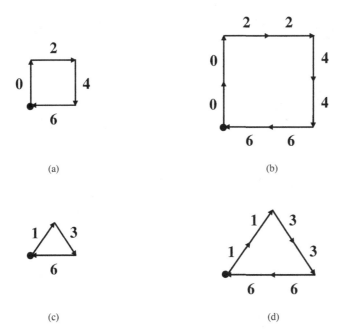

Fig. 4.3   Context-sensitive patterns.

$$S \xRightarrow{(2)}$$
$$\xRightarrow{(2)} C_{2,3}(0 \uparrow \lambda, X, 6 \uparrow \lambda) \xRightarrow{(3)}$$
$$\xRightarrow{(3)} C_{2,3}(0 \uparrow \lambda, W(S, 2 \uparrow 4), 6 \uparrow \lambda) \xRightarrow{(2)}$$
$$\xRightarrow{(2)} C_{2,3}(0 \uparrow \lambda, W(C_{2,3}(0 \uparrow \lambda, X, 6 \uparrow \lambda), 2 \uparrow 4), 6 \uparrow \lambda) \xRightarrow{(3)}$$
$$\xRightarrow{(3)} C_{2,3}(0 \uparrow \lambda, W(C_{2,3}(0 \uparrow \lambda, W(S, 2 \uparrow 4), 6 \uparrow \lambda), 2 \uparrow 4), 6 \uparrow \lambda) \xRightarrow{(1)}$$
$$\xRightarrow{(1)} C_{2,3}(0 \uparrow \lambda, W(C_{2,3}(0 \uparrow \lambda, W(C_{1,1}(\lambda \uparrow \lambda), 2 \uparrow 4), 6 \uparrow \lambda), 2 \uparrow 4), 6 \uparrow \lambda) =$$
$$= C_{2,3}(0 \uparrow \lambda, W(C_{2,3}(0 \uparrow \lambda, W(\lambda \uparrow \lambda, 2 \uparrow 4), 6 \uparrow \lambda), 2 \uparrow 4), 6 \uparrow \lambda) =$$
$$= C_{2,3}(0 \uparrow \lambda, W(C_{2,3}(0 \uparrow \lambda, 2 \uparrow 4, 6 \uparrow \lambda), 2 \uparrow 4), 6 \uparrow \lambda) =$$
$$= C_{2,3}(0 \uparrow \lambda, W(02 \uparrow 46, 2 \uparrow 4), 6 \uparrow \lambda) =$$
$$= C_{2,3}(0 \uparrow \lambda, 022 \uparrow 446, 6 \uparrow \lambda) =$$
$$= 0022 \uparrow 4466$$

Languages generated by head grammars are parsable in polynomial time [Pollard (1984)].

### 4.1.3   *Combinatory Categorial Grammars*

The combinatory categorial grammars, *CCGs*, presented in [Steedman (1987)] are an extension of the categorial grammars introduced in [Ajdukiewicz (1935); Bar-Hillel (1953)]. Before we introduce their definition, we present certain preliminary concepts and notational conventions.

A combinatory categorial grammar consists of a set of terminals $\Sigma_T$ which correspond to the lexical items of a language, a set of nonterminals $\Sigma_N$ which correspond to the atomic categories of a language,[9] a function $f$ which maps lexical items to finite subsets of the set of categories $C(\Sigma_N)$, and a set of rules $R$ which corresponds to a set of productions in a Chomsky-grammar style set.

Complex categories are defined on the basis of atomic categories with the help of the forward operator $/$ and the backward operator $\backslash$. That is, if $X$ and $Y$ are categories in $C(\Sigma_N)$, then $X/Y$ and $X\backslash Y$ are categories in $C(\Sigma_N)$ as well.[10] The complex categories $X/Y$ and $X\backslash Y$ represent mappings that return a result of type $X$ when applied to an argument of type $Y$. $X/Y$ denotes that the argument appears to the right and $X\backslash Y$ denotes that the argument appears to the left. Additionally, we assume the left associativity of the operators $/$ and $\backslash$.[11]

Now, we shall introduce four combinatory schemata which will be used for the defining of $CCG$ rules in this book. Let the vertical slash $|$ denote $/$ or $\backslash$ (the direction of the slash is of no significance). Let $x, y, z_1, \ldots, z_n$ be meta-categories which can be replaced by any categories of $C(\Sigma_N)$, $|_i \in \{\, \backslash\, ,\, /\, \}$, $i = 1, \ldots, n$.

(1) Forward application, denoted $>$

$$x/y \quad y \quad \rightarrow \quad x$$

(2) Backward application, denoted $<$

$$y \quad x/y \quad \rightarrow \quad x$$

(3) Generalized forward composition for $n \geq 1$, denoted $B_>^n$

$$x/y \quad y \mid_1 z_1 \mid_2 \cdots \mid_n z_n \quad \rightarrow \quad x \mid_1 z_1 \mid_2 \cdots \mid_n z_n$$

(4) Generalized backward composition for $n \geq 1$, denoted $B_<^n$

$$y \mid_1 z_1 \mid_2 \cdots \mid_n z_n \quad x/y \quad \rightarrow \quad x \mid_1 z_1 \mid_2 \cdots \mid_n z_n$$

> **Definition 4.4 (Combinatory Categorial Grammar):** A combinatory categorial grammar, $CCG$, is a quintuple
>
> $$G = (\Sigma_N, \Sigma_T, f, R, S), \text{ where}$$
>
> $\Sigma_N$ is a set of nonterminal symbols,
> $\Sigma_T$ is a set of terminal symbols,
> $f$ is a functor that maps elements of $\Sigma_T \cup \{\lambda\}$ to finite subsets of $C(\Sigma_N)$,
> $R$ is a finite set of rules of the form:
>
> $$c_1 c_2 \rightarrow c, \quad c_1, c_2, c \in C(\Sigma_N),$$
>
> defined according to one of four combinatory schemata $>$, $<$, $B_>^n$, $B_<^n$,
> $S$ is the start symbol (axiom), $S \in \Sigma_N$.

---

[9] A category is here understood as a syntactic type of a lexical item.
[10] The set of categories $C(\Sigma_N)$ is defined recursively in this way.
[11] That is, e.g., instead of writing $((X/Y)\backslash Z)\backslash W$ we can write $X/Y\backslash Z\backslash W$.

Now, we can define a derivational step in a combinatory categorial grammar. Let $G = (\Sigma_N, \Sigma_T, f, R, S)$ be $CCG$, $\eta_1, \eta_2 \in (C(\Sigma_N) \cup \Sigma_T)^*$, $c_1, c_2, c \in C(\Sigma_N)$, $a \in \Sigma_T$. Then

(1) $\eta_1 c \eta_2 \underset{G}{\Longrightarrow} \eta_1 c_1 c_2 \eta_2$, if $c_1 c_2 \rightarrow c \in R$.

(2) $\eta_1 c \eta_2 \underset{G}{\Longrightarrow} \eta_1 a \eta_2$, if $c \in f(a)$.

Let us note that a rule of a combinatory categorial grammar is applied "from the right-hand side of a rule to the left-hand side of a rule" during a derivation step of the form specified in point (1), i.e., contrary to the direction specified in Chomsky-style grammars. The language generated by a combinatory categorial grammar is defined in a standard way.[12]

Now, we shall define the combinatory categorial grammar $G$ which generates our exemplary language of squares $L$ (see Fig. 4.3a-b):
$G = (\Sigma_N, \Sigma_T, f, R, S)$, where:
$\Sigma_N = \{S, A, B, C, D\}$,
$R$ consists of the following rules.

$$(1) \quad (x^S/y) \ y \quad \rightarrow \quad x^S$$

$$(2) \quad y \ (x^S \backslash y) \quad \rightarrow \quad x^S$$

$$(3) \quad (A/D) \ (x^S \backslash A) \quad \rightarrow \quad (x^S/D)$$

$$(4) \quad (x^S/C) \ (C \backslash A/C \backslash B) \quad \rightarrow \quad (x^S \backslash A/C \backslash B)$$

The mapping $f$ is defined in the following way.

$$f(0) = \{(A/D)\} \qquad f(2) = \{B\} \quad f(4) = \{(C \backslash A/C \backslash B)\} \quad f(6) = \{D\}$$

$$f(\lambda) = \{(S/C), C\}$$

Let us derive the square 0246 shown in Fig. 4.3a. The first stage of the derivation is performed in the following way:

$S \xrightarrow{(1)}$
$\xrightarrow{(1)} (S/D) \ D \xrightarrow{(3)}$
$\xrightarrow{(3)} (A/D) \ (S \backslash A) \ D \xrightarrow{(1)}$
$\xrightarrow{(1)} (A/D) \ (S \backslash A/C) \ C \ D \xrightarrow{(2)}$
$\xrightarrow{(2)} (A/D) \ B \ (S \backslash A/C \backslash B) \ C \ D \xrightarrow{(4)}$
$\xrightarrow{(4)} (A/D) \ B \ (S/C) \ (C \backslash A/C \backslash B) \ C \ D$

At the second stage of the derivation, the mapping $f$ is used to the elements of the string of categories $(A/D) \ B \ (S/C) \ (C \backslash A/C \backslash B) \ C \ D$. It can be easily noticed that the terminal string 0246 is obtained.

---

[12]See Definition A.3 in Appendix A.1.

The formal properties of combinatory categorial grammars have been studied intensively in recent decades and a variety of applications have been developed on their basis [Steedman (2000); Hockenmaier *et al.* (2004); Hockenmaier and Steedman (2007); Steedman (2013)]. Combinatory categorial grammars are parsable in polynomial time [Vijay-Shanker and Weir (1994b)].

### 4.1.4 *Conjunctive and Boolean Grammars*

Conjunctive grammars were introduced in [Okhotin (2001)]. Let us introduce the following definition.

**Definition 4.5 (Conjunctive Grammar):** A conjunctive grammar is a quadruple

$$G = (\Sigma_N, \Sigma_T, P, S), \text{ where}$$

$\Sigma_N$ is a set of nonterminal symbols,
$\Sigma_T$ is a set of terminal symbols,
$P$ is a finite set of productions of the form:

$$A \to \alpha_1 \& \ldots \& \alpha_n,$$

where $A \in \Sigma_N$, $\alpha_i \in \Sigma^*$, $i = 1, \ldots, n$,
$S$ is the start symbol (axiom), $S \in \Sigma_N$.

Before we define a derivational step in a conjunctive grammar, we introduce the concept of the set of conjunctive formulae for a grammar $G$ which is defined inductively in the following way [Okhotin (2001)]:

- $\lambda$ is a conjunctive formula.
- Every symbol in $\Sigma$ is a conjunctive formula.
- If $\mathcal{A}$ and $\mathcal{B}$ are nonempty conjunctive formulae, then $\mathcal{A}\mathcal{B}$ is a conjunctive formula.
- If $\mathcal{A}_1, \ldots, \mathcal{A}_n$, $n \geq 1$ are conjunctive formulae, then $(\mathcal{A}_1 \& \ldots \& \mathcal{A}_n)$, is a conjunctive formula.

A derivational step in a conjunctive grammar is defined in the following way. Let $G = (\Sigma_N, \Sigma_T, P, S)$ be a conjunctive grammar, $\eta_1, \eta_2 \in (\Sigma \cup \{ ( , \& , ) \})^*$. Then

(1) $\eta_1 A \eta_2 \underset{G}{\Longrightarrow} \eta_1 (\alpha_1 \& \ldots \& \alpha_n) \eta_2$, if $A \to \alpha_1 \& \ldots \& \alpha_n \in P$ and $\eta_1 A \eta_2$ is a conjunctive formula.

(2) $\eta_1 (\underbrace{w \& \ldots \& w}_{n}) \eta_2 \underset{G}{\Longrightarrow} \eta_1 w \eta_2$, if $\eta_1 (\underbrace{w \& \ldots \& w}_{n}) \eta_2$, $n \geq 1$, $w \in \Sigma_T^*$, is a conjunctive formula.

The language generated by a grammar is defined in a standard way.[13]

---

[13]See Definition A.3 in Appendix A.1.

Let us define the conjunctive grammar $G$ which generates the language of triangles coded with Freeman chain codes $L = \{1^n 3^n 6^n, n > 0\}$ (see Fig. 4.3c-d). $G = (\Sigma_N, \Sigma_T, P, S)$, where:
$\Sigma_N = \{S, A, B_1, B_2, C\}$,
$P$ consists of the following productions.[14]

$$S \rightarrow AB_1 \& B_2 C \qquad B_1 \rightarrow 3B_1 6 \mid \lambda \qquad B_2 \rightarrow 1B_2 3 \mid \lambda$$

$$A \rightarrow 1A \mid \lambda \qquad C \rightarrow 6C \mid \lambda$$

The derivation of the triangle $1^2 3^2 6^2$ shown in Fig. 4.3d is performed in the following way:

$$S \Longrightarrow (AB_1 \& B_2 C) \Longrightarrow (1AB_1 \& B_2 C) \Longrightarrow (11AB_1 \& B_2 C) \Longrightarrow (11B_1 \& B_2 C) \Longrightarrow$$
$$\Longrightarrow (113B_1 6 \& B_2 C) \Longrightarrow (1133B_1 66 \& B_2 C) \Longrightarrow (113366 \& B_2 C) \Longrightarrow$$
$$\Longrightarrow (113366 \& 1B_2 3C) \Longrightarrow (113366 \& 11B_2 33C) \Longrightarrow (113366 \& 1133C) \Longrightarrow$$
$$\Longrightarrow (113366 \& 11336C) \Longrightarrow (113366 \& 113366C) \Longrightarrow (113366 \& 113366) \Longrightarrow 113366$$

Boolean grammars defined in [Okhotin (2004)] are an extension of conjunctive grammars. The negation operator is introduced in addition to the conjunction, so every Boolean operation over sets of languages can be expressed. Polynomial parsing algorithms were defined for conjunctive grammars [Okhotin (2003)] and Boolean grammars [Okhotin (2010)].

### 4.1.5 *Remarks on Mildly Context-Sensitive Grammars*

Linear indexed grammars (*LIG*), head grammars (*HG*), combinatory categorial grammars (*CCG*) and Tree Adjoining Grammars (*TAG*)[15] belong to the class of Mildly Context-Sensitive Grammars (*MCSG*). *MCSGs* generate Mildly Context-Sensitive Languages which fulfill the following conditions [Kallmeyer (2010)]. Firstly, they contain all context-free languages. Secondly, they describe *a limited amount of cross-serial dependencies*, i.e., there is $n \geq 2$ such that $\{w^k : w \in \Sigma_T^*\} \in \mathcal{L}(MCSG)$ for all $k \leq n$. Thirdly, they are of *a constant growth*, i.e., if we order the words of a language according to their length, then the length grows in a linear way. Finally, they are polynomially parsable.

On the basis of the theorems presented in [Vijay-Shanker and Weir (1994a); Joshi and Schabes (1997); Okhotin (2004)] we can define the diagram which presents the relations among the classes of enhanced *CF* languages as in Fig. 4.4.[16]

---

[14]We use the following notational convention. If $A \rightarrow \beta_1, A \rightarrow \beta_2, \ldots, A \rightarrow \beta_k$ are the productions which start with the same nonterminal $A$, then we denote this by $A \rightarrow \beta_1 \mid \beta_2 \mid \ldots \mid \beta_k$.

[15]Tree Adjoining Grammars are presented in Sec. 7.5. Although from the point of view of the theory of abstract rewriting systems *TAGs* are tree generating systems, they can also be used for generating enhanced string context-free languages.

[16]Boolean grammars are denoted by *Bool* while conjunctive grammars are denoted by *Conj*.

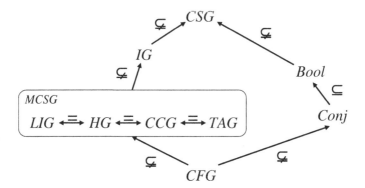

Fig. 4.4   The relations among the classes of languages generated by enhanced *CF* grammars.

## 4.2   Grammars with Programmed Derivations

In the second approach to the controlling of derivations, the control mechanism is not embedded ("hidden") in the left- or right-hand sides of grammar productions but it is specified separately. The grammars which belong to this approach include: programmed grammars and dynamically programmed grammars.

### 4.2.1   *Programmed Grammars*

Programmed grammars were introduced in [Rosenkrantz (1969)]. Let us introduce the following definition.[17]

> **Definition 4.6 (Programmed Grammar):** A programmed grammar is a quintuple
>
> $$G = (\Sigma_N, \Sigma_T, J, P, S), \text{ where}$$
>
> $\Sigma_N$ is a set of nonterminal symbols,
> $\Sigma_T$ is a set of terminal symbols,
> $J$ is a set of production labels,
> $P$ is a finite set of productions of the form:
>
> $$(r) \quad \alpha \to \beta \ \ S(U) \ \ F(W), \text{ in which}$$
>
> $\alpha \to \beta$, $\alpha \in \Sigma^*\Sigma_N\Sigma^*$, $\beta \in \Sigma^*$, is called the *core*, $(r)$ is the production label, $r \in J$, $U \subset J$ is the success field and $W \subset J$ is the failure field,
> $S$ is the start symbol (axiom), $S \in \Sigma_N$.

A derivation in a programmed grammar can be described in the following way: firstly, the production labelled with (1) is applied. If a production $(r)$ can be applied, then after its application the next production is chosen from its success

---

[17]We introduce the programmed *phrase-structure* grammar according to [Rosenkrantz (1969)]. However, we are interested in programmed *context-free* grammars in this chapter.

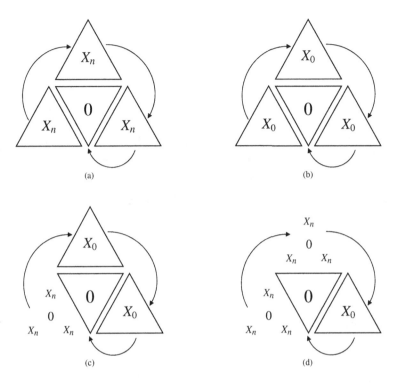

Fig. 4.5 The generation of the Sierpiński Triangle by the programmed grammar.

field $U$. Otherwise, the next production is chosen from the failure field $W$.

Let us define the programmed grammar $G$ which generates the Sierpiński Triangle used as the example of indexed grammar derivations in Sec. 4.1.1 (see Fig. 4.1). We assume the representation scheme defined in Fig. 4.2a.

The set of productions $P$ is defined as follows.

$$(1)\ S \to (X_n X_n X_n 0)\quad S(\{2,4\})\quad F(\emptyset)$$

$$(2)\ X_n \to (X_0)\qquad\qquad S(\{2\})\qquad F(\{3\})$$

$$(3)\ X_0 \to X_n X_n X_n 0\quad S(\{3\})\qquad F(\{2,4\})$$

$$(4)\ X_n \to 1\qquad\qquad\quad S(\{4\})\qquad F(\emptyset)$$

Let us generate, e.g., the Sierpiński Triangle shown in Fig. 4.1c. (The graphical interpretation of the main phases of the derivation is shown in Fig. 4.5).

$$S \xrightarrow{(1)} (X_n X_n X_n 0) \xrightarrow{(2)} ((X_0)X_n X_n 0)$$
$$\xrightarrow{2\times(2)} ((X_0)(X_0)(X_0)0)$$
$$\xrightarrow{(3)} ((X_n X_n X_n 0)(X_0)(X_0)0)$$
$$\xrightarrow{2\times(3)} ((X_n X_n X_n 0)(X_n X_n X_n 0)(X_n X_n X_n 0)0)$$
$$\xrightarrow{9\times(4)} ((1110)(1110)(1110)0)$$

Two deterministic subclasses of context-free programmed grammars which are parsable in polynomial time were defined in [Sebesta (1989)].

### 4.2.2  *Dynamically Programmed Grammars*

The controlling of derivations in programmed grammars is done with the help of the fields which are pre-specified when a grammar is defined, i.e., these fields are, somehow, static. The concept of the use of (dynamic) "fields" which can be filled with indices of grammar productions during a derivation for the purpose of a derivation control was introduced in [Flasiński (1995a)].

> **Definition 4.7 (Dynamically Programmed Grammar):** A dynamically programmed (context-free), $DP$, grammar is a quintuple
>
> $$G = (\Sigma_N, \Sigma_T, O, P, S), \text{ where}$$
>
> $\Sigma_N$ is a set of nonterminal symbols,
> $\Sigma_T$ is a set of terminal symbols,
> $O$ is the set of tape operations: *add, read, move*,
> $P$ is a set of $n$ productions of the form:
>
> $$p_i = (\pi_i, L_i, R_i, A_i, DCL_i), \text{ in which}$$
>
> $\pi_i : \bigcup_{k=1,\ldots,n} DCL_k \rightarrow \{TRUE, FALSE\}$ is the predicate of applicability of $p_i$,
> $L_i \in \Sigma_N$ and $R_i \in \Sigma^*$ are the left- and right-hand sides of $p_i$, respectively,
> $A_i$ is the sequence of actions *add, move* performed over $\bigcup_{k=1,\ldots,n} DCL_k$,
> $DCL_i$ is the derivation control tape for $p_i$,
> $S$ is the start symbol (axiom), $S \in \Sigma_N$.

The pair $(L_i, R_i)$ is called the core of $p_i$. For each two productions $p_i, p_j \in P$, $i \neq j$, the core of $p_i$ is different from the core of $p_j$, i.e., $L_i \neq L_j$ or $R_i \neq R_j$. In $DP$ grammars, instead of success and failure fields, the derivation control tape $DCL_i$ with the head operations *add, read, move* is assigned to each production $p_i$. The operation $add(k, m)$ writes the symbol $m$ on the cell of $DCL_k$ which is under the head.[18] The operation $read(k)$ gives the value which has been read by the head of $DCL_k$. The operation $move(k)$ moves the head of $DCL_k$ right.

A derivation in a $DP$ grammar is defined in the following way: firstly, the production (1) is applied. Then, a production (i) is applied if its predicate of applicability $\pi_i$ is true. (The predicate of applicability is formulated with the help of the operation *read*.) After the application of the syntactic part of the production, i.e., its core $L_i \rightarrow R_i$, the sequence of actions *add, move* (i.e., $A_i$) is performed for some tapes.

For example, let us define the $DP$ grammar $G = (\Sigma_N, \Sigma_T, O, P, S)$, which generates the language $L = \{a^n b^n a^n b^n, n > 0\}$. $\Sigma_T = \{a, b\}$ and $\Sigma_N = \{S, A, B, C, D\}$.

---

[18]The labels of the productions are written on the tapes.

$P$ consists of the following productions.

| $(i):$ | $\pi_i:$ | $(L_i, R_i):$ | $A_i:$ |
|--------|----------|---------------|--------|
| (1) | $TRUE$ | $S \to ABCD$ | $\perp$ |
| (2) | $TRUE$ | $A \to aA$ | $add(4,4); add(6,6); add(8,8);$ |
| (3) | $TRUE$ | $A \to \lambda$ | $add(4,5); add(6,7); add(8,9);$ |
| (4) | $read(4) = 4$ | $B \to bB$ | $move(4);$ |
| (5) | $read(4) = 5$ | $B \to \lambda$ | $move(4);$ |
| (6) | $read(6) = 6$ | $C \to aC$ | $move(6);$ |
| (7) | $read(6) = 7$ | $C \to \lambda$ | $move(6);$ |
| (8) | $read(8) = 8$ | $D \to bD$ | $move(8);$ |
| (9) | $read(8) = 9$ | $D \to \lambda$ | $move(8);$ |

Let us derive the string $a^2b^2a^2b^2$. (Current head positions are underlined.)

| | $DCL_4:$ | $DCL_6:$ | $DCL_8:$ |
|---|---|---|---|
| $S \overset{(1)}{\Longrightarrow}$ | | | |
| $ABCD \overset{(2)}{\Longrightarrow}$ | | | |
| $aABCD \overset{(2)}{\Longrightarrow}$ | $\underline{4}$ | $\underline{6}$ | $\underline{8}$ |
| $aaABCD \overset{(3)}{\Longrightarrow}$ | $4\underline{4}$ | $6\underline{6}$ | $8\underline{8}$ |
| $aaBCD \overset{(4)}{\Longrightarrow}$ | $44\underline{5}$ | $66\underline{7}$ | $88\underline{9}$ |
| $aabBCD \overset{(4)}{\Longrightarrow}$ | $\#\underline{4}5$ | $66\underline{7}$ | $88\underline{9}$ |
| $aabbBCD \overset{(5)}{\Longrightarrow}$ | $\#\#\underline{5}$ | $66\underline{7}$ | $88\underline{9}$ |
| $aabbCD \overset{(6)}{\Longrightarrow}$ | $\#\#\#_-$ | $6\underline{6}7$ | $88\underline{9}$ |
| $aabbaCD \overset{(6)}{\Longrightarrow}$ | $\#\#\#_-$ | $\#\underline{6}7$ | $88\underline{9}$ |
| $aabbaaCD \overset{(7)}{\Longrightarrow}$ | $\#\#\#_-$ | $\#\#\underline{7}$ | $88\underline{9}$ |
| $aabbaaD \overset{(8)}{\Longrightarrow}$ | $\#\#\#_-$ | $\#\#\#_-$ | $88\underline{9}$ |
| $aabbaabD \overset{(8)}{\Longrightarrow}$ | $\#\#\#_-$ | $\#\#\#_-$ | $\#\underline{8}9$ |
| $aabbaabbD \overset{(9)}{\Longrightarrow}$ | $\#\#\#_-$ | $\#\#\#_-$ | $\#\#\underline{9}$ |
| $aabbaabb$ | $\#\#\#_-$ | $\#\#\#_-$ | $\#\#\#_-$ |

In order to define a polynomial parsing algorithm, the concepts of $DP$ grammars and $LL(k)$ grammars[19] have been incorporated into $DPLL(k)$ grammars. Let us introduce the following definition [Flasiński and Jurek (1999)].[20]

**Definition 4.8 ($DPLL(k)$ Grammar):** Let $G = (\Sigma_N, \Sigma_T, P, S)$ be a (context-free) dynamically programmed grammar, $\underset{\text{core}}{\overset{*}{\Longrightarrow}}$ denotes a sequence of derivation steps consisting in the applying of production cores only. $G$ is called a $DPLL(k)$ grammar iff the following two conditions are fulfilled.

(1) For every two leftmost derivations in $G$

$$S \overset{*}{\Longrightarrow} \alpha A\theta \Longrightarrow \alpha\beta\theta \underset{\text{core}}{\overset{*}{\Longrightarrow}} \alpha x$$

$$S \overset{*}{\Longrightarrow} \alpha A\theta \Longrightarrow \alpha\gamma\theta \underset{\text{core}}{\overset{*}{\Longrightarrow}} \alpha y,$$

where $\alpha, x, y \in \Sigma_T^*$, $\beta, \gamma, \theta \in \Sigma^*$, $A \in \Sigma_N$, the following condition holds.

If $FIRST_k(x) = FIRST_k(y)$, then $\beta = \gamma$.

(2) For $G$ there exists $m > 0$ such that for any leftmost derivation $S \overset{*}{\Longrightarrow} \alpha A\theta \overset{\sigma}{\Longrightarrow} \alpha\beta\theta$, where $\sigma$ is the string of the indices of productions applied, if $|\sigma| \geq m$ then the first symbol of $\beta\theta$ is terminal.

$DPLL(k)$ grammars generate the considerable subclass of context-sensitive languages, e.g., $L_1 = \{a^n b^n c^n : n \geq 0\}$, $L_2 = \{a^n b^m c^n d^m : n, m \geq 0\}$, $L_3 = \{a^{2^n} : n \geq 0\}$. The $DPLL(k)$ parser of the $\mathcal{O}(n^2)$ time complexity was presented in [Flasiński and Jurek (1999)]. The parser time complexity was improved to the linear in [Jurek (2000)]. The grammatical inference algorithm of the $\mathcal{O}(m^3 \cdot n^3)$ time complexity, where $m$ is the sample size, $n$ is the maximum length of a string in the sample was proposed in [Jurek (2004)]. *Generalized $DPLL(k)$ grammars*, $GDPLL(k)$, were presented in [Jurek (2005)].

## 4.3 Augmented Regular Expressions

*Augmented Regular Expressions, AREs*, were introduced in [Sanfeliu and Alquézar (1996); Alquézar and Sanfeliu (1996); Sanfeliu and Sainz (1996); Alquézar and Sanfeliu (1997)].

Let us introduce the main notions of this model. Let $R$ be a regular expression[21] which contains $ns$ Kleene star symbols, $ns \geq 0$. The *set of star variables* $V$ associated with $R$ is an ordered set of natural-valued variables $\{v_1, \ldots, v_{ns}\}$ which are associated one-to-one with the Kleene star symbols that appear in $R$ (from left to right). For example, for the regular expression $a(bc^* + d^*e)^* f^*$ the corresponding star variable expression, denoted $R(V/*)$, $V = \{v_1, v_2, v_3, v_4\}$, is defined as follows:

---

[19] $LL(k)$ grammars are presented in Sec. 3.2.1.
[20] The definition of $FIRST_k$ is presented in Sec. 3.2.1.
[21] Regular expressions are introduced in the preliminaries of Appendix A.1.

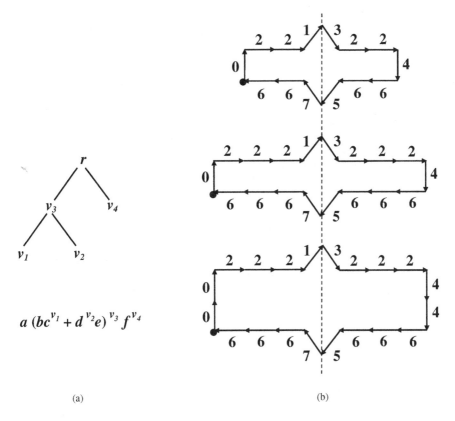

$a\,(bc^{v_1} + d^{v_2}e)^{v_3}\,f^{v_4}$

(a)                                                (b)

Fig. 4.6    (a) Example of a star tree. (b) Context-sensitive patterns.

$a(bc^{v_1} + d^{v_2}e)^{v_3} f^{v_4}$. In order to represent the nesting of star variables a *star tree* representation is introduced in the model as is shown in Fig. 4.6a.

Now, we can introduce the following definition [Alquézar and Sanfeliu (1997)].

**Definition 4.9 (Augmented Regular Expression):** An *Augmented Regular Expression*, *ARE*, is a quadruple

$$ARE = (R, V, \mathcal{T}, C), \text{ where}$$

$R$ is a regular expression over an alphabet $\Sigma_T$,
$V$ is its associated set of star variables,
$\mathcal{T}$ is its associated star tree,
$C$ is a set of linear combinations $\{c_1, \ldots, c_{nc}\}$ defined as follows. Let $V$ be partitioned into two subsets $V^{ind}$ and $V^{dep}$ of $ni$ independent and $nc$ dependent star variables, respectively. The dependent star variables are expressed as linear combinations of the independent star variables in the following way.

$$c_i \equiv v_i^{dep} = \alpha_{i1}v_1^{ind} + \ldots + \alpha_{ij}v_j^{ind} + \ldots + \alpha_{i(ni)}v_{ni}^{ind} + \alpha_{i0}, \ 1 \leq i \leq nc$$

For example, let us define the *Augmented Regular Expression ARE* which represents the (context-sensitive) language of symmetric contours coded with Freeman
chain codes and shown in Fig. 4.6b, i.e., $L = \{0^n2^k132^k4^n6^k576^k, \ n \geq 1, \ k \geq 1\}$.
$ARE = (R, V, \mathcal{T}, C)$, where:
$R = 00^*22^*1322^*44^*66^*5766^*$ (the starting point for the defining of $ARE$),
$V = \{v_1, v_2, v_3, v_4, v_5, v_6\}$,
$R(V/*) = 00^{v_1}22^{v_2}1322^{v_3}44^{v_4}66^{v_5}5766^{v_6}$,
$\mathcal{T}$ is the star tree which consists of the root labelled with $r$ and its child nodes
labelled with $v_1, v_2, v_3, v_4, v_5$ and $v_6$,
$C$ consists of the following constraints:

$$v_4 = v_1 \qquad v_5 = v_2$$

$$v_3 = v_2 \qquad v_6 = v_2$$

Although regular languages are the starting point for the defining of this model,
many context-sensitive languages expressing multiple and complex context constraints are recognized with the help of *AREs*. The recognition method is efficient
(the linear time complexity). Moreover, an efficient inference algorithm for *AREs*
was proposed in [Alquézar and Sanfeliu (1997)].

## 4.4   Attributed Grammars

The use of attributes for primitives represented by terminals[22] seems to be the
most natural way to increase the descriptive power of formal grammars. In
syntactic pattern recognition, an attribute constitutes any property of a primi-
tive/substructure/structure such as the length of the primitive, the slope of the
primitive etc. Of course, an attributed grammar has to be applied in this case.
Attributed grammars were proposed in [Knuth (1968)] in the area of compiler design.[23] Then, they were adopted for syntactic pattern recognition [Shaw (1969);
Tsai and Fu (1980); Stiny (1980); Jakubowski (1985)].

Let $A_X$ denote the set of attributes of the symbol $X \in \Sigma$, $X_{\bullet}\alpha$ denote the
attribute $\alpha$ of $X$, $D_\alpha$ denote the set of possible values for the attribute $\alpha$.

Let $(p) \ X^0 \rightarrow X^1X^2 \ldots X^m$ be a production of a context-free grammar and
$A^{(p)} = A_{X^0} \cup A_{X^1} \cup A_{X^2} \cup \ldots \cup A_{X^m}$. A *semantic rule* for the production $(p)$ is an
expression of the following form

$$\beta := f(\gamma_1, \gamma_2, \ldots, \gamma_k), \text{ where}$$

$\beta, \gamma_1, \gamma_2, \ldots, \gamma_k \in A^{(p)}$,
$f : D_{\gamma_1} \times D_{\gamma_2} \times \ldots \times D_{\gamma_k} \rightarrow D_\beta$ is a function. The set of semantic rules for the
production $(p)$ is denoted by $R^{(p)}$.

---

[22]Of course, attributes have to be ascribed to the nonterminals of a grammar as well.
[23]We do not present here the details of the concept of attributed grammars since this is a standard
issue of compiler design theory. The reader is referred to [Aho *et al.* (2007)].

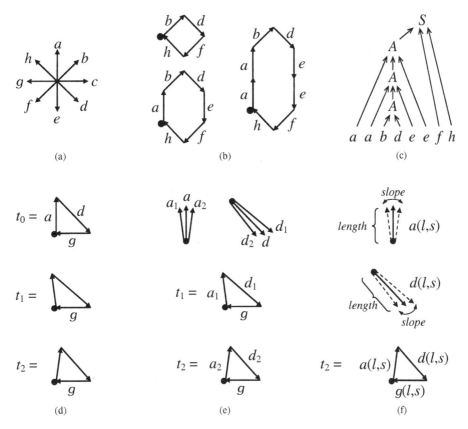

(a)                (b)                (c)

(d)                (e)                (f)

Fig. 4.7   (a) The set of primitives $PS$, (b) patterns generated by the attributed grammar $G$ and (c) the derivation tree for the pattern $aabdeefh$. (d) The pattern $t_0$ and its variants $t_1$ and $t_2$, (e) the description of variants $t_1$ and $t_2$ with the help of the extended set of primitives $EPS$ and (f) the description of variant $t_2$ with the help of the attributed primitives.

Now we can introduce the following definition [Knuth (1968); Fu (1982)].

**Definition 4.10 (Attributed *CF* Grammar):** An attributed context-free grammar is a sextuple

$$G = (\Sigma_N, \Sigma_T, P, S, A, R), \text{ where}$$

$\Sigma_N, \Sigma_T, P, S$ are defined as for a context-free grammar,
$A = \bigcup_{X \in \Sigma} A_X$ is a finite set of attributes,
$R = \bigcup_{p \in P} R^{(p)}$ is a finite set of semantic rules.

Let us consider the following example. The set of primitives $PS$ is shown in Fig. 4.7a. Let the language $L$ consist of symmetric contours as shown in Fig. 4.7b, i.e., $L = \{a^n bde^n fh, \; n \geq 0\}$. With the help of an attributed grammar, not only can we check whether a contour fulfills the syntactic conditions, which are defined by the productions of this grammar, but we can also verify some numerical

properties. Numerical properties are defined with the help of the semantic rules of this grammar. We will define the semantic rules which allow us to compute the length of a generated contour. The attributed grammar $G = (\Sigma_N, \Sigma_T, P, S, A, R)$ for our example is defined in the following way. $\Sigma_T = \{a, b, d, e, f, h\}$, $\Sigma_N = \{S, A\}$ and $A = \{\ length\ \}$, where *length* is the attribute of each element of $\Sigma$.
$P$ and $R$ are defined in the following way. (The index is used for the nonterminal $A$ in order to distinguish among various occurrences of $A$ in the second production.)

$(i):$    Productions $(P):$    Semantic rules $(R):$

(1)    $S \rightarrow Afh$         $S_{\bullet}length := A_{\bullet}length + f_{\bullet}length + h_{\bullet}length$

(2)    $A \rightarrow aA_1e$        $A_{\bullet}length := a_{\bullet}length + A_{1\bullet}length + e_{\bullet}length$

(3)    $A \rightarrow bd$           $A_{\bullet}length := b_{\bullet}length + d_{\bullet}length$

Now, let us assume that the bottom-up parsing strategy is applied to parse the word *aabdeefh* which represents the third contour in Fig. 4.7b. The corresponding parse/derivation tree is shown in Fig. 4.7c. The arrows show the direction of the computing of the attributes. One can easily notice that the length of this contour is stored in $S_{\bullet}length$ at the parsing completion.

As we have mentioned, the use of attributes enhances the descriptive power of a formal grammar. Attributes can be applied to express variants of structural patterns. For example, let us consider the "ideal" pattern $t_0$ and its two variants (or distortions) $t_1$ and $t_2$ which are shown in Fig. 4.7d. In order to describe patterns $t_1$ and $t_2$, the variants of the primitive $a$ and the primitive $d$ can be defined as shown in Fig. 4.7e. We have already used such a strategy when introducing stochastic languages in Sec. 3.3.1 (cf. Fig. 3.15). However, if many variants are to be defined, this strategy is, obviously, cumbersome. Then, the use of attributes, as shown in Fig. 4.7f, is a much better strategy.

If we use an attribute grammar, we should modify the recognition method as well. Parsers/automata should compute the values of key attributes additionally. These values are used in order to verify whether a pattern analyzed belongs to the corresponding language. For example, thresholds (or tolerance intervals) can be defined and, then, used for the accepting of attributed structural patterns in an analogous way as the acceptance with thresholds by stochastic automata is made (cf. Definition 3.7 in Sec. 3.3.1).

Since D. E. Knuth named the defining of attributes of grammar symbols as the assigning "meaning" to strings generated by the grammar [Knuth (1968)], we say about *semantic information*, or simply *semantics*, when we refer to the attributes in computer science.

If $A_X = (\alpha_1, \alpha_2, \ldots, \alpha_n)$ is defined as the vector of attributes and $z_i$ is the value of $\alpha_i$, $i = 1, 2, \ldots, n$, then $(z_1, z_2, \ldots, z_n)$ can be interpreted as a feature vector in the sense of the decision-theoretic approach to pattern recognition (see Sec.

1.3). Then, instead of the use of acceptance thresholds and intervals for separated attributes, the decision-theoretic methods for the feature/attribute vectors can be used. Indeed, attributed grammars are the basic formal tool for the constructing of hybrid syntactic-semantic pattern recognition systems. The so-called *syntactic-semantic issue* will be discussed in Sec. 13.2.

In our example above, only *synthesized attributes* [Knuth (1968)] have been considered. A synthesized attribute is an attribute of a derivation tree node $v$ which is computed from the values of the attributes of the child nodes of the node $v$.[24] *Inherited attributes* [Knuth (1968)] are the second type of attributes. An inherited attribute is an attribute of a derivation tree node which is computed from the values of the attributes of the parent node and/or the sibling nodes of the node $v$. The use of inherited attributes allows one to express the dependence of a substructure on its context in syntactic pattern recognition.

The use of attributes remarkably increases the descriptive power of grammars. Therefore, in practical applications such a syntactic-semantic approach is often applied. For *PDL* grammars, shape grammars and *SFL* grammars introduced in the next section the attributed extensions have been proposed in [Shaw (1969)], [Stiny (1980)] and [Jakubowski (1985)], respectively.

## 4.5 Picture Languages

As we have mentioned at the beginning of this chapter, the increasing of the descriptive power of string grammars is achieved by the enhancement of the representation scheme (representation mapping) in syntactic pattern recognition. *Picture languages*, which are "a generalization of string languages to two dimensions" [Rosenfeld (1979)], are the best example of such a methodological strategy. The first fundamental pattern analysis models based on picture languages were published in [Freeman (1961); Kirsch (1964); Narasimhan (1964); Feder (1968); Shaw (1969); Pavlidis (1968); Stiny and Gips (1972); Siromoney *et al.* (1972); Rosenfeld (1973)]. Freeman chain codes have been already introduced in Sec. 3.1. In the following sections *Picture Description Languages*, *PDLs*, two-dimensional automata, Siromoney matrix/array grammars, shape grammars, *Shape Feature Languages*, *SFLs*, and the grammars for visual languages will be presented.

### 4.5.1 *Picture Description Languages*

*Picture Description Languages*, *PDLs*, were introduced for the analysis of particle tracks in high energy particle physics experiments in [Shaw (1968)]. An arbitrary set of structural primitives can be defined in this approach, assuming that two

---

[24]This property of synthesized attributes results from the form of semantic rules defined for productions. Let us notice that the attributes of the left hand side symbols are defined on the basis of the attributes of the symbols which belong to the right-hand sides of the productions in the semantic rules defined in our examples.

distinguished points, called here a *head* and a *tail*, are identified in each primitive.[25]
Additionally, the *null primitive* $\lambda$ having an identical tail and head is defined. The
exemplary set of primitives is shown in Fig. 4.8a. The heads of the primitives are
marked with arrows, whereas their tails are marked with dots.

Heads and tails are used for the concatenating of primitives. The following
four binary concatenation operations are defined for *PDLs*. (The set of primitives
shown in Fig. 4.8a is used for the interpreting of these operations. *CONCAT* means
concatenating. *H* and *T* in Figs 4.8b-d mean the new head and the new tail of the
constructed structure.)

- $b + a$ iff *head*($b$) *CONCAT tail*($a$) (see Fig. 4.8b).
- $b \times a$ iff *tail*($b$) *CONCAT tail*($a$) (see Fig. 4.8c).
- $b - a$ iff *head*($b$) *CONCAT head*($a$) (see Fig. 4.8d).
- $c * e$ iff *head*($c$) *CONCAT head*($e$) *AND tail*($c$) *CONCAT tail*($e$) (see Fig. 4.8e).

The unary operator $\sim$ is a head/tail reverser (see Fig. 4.8f). In order to allow
cross reference to the primitive $p$, this primitive is labelled with the so-called *label
designator*, e.g., $n$, which is denoted by $p^n$. The / operator allows the tail and
the head of the primitive $p^n$ to be located arbitrarily. (We shall illustrate these
operations with an example later.)

Let us introduce the definition of a *PDL* grammar [Shaw (1969)].

**Definition 4.11 (*PDL* Grammar):** Let $\Sigma_{PDL}$ be a set of *PDL* structural
primitives. A *PDL* grammar is a context-free grammar

$$G = (\Sigma_N, \Sigma_T, P, S), \text{ where}$$

$\Sigma_N = \{S, SL\}$,
$\Sigma_T = \Sigma_{PDL} \cup \{+, \times, -, *, \sim, /, (,)\} \cup L$, in which $L$ is a set of label designators,
$P$ is a set of productions of the form:

$$S \rightarrow (S\phi S), \qquad S \rightarrow (\sim S), \qquad S \rightarrow SL, \qquad S \rightarrow (/SL),$$

$$SL \rightarrow S^n, \; n \in L, \qquad SL \rightarrow (SL\phi SL), \qquad SL \rightarrow (\sim SL), \qquad SL \rightarrow (/SL),$$

$$\phi \rightarrow +, \qquad\qquad \phi \rightarrow \times, \qquad\qquad \phi \rightarrow -, \qquad\qquad \phi \rightarrow *,$$

$$S \rightarrow p, \; p \in \Sigma_{PDL},$$
$S$ is the start symbol.

The example of an expression generated according to a *PDL* grammar is shown
in Fig. 4.8g. This expression represents the structural pattern which is shown at the
bottom of the figure. Firstly, three substructures described with the expressions:
$((d^m + b) * c)$, $((((/d^m) + a) + (/d^n)))$ and $((b + d^n) * e)$ are constructed. The
primitives $(/d^m)$ and $(/d^n)$ in the (middle) substructure $((((/d^m) + a) + (/d^n)))$ are,

---

[25]Structural primitives of *Picture Description Languages* can be treated as specific N attaching
point entities (NAPEs) of plex languages, introduced in Sec. 10.5, for N = 2.

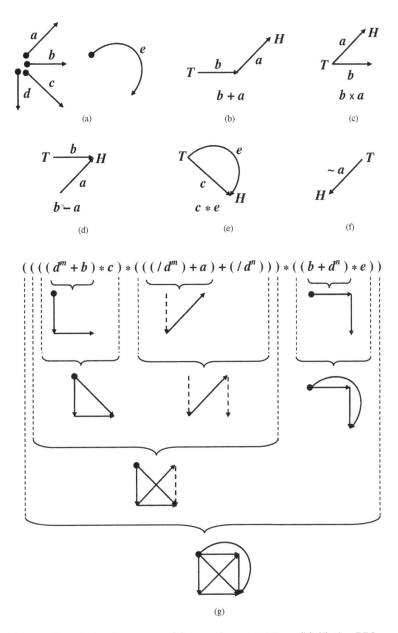

$$( ( ( ( d^m + b ) * c ) * ( ( ( / d^m ) + a ) + ( / d^n ) ) ) * ( ( b + d^n ) * e ) )$$

Fig. 4.8  Picture Description Languages: (a) exemplary primitives, (b)-(f) the *PDL* operations, (g) the example of a pattern generation.

somehow, "virtual" primitives.[26] They are marked with dashed arrows in Fig. 4.8g and they are used to "glue" these three substructures. As we can see in the figure,

---

[26]The primitives $(/d^m)$ and $(/d^n)$ are "virtual" counterparts of the primitives $d^m$ and $d^n$, respectively.

the primitive $(/d^m)$ is glued to the primitive $d^m$ of the first substructure and the new substructure is created. (Let us note that these primitives should have the same label designator.) At the end, this newly created substructure is joined with the third substructure by a gluing of the primitives $(/d^n)$ and $d^n$, and the whole structural pattern is defined.

The formal foundations of *Picture Description Languages* were presented in [Shaw (1969, 1970)].

### 4.5.2 *Two-Dimensional Automata*

Before we define two-dimensional automata we shall introduce the basic notions concerning the representation of pictures in this approach.

Let $\Sigma_T$ be a finite set of symbols. A two-dimensional matrix $P = [p_{ij}]_{k \times n}$, $p_{ij} \in \Sigma_T$, $i = 1, \ldots, k$, $j = 1, \ldots, n$ is called a *picture*. The set of all pictures over $\Sigma_T$ is denoted $\Sigma_T^{**}$. The set of all pictures over $\Sigma_T$ of size $k \times n$ is denoted $\Sigma_T^{k \times n}$. For practical reasons, we add the boundary to a picture. The boundary surrounds a picture and each cell of the boundary is labelled by a special symbol $\# \notin \Sigma_T$. Thus, the bounded picture $\hat{P}$ is defined in the following way.

$$\hat{P} = \begin{bmatrix} \# & \# & \cdots & \# & \# \\ \# & p_{11} & \cdots & p_{1n} & \# \\ \vdots & \vdots & \ddots & \vdots & \vdots \\ \# & p_{k1} & \cdots & p_{kn} & \# \\ \# & \# & \cdots & \# & \# \end{bmatrix}$$

Now, we can introduce two-dimensional automata. We shall present a four-way deterministic finite automaton (*4DFA*) [Blum and Hewitt (1967)].

---

**Parsing Scheme 4.1: Four-Way Finite Automaton**

A deterministic four-way finite automaton, *4DFA*, is a septuple

$$A = (Q, \Sigma_T, W, \delta, q_0, q_a, q_r), \text{ where}$$

$Q$ is a finite set of states,
$\Sigma_T$ is a set of input symbols,
$W = \{L, R, U, D\}$ is the set of directions,
$\delta : (Q \setminus \{q_a, q_r\}) \times (\Sigma_T \cup \{\#\}) \longrightarrow Q \times W$ is the state-transition function,
$q_0 \in Q$ is the initial state,
$q_a \in Q$ is the accepting state,
$q_r \in Q$ is the rejecting state.

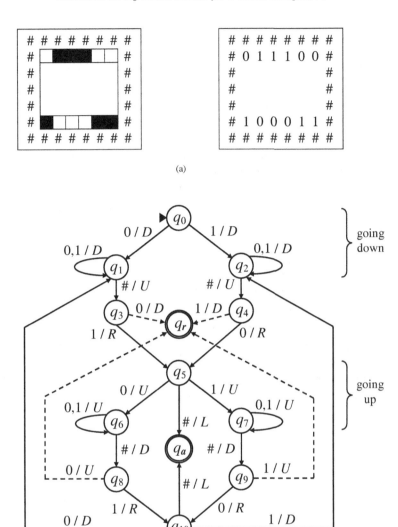

Fig. 4.9  (a) The exemplary picture and (b) the four-way finite automaton $A$.

*4DFA* is an extension of a deterministic finite automaton. The automaton reads symbols from the input picture $\hat{P}$ (instead of the input tape) and it can move in four directions, namely *Left, Right, Up, Down*. It starts the reading of the input picture from the cell $p_{11}$. The transition function not only determines the next state but also the direction of movement.

Let us consider the following example of binary pictures $\Sigma_T^{k \times n}$, i.e., $\Sigma_T = \{0, 1\}$. Let us define the language $L$ of pictures $\Sigma_T^{k \times n}$ such that the first row is the inverse of the last one, as it is shown, e.g., in Fig. 4.9a. Formally, the language $L$ is defined as $L = \{p \in \Sigma_T^{k \times n} : p_{1i} = I(p_{ki}), \ i = 1, \ldots n, \ I$ is the inverting operation $\}$.

Now, we shall define the deterministic four-way finite automaton $A$ which recognizes the language $L$. The automaton scans the input picture $\hat{P}$ column by column, proceeding from left to right. The first column is scanned from top to bottom, the second column is scanned from bottom to top, the third column is scanned from top to bottom, etc.

A diagram of the automaton $A$ is shown in Fig. 4.9b. If the transition function is defined as $\delta(q, a) = (\bar{q}, W)$ then the transition from state $q$ to state $\bar{q}$ is labelled by $a/W$. The upper part of the diagram corresponds to the scanning of $\hat{P}$ from top to bottom. The transition to state $q_1$ means that the first cell in the column is labelled by 0. (This means that the last cell in this column should be labelled by 1.) Then, the automaton goes down in $\hat{P}$ until the bottom boundary is recognized. If so, the automaton goes to state $q_3$ and makes one move up to the last (non-boundary) cell of the column. This cell should be labelled by 1 (the inverse of the first cell of the column). If so, the automaton moves to the next column and goes to state $q_5$ in order to scan this column from bottom to top. Otherwise, the automaton goes into the rejecting state $q_r$. If after going to the next column it has turned out that this column is the right boundary, the automaton goes to the accepting state $q_a$.

The right part of the diagram is analogous to the left one we have just presented. The bottom part of the diagram, i.e., form state $q_5$ to state $q_{10}$ is analogous to the upper one and it corresponds to the scanning of a column of $\hat{P}$ from bottom to top.

Two- and multi-dimensional automata were studied in [Milgram and Rosenfeld (1971); Mylopoulos (1972a,b); Rosenfeld (1973); Shah (1974); Nakamura (2001); Mäurer (2007); Fernau *et al.* (2018)].

### 4.5.3  *Siromoney Matrix/Array Grammars*

Matrix grammars were introduced in [Ábrahám (1965)]. Siromoney matrix/array grammars, called also kolam[27] array grammars, were presented in [Siromoney (1969); Siromoney *et al.* (1972)]. The derivation of a picture (matrix) is performed in the following two phases:

- In the *horizontal phase*, the string of *intermediate symbols* is generated by the so-called *horizontal productions*.[28] This string can be treated as the first row of a matrix generated. An intermediate symbol can be treated as a terminal symbol for this phase. At the same time, intermediate symbols are the start symbols for the second (vertical) phase. Horizontal productions can be context-sensitive, context-free or right-regular. However, for a given Siromoney grammar the type of horizontal productions is fixed.
- In the *vertical phase*, the *vertical productions* are applied in parallel (i.e., si-

---

[27]Kolam is an art form composed of curved lines. The kolam patterns are created in India, Sri Lanka, Indonesia, Malaysia and some other Asian countries.

[28]In Siromoney grammars, productions are usually called *rules*.

multaneously), in order to derive the columns of the matrix. The columns are generated in the downward direction. Vertical productions are right-regular.

Let us introduce Siromoney matrix grammars.

**Definition 4.12 (Siromoney Matrix Grammar):** A context-sensitive (context-free, right-regular) matrix grammar is a septuple

$$G = (\Sigma_N^h, \Sigma_N^v, \Sigma_I, \Sigma_T, P^h, P^v, S), \text{ where}$$

$\Sigma_N^h$ is a finite set of horizontal nonterminal symbols,
$\Sigma_N^v$ is a finite set of vertical nonterminal symbols,
$\Sigma_I$ is a finite set of intermediate symbols, $\Sigma_I \subseteq \Sigma_N^v$,
$\Sigma_T$ is a finite set of terminal symbols,
$P^h$ is a finite set of horizontal context-sensitive (context-free, right-regular) productions,
$P^v$ is a finite set of vertical right-regular productions,
$S$ is the start symbol, $S \in \Sigma_N^h$.

For example, let us define the right-regular matrix grammar $G = (\Sigma_N^h, \Sigma_N^v, \Sigma_I, \Sigma_T, P^h, P^v, S)$ which generates the language of pictures such that the first column and the last one are black, whereas the remaining columns are white. The exemplary picture $P$ is shown in Fig. 4.10a. $\Sigma_N^h = \{S, B, W, X\}$, $\Sigma_N^v = \Sigma_I = \{B, W\}$, $\Sigma_T = \{0, 1\}$.
$P^h$ consists of the following horizontal productions.

$$(1)\ S \rightarrow BX \quad (2)\ X \rightarrow WX \quad (3)\ X \rightarrow B$$

$P^v$ consists of the following vertical productions.

$$(4)\ B \rightarrow 1B \quad (5)\ B \rightarrow 1 \quad (6)\ W \rightarrow 0W \quad (7)\ W \rightarrow 0$$

The picture $P$ is derived in the following way.

$$S \underset{G}{\Rightarrow} \begin{bmatrix} B & X \end{bmatrix} \underset{G}{\Rightarrow} \begin{bmatrix} B & W & X \end{bmatrix} \underset{G}{\overset{+}{\Rightarrow}} \begin{bmatrix} B & W & W & W & X \end{bmatrix} \underset{G}{\Rightarrow} \begin{bmatrix} B & W & W & W & B \end{bmatrix}$$

$$\underset{G}{\overset{+}{\Rightarrow}} \begin{bmatrix} 1 & 0 & 0 & 0 & 1 \\ B & W & W & W & B \end{bmatrix} \underset{G}{\overset{+}{\Rightarrow}} \begin{bmatrix} 1 & 0 & 0 & 0 & 1 \\ 1 & 0 & 0 & 0 & 1 \\ 1 & 0 & 0 & 0 & 1 \\ 1 & 0 & 0 & 0 & 1 \\ B & W & W & W & B \end{bmatrix} \underset{G}{\overset{+}{\Rightarrow}} \begin{bmatrix} 1 & 0 & 0 & 0 & 1 \\ 1 & 0 & 0 & 0 & 1 \\ 1 & 0 & 0 & 0 & 1 \\ 1 & 0 & 0 & 0 & 1 \\ 1 & 0 & 0 & 0 & 1 \end{bmatrix}$$

Matrix/array grammars were investigated in [Siromoney *et al.* (1972); Salomaa (1972); Siromoney *et al.* (1982); Subramanian *et al.* (1989); Wang (1989); Yamamoto *et al.* (1989); Nivat and Saoudi (1992); Crespi-Reghizzi and Pradella (2008)].

### 4.5.4   *Shape Grammars*

Let us introduce shape grammars [Stiny and Gips (1972)].

**Definition 4.13 (Shape Grammar):** A shape grammar is a quadruple

$$G = (\Sigma_M, \Sigma_T, P, I), \text{ where}$$

$\Sigma_M$ is a finite set of nonterminal shapes, called *markers*,
$\Sigma_T$ is a finite set of terminal shapes, $\Sigma_M \cap \Sigma_T = \emptyset$,
$P$ is a finite set of productions $L \rightarrow R$, in which $L$ is a shape consisting of an element of $\Sigma_T^+$ combined with an element of $\Sigma_M^+$, $R$ is a shape consisting of an element of $\Sigma_T^*$ combined with an element of $\Sigma_M^*$,
$I$ is the initial shape consisting of an element of $\Sigma_T^+$ combined with an element of $\Sigma_M^+$.

Markers define the characteristic points of shapes. A marker is used to match the left-hand side of the production to be applied to the shape which is to be transformed during a derivational step.

Let us consider the following example. Let $G = (\Sigma_M, \Sigma_T, P, I)$ be a shape grammar. The initial (triangular) shape $I$ is shown in Fig. 4.10b. The shape markers are denoted with black dots. The grammar $G$ consists of two productions depicted in Figs. 4.10c and d. The exemplary derivation of the shape $S$ is shown in Fig. 4.10e. Each derivational step is performed in the following way. Firstly, the left-hand side $L$ of the production to be applied is matched, also with the help of its markers, to the part of the shape which is to be expanded.[29] During matching, the geometric transformations, such as translation, reflection, rotation and scaling, can be made to $L$. Then, the transformations, which have been made to $L$, are applied to the right-hand side $R$ of the production. Secondly, the part of the shape which corresponds to $L$ is replaced by $R$. Let us notice that no geometric transformation has been used during the first derivational step. However, during the second step, rotation and scaling have been applied.

The language of a shape grammar is the set of shapes which do not contain markers.

Shape grammars were investigated in [Gips (1975); Stiny (1975, 1980, 1982, 2006)]. *Split grammars* [Wonka *et al.* (2003)] introduced for the 3D modelling of architectural objects are a modification of shape grammars. Additional split productions are used in split grammars for the decomposing of shapes into sets of smaller shapes.

### 4.5.5   *Shape Feature Languages*

*Shape Feature Languages, SFLs,* were introduced in [Jakubowski and Kasprzak (1977); Jakubowski (1982)] for the analyzing of machine parts modelled in the area

---

[29]There is only one marker to be matched in our example.

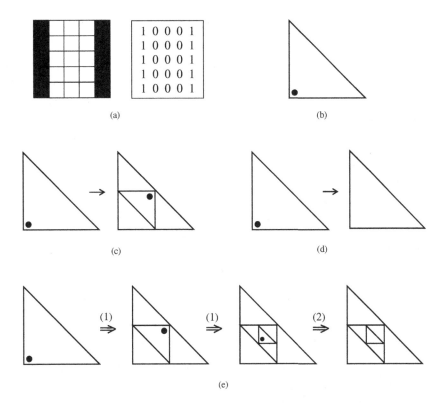

Fig. 4.10 (a) The picture $P$ generated by the matrix grammar $G$, (b) the initial shape of the shape grammar $G$, (c)-(d) the productions of the shape grammar $G$ and (e) the derivation of the shape $S$ in the shape grammar $G$.

of computer-aided manufacturing. In fact, *SFLs* describe contours which are cross sections of 3D solids. (Cross-sections are rotated or swept in 3D in order to obtain modelled solids.)

Solids/contours can be described at the several levels of abstraction in the *SFLs*, depending on the specific goal of the pattern analysis. At the lowest level, a contour is described with the help of the set of *SFL* primitives shown in Fig. 4.11a. The *axial primitives* $s_{1i}$, $i = 1, 2, 3, 4$, divide 2D space into four quadrants $Q_i$. Let us note that each axial primitive belongs to both adjacent quadrants. The primitives of the form $s_{2i}$ are called *sloped primitives*. The primitives of the form $s_{3i}$ are called *concave primitives*, whereas the primitives of the form $s_{4i}$ are called *convex primitives*. (The interior of contours described is marked in grey in Fig. 4.11a.)

Let us analyze the example of the two rotational machine parts shown in Figs. 4.11c and d. Their (lowest-level) descriptions are defined as follows:[30]

- $s_{12}s_{11}s_{12}s_{11}s_{34}s_{31}s_{11}s_{14}s_{11}s_{14}s_{13}$ (Fig. 4.11c) and

---

[30]The defining of the description begins with the left-most lowest point of the contour which is marked with the black dot in the figures.

- $s_{12}s_{11}s_{12}s_{11}s_{24}s_{11}s_{21}s_{11}s_{14}s_{11}s_{14}s_{13}$ (Fig. 4.11d).

The extraction of machine part features starts at the lowest-level description of a solid and the syntax analysis is performed with the help of $LR(k)$ parsing in the *SFL* model [Jakubowski (1982)]. At the same time, the grouping of similar machine parts into *part families*[31] is possible in the *SFL* model due to the introducing of higher level descriptions.

The second-level description is obtained from the lowest-level description with the help of a (deterministic) finite-state transducer [Harrison (1978); Rozenberg and Salomaa (1997)] in the *SFL* model.[32] Let us introduce the following definition [Jakubowski (1985)].

---

**Parsing Scheme 4.2:** *SFL* **Finite-State Transducer**

A (deterministic) *SFL* finite-state transducer is a quintuple

$$A = (Q, \Sigma_T^I, \Sigma_T^O, \delta, Q_0), \text{ where}$$

$Q = \{q_0, q_1, q_3, q_4\}$ is the set of states,
$\Sigma_T^I$ is the set of input symbols corresponding to *SFL* primitives,
$\Sigma_T^O = \{12, 13, 14, 21, 23, 24, 31, 32, 34, 41, 42, 43\}$ is the set of output symbols, called *switches*,
$\delta : Q \times \Sigma_T^I \longrightarrow Q \times (\Sigma_T^O \cup \{\lambda\})$ is the transition-output function defined by the diagram shown in Fig. 4.11b,
$Q_0 = \{q_0, q_1, q_3, q_4\}$ is the set of initial states.

---

The *SFL* finite-state transducer reads the succeeding symbols of the lowest-level description and generates the sequence of *switches*.[33] A switch $ij$ denotes the occurring of the primitive $s_{kj}$ during the reading, i.e., the primitive which belongs to the quadrant $Q_j$, whereas the preceding primitives belong to the quadrant $Q_i$. The corresponding transition of the *SFL* transducer is labelled by $Q_j \setminus Q_i / ij$. The transition labelled by $Q_j^0 / ij$ means that the primitive $s_{kj}$ is not an axial primitive. As long as the *SFL* transducer reads the primitives belonging to the same quadrant $Q_i$, it remains in the state $q_i$ and does not write any output symbol.

Let us come back to our example shown in Figs. 4.11c and d. As we can see in these figures, the *SFL* transducer generates, for both (similar) machine parts, the same second-level description of the form:[34]

$$32 \cdot 21 \cdot 14 \cdot 41 \cdot 14 \cdot 43.$$

---

[31]Part families are a basic concept of the group technology (GT) approach in the theory of manufacturing processes.
[32]A finite-state transducer is, somehow, a finite-state automaton with output. The *SFL* finite-state transducer will be introduced in this book as an automaton with no final states (i.e., according to [Harrison (1978)]).
[33]We introduce here the simple form of switches, i.e., without the 0-1 concavity/convexity markers.
[34]The switches are marked with thick arrows.

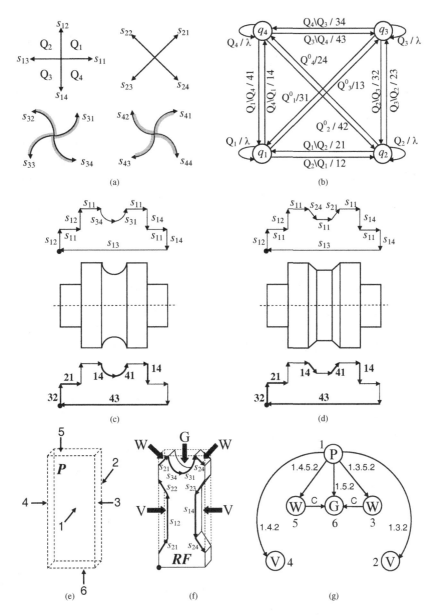

Fig. 4.11 (a) The *SFL* primitives, (b) the *SFL* transducer, (c)-(d) *SFL* descriptions (e)-(f) the constructing of the exemplary *SFL/IE Graph* representation [Jakubowski and Flasiński (1992)] and (g) the *IE Graph* representation of the part *RF* [Flasiński (1995b)].

The hierarchical (multi-level) *SFL* model allows one to recognize a variety of complex shape features which are important from the technological point of view [Jakubowski (1986, 1990)]. Moreover, the hybrid CAD/CAM model which consists of the (string) *SFL* model at the lower layer and the (graph grammar-based)

*ETPL(k)* model [Flasiński (1988, 1993)][35] at the higher level was presented in [Jakubowski and Flasiński (1992)]. Let us consider the example of the construction of the so-called *SFL/IE Graph* representation (see Figs. 4.11e-g). The machine part *RF* (*reversing fork*) is modelled in the following two stages.

In the first stage, the contour of the part *RF* is described with the help of the shape feature language *SFL* as it is shown in Fig. 4.11f.[36]

In the second stage, the contour is embedded in the rectangular prism *P* having faces indexed as shown in Fig. 4.11e according to the method introduced in [Flasiński (1995b)]. Then, the contour is swept in 3D space as shown in Fig. 4.11f. The *SFL* syntax analyzer recognizes/extracts features on the basis of the lowest-level *SFL* description. As we can see in Fig. 4.11f, one groove (G), two wedges (W) and two V-slots (V) have been recognized. As a result, the *IE Graph* representation of the part *RF* is generated,[37] as shown in Fig. 4.11g. Finally, the IE Graph representation is analyzed by the *ETPL(k)* graph grammar parser.[38]

### 4.5.6   *Remarks on Picture and Visual Languages*

There are other important picture language-based models which include: isometric array grammars [Milgram and Rosenfeld (1971); Rosenfeld (1971, 1973, 1976, 1979, 1989); Thompson and Rosenfeld (1999)], tessellation automata [Yamada and Amoroso (1969)], 2-D on-line tessellation automata [Inoue and Nakamura (1977); Inoue and Takanami (1991)], Wang systems [Wang (1960, 1961); Prophetis De and Varricchio (1997); Lonati and Pradella (2010)], drawn picture languages [Maurer *et al.* (1982, 1983); Kim and Sudborough (1987); Brandenburg and Chytil (1991); Costagliola *et al.* (2003, 2005)], tiling systems [Giammarresi and Restivo (1992); Giammarresi *et al.* (1996); Pradella and Crespi-Reghizzi (2008); Anselmo *et al.* (2009)], tile rewriting grammars [Crespi-Reghizzi and Pradella (2005); Cherubini *et al.* (2006); Thomas *et al.* (2008)], puzzle grammars [Nivat *et al.* (1991); Laroche *et al.* (1994); Siromoney *et al.* (1992); Subramanian *et al.* (1995); Siromoney *et al.* (1999); Subramanian *et al.* (2001)], array-rewriting P systems [Ceterchi *et al.* (2003)] based on P systems [Păun (2000)], contextual array grammars [Freund *et al.* (2007)] based on contextual grammars [Marcus (1969)], contextual array P systems [Fernau *et al.* (2015)], pure 2D grammars [Subramanian *et al.* (2009)] based on pure grammars [Maurer *et al.* (1980)], grid grammars [Drewes (1996)], tree-based picture systems [Drewes (2000)], generalized operator picture grammars [Matz (1997)].

The theoretical foundations of picture languages were presented in [Rosenfeld (1979); Giammarresi and Restivo (1997); Matz (2002); Pradella *et al.* (2011)].

---

[35]The graph grammar-based *ETPL(k)* model will be presented in Sec. 10.4.

[36]Only those primitives which define features in the solid are marked with thick arrows and described with $s_{ij}$ codes in this figure.

[37]The labels of the graph edges denote the interactions of extracted features with the faces of the prism *P* according to the method introduced in [Flasiński (1995b)].

[38]The *ETPL(k)* graph grammar parser will be introduced in Sec. 10.4.

As we have mentioned in Sec. 2.3, *visual languages* have been developed in the area of software/system engineering since the 1970s [Chang (1971, 1986)]. They are used for such important applications as the development of visual programming languages, the constructing of (graphical) software development tools and the designing of graphical user interfaces. Visual (programming) languages allow users to construct programs, interact with software systems and process visual information by manipulating visual objects. Although they are applied in syntactic pattern recognition relatively seldom[39], it seems that they have the great potential which could be successfully used in this area.

*Picture processing grammars*, introduced in [Chang (1971)] and studied in [Chang and Liu (1984); Chang *et al.* (1987); Chang (1990)], were the first model in this area. In this model an arbitrary number of spatial attributes can be ascribed to an object.

The ability to express numerous spatial (2D) relations is the immanent property of visual languages since they merely represent the spatial arrangements of graphical objects. On the other hand, standard Chomsky languages are able to express the rigid linear structures only, i.e., only the concatenation relation is used for the defining of string structures in the Chomsky approach. Therefore, Chomsky languages have to be modified/enhanced when applied in this area. There are several strategies to solve this problem. Let us present the most important ones.

Multisets[40] can be treated as strings in which the order of the symbols is insignificant. *Multiset grammars*, called *commutative*[41] *grammars*, were introduced in [Crespi-Reghizzi and Mandrioli (1976)]. A set of all the multisets over an alphabet $\Sigma$ is denoted with $\Sigma^{\oplus}$.

*Attributed*[42] *multiset grammars*, *AMGs*, were introduced in [Golin and Reiss (1990); Golin (1991a,b)].[43] A production of *AMG* is of the following form:[44]

$$A \rightarrow \alpha \ , \ R \ , \ C \ , \text{where}$$

$A \in \Sigma_N$, $\alpha \in \Sigma^{\oplus}$,
$R$ is a semantic rule which computes (synthesized) attributes of $A$,
$C$ is a constraint defined over the attributes of $\alpha$ which verifies the applicability of

---

[39]For example, multiset grammars are used for the analysis of visual events and activities, positional grammars are applied in optical character recognition and adjacency grammars are used for the interpretation of sketched diagrams (see Chap. 6).

[40]Let us remind ourselves that in a multiset the elements are allowed to occur more than once.

[41]In the theory of formal languages, string languages are sometimes viewed as free monoids, in which the concatenation is the monoid operation and the empty word is the identity element. Thus, grammars which generate multisets, instead of strings, can be viewed as free *commutative* monoids.

[42]Attributed grammars were presented in Sec. 4.4.

[43]If productions of an attributed multiset grammar correspond to picture composition operators, the grammar is called a *picture layout grammar*.

[44]We shall unify denotations which are used for various visual languages according to the conventions assumed in this book.

the production.[45]

The idea of *constraint multiset grammars, CMGs,* was presented in [Helm *et al.* (1991)], whereas the formal definition of *CMGs* was introduced in [Marriott (1994)]. Constraint multiset grammars were studied in [Marriott (1995); Marriott and Meyer (1997)]. A production of *CMG* is defined as follows:

$$A, \beta \rightarrow \alpha, \beta \parallel C , \ \vec{\mathbf{V}} := E \ , \text{ where}$$

$A \in \Sigma_N$ is replaced by $\alpha \in \Sigma^\oplus$ if a multiset which is rewritten contains the context $\beta \in \Sigma^\oplus$ such that the attributes of the elements of $\beta$ satisfy the constraint $C$, $\vec{\mathbf{V}}$ is the vector of attributes of $A$ whose values are determined by the vector expression $E$ over other symbols which occur in the production.

*Relation grammars,* called also *SR grammars,* were defined in [Crimi *et al.* (1991)] and they were studied in [Tucci *et al.* (1994); Ferruci *et al.* (1996)]. Apart from (standard) symbol sets $\Sigma_N$ and $\Sigma_T$, a relation grammar contains also a set of relation symbols $\Sigma_R$.[46] A sentential form over $\Sigma$, $\Sigma = \Sigma_N \cup \Sigma_T$, and $\Sigma_R$ is a pair $(\mathbf{M}, \mathbf{R})$, where:

- $\mathbf{M}$ is a set of the so-called *s-items*[47] of the form $(Y, i)$, in which $Y \in \Sigma$ and $i \in \mathbb{N}$ is the index[48] (instead of $(Y, i)$, we will write $Y^i$),
- $\mathbf{R}$ is a set of the so-called *r-items*[49] of the form $r(m_1, m_2)$, in which $m_1, m_2 \in \mathbf{M}$ and $r \in \Sigma_R$ denotes the relation which holds between $m_1$ and $m_2$.

A relation grammar contains two sets of productions. A set of *s-productions $P$,* which is used for the rewriting of s-items, is of the following form:

$$l : \ A^0 \rightarrow (\mathbf{M}, \mathbf{R}) \ , \text{ where}$$

$l \in \mathbb{N}_+$ is the label of the production, $A \in \Sigma_N$, $A^0 \notin \mathbf{M}$ and $(\mathbf{M}, \mathbf{R})$ is a sentential form over $\Sigma$ and $\Sigma_R$.

A set of *r-productions $R$,* which is used for the rewriting of r-items, is of the form:

$$r(A^0, X^1) \rightarrow [\, l\, ]\mathbf{Q} \quad \text{or} \quad r(X^1, A^0) \rightarrow [\, l\, ]\mathbf{Q} \ , \text{ where}$$

$r \in \Sigma_R$, $l$ is the label of the corresponding s-production $A^0 \rightarrow (\mathbf{M}, \mathbf{R})$, $X \in \Sigma$, $X^1 \notin \mathbf{M}$ and $\mathbf{Q} \neq \emptyset$ is a finite set of r-items of the form $r'(Z, X^1)$ or $r'(X^1, Z)$, in which $Z \in \mathbf{M}$.

A derivational step is performed in two parts.[50] During the first stage, a nonterminal $A$ in the current sentential form, which corresponds to the left-hand side of

---

[45]Constraints $C$ in visual languages play a similar role to predicates of applicability $\pi$ used for attributed programmed grammars.

[46]Relation grammars simulate, somehow, graph grammars (see Chap. 10).

[47]S-items represent objects of a picture.

[48]Indices are used to distinguish among multiple occurrences of symbols.

[49]R-items represent relations between the pairs of objects.

[50]A derivational step in relation grammars is performed in an analogous way to a derivational step in edNLC graph grammars (see Sec. 10.4 and Definition A.15 in Appendix A.)

an s-production, is replaced by the right-hand side of this s-production. During the second stage, r-productions which correspond to the s-production[51] are applied.[52] The application of an r-production consists in the replacing of the r-item which corresponds to its left-hand side by the r-items of **Q**.

*Positional grammars*, *PGs*, were introduced in [Costagliola and Chang (1990)] and they were studied in [Costagliola *et al.* (1997); Costagliola and Chang (1999)]. A production of *PG* is of the following form:

$$A \rightarrow v_1 R_1 v_2 R_2 \ldots R_{(k-1)} v_k \quad , \text{ where}$$

$A \in \Sigma_N$, $v_i \in \Sigma$, $i = 1, \ldots, k$ and $R_j$, $j = 1, \ldots, k-1$ is a *positional relation identifier* which defines the relative position of $v_m$ with respect to $v_{m-1}$. For example, if the positional relation identifier $R$ defines the 2D relation of the form $(dx, dy)$, $u \in \Sigma$ is located at $(x_u, y_u)$ and $uRw$, then $w \in \Sigma$ is located at $(x_u + dx, \ y_u + dy)$.

*Unification grammars* were introduced in [Wittenburg and Weitzman (1990); Wittenburg *et al.* (1991)] and they were extended to *atomic relational grammars*, *ARGs*, in [Wittenburg (1992)]. A production of *ARG* is defined as follows:

$$A \rightarrow \alpha \ , \ C \ , \ F \quad , \text{ where}$$

$A \in \Sigma_N$, $\alpha \in \Sigma^+$,
$C$ is a set of constraints of the form $r(x, y)$, in which $r$ is a relation symbol, $x$ and $y$ refer either to symbols in $\alpha$ or to the attributes of these symbols,
$F$ is a set of assignments of the form $a := x$, in which $a$ is an attribute of $A$, $x$ refers either to a symbol in $\alpha$ or to the attribute of such a symbol.

Atomic relational grammars were studied in [Wittenburg (1993); Wittenburg and Weitzman (1998)].

*Adjacency grammars*, *AG*, were proposed in [Jorge and Glinert (1995)] and they were studied in [Mas *et al.* (2008, 2010)]. A production of *AG* is defined in the following way:

$$A \rightarrow \alpha \ , \ C \ , \ R \quad , \text{ where}$$

$A \in \Sigma_N$, $\alpha \in \Sigma^{\oplus}$,
$C$ is an *adjacency constraint* defined over the attributes of $\alpha$,
$R$ is a semantic rule which computes (synthesized) attributes of $A$.

Three main kinds of adjacency are distinguished in this model [Jorge and Glinert (1995)]. *Spatial adjacency* concerns objects which are "close enough". *Algebraic adjacency* $R$ is defined in the following way. Two objects $x$ and $y$ are adjacent, i.e. $xRy$, iff $\neg \exists z$ such that $xRz \land zRy$. *Logical adjacency* involves the use of labelled connection points which are applied to join adjacent parts (e.g., in electrical networks, flowcharts).

---

[51] This correspondence is established by the label *l*
[52] R-productions play an analogous role to items of the embedding transformation in edNLC graph grammars (see Sec. 10.4 and Definition A.15 in Appendix A.)

Formal properties of multiset (commutative) grammars were investigated in [Huynh (1983, 1985)]. The foundations of visual languages are presented in the monograph [Marriott and Meyer (1998)].

## 4.6   Timed Automata

In the previous sections, formal grammars and the corresponding automata were enhanced in order to increase the descriptive power in the sense of the expressing of spatial (2D, 3D) relations among primitives/substructures. However, in modelling (and recognizing) physical phenomena, we have to sometimes take into account the "fourth dimension" of spacetime, i.e. time. As we will see in Chap. 6, which contains a survey of the applications of string methods, timed automata and real-time automata are frequently used for signal analysis in the area of process monitoring and control.

A timed automaton is a finite-state automaton which is controlled with a finite set of real-valued clocks. The clocks are initialized with zero when the automaton starts the analyzing of a word and they increase with the same rate. A transition in the automaton is permitted only if the time constraint for this transition, called a *guard*, is fulfilled. When a transition is performed some clocks may be reset to zero.

Timed automata were introduced in [Alur and Dill (1994)]. Let us present the following definition.

---

**Parsing Scheme 4.3: Timed Automaton**

A timed automaton is a quintuple

$$A = (Q, \Sigma_T, C, \delta, q_0), \text{ where}$$

$Q$ is a finite set of states,
$\Sigma_T$ is a finite set of input symbols,
$C$ is a finite set of clocks,
$\delta : Q \times \Sigma_T \times B(C) \longrightarrow Q \times 2^C$ is the state-transition function, in which $B(C)$ is the set of Boolean constraints, called *guards*, defined for the clocks of $C$,
$q_0 \in Q$ is the initial state.

---

$\delta(q, a, G) = (q', R)$ defines the transition from the state $q$ to the state $q'$ after reading the symbol $a$, assuming that the set of constraints $G$ is fulfilled. After the performing of the transition, the clocks which belong to the set $R$ are reset.

Let us consider the following example. The timed automaton $A$ is shown in Fig. 4.12a. Let the set of input symbols $\Sigma_T$ define three events $a$, $b$ and $c$. The automaton $A$ recognizes the sequences of events *abcabcabc*.... The *guards* of the automaton transitions define when the events should occur with the help of two

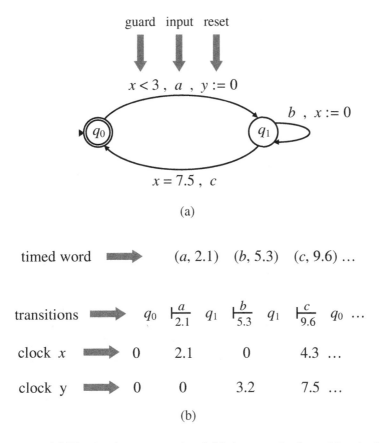

guard input reset

$$x < 3 , \; a , \; y := 0$$

$b , \; x := 0$

$q_0$       $q_1$

$$x = 7.5 , \; c$$

(a)

timed word ➡ $(a, 2.1)$   $(b, 5.3)$   $(c, 9.6)$ ...

transitions ➡ $q_0 \vdash_{\!\! 2.1}^{\!\! a} q_1 \vdash_{\!\! 5.3}^{\!\! b} q_1 \vdash_{\!\! 9.6}^{\!\! c} q_0$ ...

clock $x$ ➡   0     2.1     0     4.3 ...

clock $y$ ➡   0     0     3.2     7.5 ...

(b)

Fig. 4.12   (a) The timed automaton $A$ and (b) the example of transitions in $A$.

*clocks* $x$ and $y$. The clock $y$ is reset, if the transition from the state $q_0$ to the state $q_1$ takes place (i.e. the event $a$ has occurred), whereas the clock $x$ is reset, if the transition from the state $q_1$ to itself takes place (i.e. the event $b$ has occurred).

The analysis of the sequence of events by the automaton $A$ is shown in Fig. 4.12b. The part of the timed word $(a, 2.1)$ $(b, 5.3)$ $(c, 9.6)$ ... represents the following sequence of events. Firstly, the event $a$ occurred at time $t = 2.1s$, then the event $b$ occurred at time $t = 5.3s$ etc. The values of the clocks $x$ and $y$ are shown in Fig. 4.12b as well.

Timed automata were applied, e.g., for fault diagnosis of discrete event systems in [Tripakis (2002); Bouyer *et al.* (2005)], static scheduling problems and air-traffic control problems in [Torre La *et al.* (2002)], timed controller synthesis in [Bouyer *et al.* (2003)]. The inference methods for timed automata were defined in [Grinchtein *et al.* (2005, 2006)].

Whereas in a timed automaton, timing constraints are defined with the help of a set of clocks and a guard for each transition, a *real-time automaton* has one clock which is used for the defining of the time delay between succeeding events. Let us introduce the following definition [Dima (2001)].

---

### Parsing Scheme 4.4: Real-Time Automaton

A real-time automaton is a quintuple

$$A = (Q, \Sigma_T, \delta, q_0, F), \text{ where}$$

$Q$ is a finite set of states,
$\Sigma_T$ is a finite set of input symbols,
$\delta : Q \times \Sigma_T \times G \longrightarrow Q$ is the state-transition function, in which
$G = \{[n, n'] \cap \mathbb{N} \, , \, n, n' \in \mathbb{N}\}$ is the family of delay guards,
$q_0 \in Q$ is the initial state,
$F \subseteq Q$ is a set of accepting states.

---

$\delta(q, a, [n, n']) = q'$ defines the transition from the state $q$ to the state $q'$ after reading the symbol $a$, assuming that the symbol $a$ occurred at time $t \in [n, n']$, $t \in \mathbb{N}$.

Timed automata were applied, e.g., for the modelling of the driving behavior of truck drivers [Verwer *et al.* (2011); Zhang *et al.* (2017)] and anomaly detection in industrial control systems [Lin *et al.* (2018)]. The inference methods for timed automata were defined in [Verwer *et al.* (2012); Klerx *et al.* (2014); Schmidt and Kramer (2014)].

After introducing timed automata, we complete our presentation of the methods of the generative/descriptive power enhancement for string grammars. Further enhancement is possible with the use of the tree grammars and graph grammars which will be presented in Part III and Part IV, respectively, of this book.

# Chapter 5

# Inference (Induction) of String Languages

As we have discussed in Chap. 2 formal languages used in syntactic pattern recognition are represented with generative grammars and automata/parsers.[1] The term *grammatical* inference (induction) is usually used in syntactic pattern recognition, although the induction schemes applied here can generate grammars or (the corresponding) automata. In this chapter introduced are the classic methods which belong to two approaches in the field of grammatical inference, *text learning* and *informed learning*.

Before we present inference methods we shall introduce the basic notions involved [Feldman (1967, 1972); Gold (1978); Angluin (1978, 1982)].

A *sample* of a language $L$ over an alphabet $\Sigma_T$ is an ordered pair $(S_+, S_-)$, where a finite set $S_+ \subseteq L$, $S_+ \neq \emptyset$ is called a *positive sample* and a finite set $S_- \subseteq (\Sigma_T^* \setminus L)$ is called a *negative sample* (i.e., $S_+ \cap S_- = \emptyset$).

We talk about *text learning* (inference from a positive sample), if $S_- = \emptyset$. We talk about *informed learning* (inference from positive and negative samples), if $S_- \neq \emptyset$.

The problem of grammatical inference consists in looking for a grammar $G$ (an automaton $A$) which generates (recognizes) the language $L$.[2] It is said also that we look for a grammar/automaton which is *consistent* with the sample $(S_+, S_-)$.

In the case of text learning, $G$ is *consistent* with $(S_+, S_-)$ iff $\forall x \in \Sigma_T^* : x \in S_+ \Rightarrow x \in L(G)$. $A$ is consistent with $(S_+, S_-)$ iff $\forall x \in \Sigma_T^* : x \in S_+ \Rightarrow x \in L(A)$.

In order to define consistency for informed learning we have to extend the set of final states $F$[3] of an automaton $A$ into $F = (F_A, F_R)$, $F_A \cap F_R = \emptyset$, where $F_A$ is a set of accepting states and $F_R$ is a set of rejecting states. Now, $G$ is *consistent* with $(S_+, S_-)$ iff $\forall x \in \Sigma_T^* : x \in S_+ \Rightarrow x \in L(G)$ and $\forall x \in \Sigma_T^* : x \in S_- \Rightarrow x \notin L(G)$. $A$ is (strongly) *consistent* with $(S_+, S_-)$ iff $\forall x \in \Sigma_T^* : x \in S_+ \Rightarrow \delta(q_0, x) \in F_A$ and $\forall x \in \Sigma_T^* : x \in S_- \Rightarrow \delta(q_0, x) \in F_R$. In the case of *weak consistency* the second condition is $\forall x \in \Sigma_T^* : x \in S_- \Rightarrow \delta(q_0, x) \notin F_A$.

---

[1]In general, formal languages can be represented with other formalisms as well. For example, regular languages can be represented with formalisms of monadic second-order logic, abstract algebra (semigroup theory).

[2]We also assume a class $X$ of languages $\mathcal{L}(X)$ such that $L \in \mathcal{L}(X)$.

[3]See the definitions in Appendix A.2.

Let $w = uv \in \Sigma_T^*$. $u$ is called a *prefix* of $w$ and $v$ is called a *suffix* of $w$.

$\| Y \|$ denotes the sum of the lengths of strings which belong to the set of strings $Y$.

The methods of grammatical inference for regular languages which are based on text learning are introduced in Sec. 5.1, whereas those based on informed learning are presented in Sec. 5.2. The inference of context-free languages is discussed in Sec. 5.3 and *HMMs* learning is presented in Sec. 5.4. The bibliographical notes and remarks on the field of grammatical inference are included in the last section.

## 5.1    Text Learning Methods for Regular Languages

The classic methods of inference using positive samples which are based on: Brzozowski derivatives, $k$-tails, $k$-testable languages and reversible languages are presented in this section.

### 5.1.1    *Brzozowski-Derivative-Based Inference*

The text learning method which is based on Brzozowski derivatives [Brzozowski (1964)] is one of the first models in the field. Although in general the Brzozowski derivative concerns regular expressions we define it here with respect to finite strings only.

> **Definition 5.1 (Brzozowski Derivative):** Let $Y$ be a set of strings over an alphabet $\Sigma_T$. The Brzozowski derivative of $Y$ with respect to the string $u \in \Sigma_T^*$ is defined as
>
> $$\partial_u Y = \{v \in \Sigma_T^* : uv \in Y\} .$$

Let us note that $\partial_\lambda Y = Y$, $\partial_u \lambda = \emptyset$.

The method consists of two steps. For a sample $S_+$ derivatives with respect to symbols of $\Sigma_T$ are calculated in the first step. Then, a derivative canonical grammar is constructed on the basis of these derivatives.

Let the sample $S_+ = \{aaba, abba, baab, bbab, bbbb\}$. Derivatives for $S_+$ are calculated as follows: we set $X_0 := S_+$.

$$\partial_a X_0 = \{aba, bba\} = X_1 \quad \partial_a X_3 = \{\lambda\} \qquad\qquad \partial_a X_5 = \{b\} = X_7$$

$$\partial_a X_1 = \{ba\} = X_2 \qquad \partial_b X_0 = \{aab, bab, bbb\} = X_4 \quad \partial_b X_7 = \{\lambda\}$$

$$\partial_b X_1 = \{ba\} = X_2 \qquad \partial_a X_4 = \{ab\} = X_5 \qquad\qquad \partial_a X_6 = \{b\} = X_7$$

$$\partial_b X_2 = \{a\} = X_3 \qquad \partial_b X_4 = \{ab, bb\} = X_6 \qquad\quad \partial_b X_6 = \{b\} = X_7$$

A *derivative canonical grammar* (*DCG*) $G = (\Sigma_N, \Sigma_T, P, S)$ generating $S_+$ is inferred on the basis of Brzozowski derivatives with the following scheme:

---

### Induction Scheme 5.1: Derivative Canonical Grammar Inference

$/ * \ T$ - set of terminals in strings of $S_+$ $* /$
$/ * \ X = \{X_0, \ldots, X_n\}$ - set of distinct derivatives of $S_+$ not equal to $\emptyset$ $* /$
$\Sigma_N := X; \ \Sigma_T := T; \ S := X_0;$
$P := \emptyset;$
**for each** $\partial_a X_i = X_j$ **do**
  $P := P \cup \{X_i \ \to \ aX_j\};$
**for each** $\partial_a X_i = X_j \ni \lambda$ **do**
  $P := P \cup \{X_i \ \to \ a\};$

---

At the end of the section we shall define the derivative canonical grammar $G$ for our sample $S_+$ according to the Induction Scheme 5.1.
$\Sigma_N = \{X_0, \ldots X_7\}, \ \Sigma_T = \{a, b\}, \ S = X_0.$
$P$ consists of the following productions.

| | | |
|---|---|---|
| (1) $X_0 \ \to \ aX_1$ | (5) $X_3 \ \to \ a$ | (9) $X_5 \ \to \ aX_7$ |
| (2) $X_1 \ \to \ aX_2$ | (6) $X_0 \ \to \ bX_4$ | (10) $X_7 \ \to \ b$ |
| (3) $X_1 \ \to \ bX_2$ | (7) $X_4 \ \to \ aX_5$ | (11) $X_6 \ \to \ aX_7$ |
| (4) $X_2 \ \to \ bX_3$ | (8) $X_4 \ \to \ bX_6$ | (12) $X_6 \ \to \ bX_7$ |

### 5.1.2  *k-Tail-Based Inference*

The method introduced in [Biermann and Feldman (1972)] allows one to define equivalence classes on the states of an automaton inferred. For a sample $S_+$, $k$-tails[4] which correspond to the automaton states are calculated in the first step.

**Definition 5.2 ($k$-Tail):** Let $Y$ be a set of strings over an alphabet $\Sigma_T$, $z \in \Sigma_T^*$, $k \geq 0$. The $k$-tail of $z$ with respect to $Y$ is defined in the following way:

$$g(z, Y, k) = \{w \in \Sigma_T^* : zw \in Y \text{ and } | \ w \ | \leq k\} .$$

$g(z, Y, k)$ is undefined if $z$ and $k$ are outside of the domains assumed.

Let the sample $S_+ = \{a, ab, abb, c, cd, cdd\}$ and $k = 1$. $k$-tails for $S_+$ are calculated as follows:

$g(\lambda, S_+, 1) = \{a, c\} = q_0 \quad g(ab, S_+, 1) = \{\lambda, b\} = q_1 \quad g(abb, S_+, 1) = \{\lambda\} = q_3$

$g(a, S_+, 1) = \{\lambda, b\} = q_1 \quad g(cd, S_+, 1) = \{\lambda, d\} = q_2 \quad g(cdd, S_+, 1) = \{\lambda\} = q_3$

$g(c, S_+, 1) = \{\lambda, d\} = q_2$

---

[4]$k$ is a parameter of the method.

A *k-tail-based (non-deterministic) automaton* $A(S_+, k) = (Q, \Sigma_T, \delta, q_0, F)$ is inferred according to the following scheme.[5]

**Induction Scheme 5.2: $k$-Tail-Based Automaton Inference**

$/ * \ T$ - set of terminals in strings of $S_+$ $* /$
$/ * \ G = \{g(z_0, S_+, k), \ldots, g(z_n, S_+, k)\}$ - set of distinct $k$-tails for $S_+$ $* /$
$Q := G$; $\Sigma_T := T$; $q_0 := g(\lambda, S_+, k)$; $F := \{q \in Q : \lambda \in q\}$;
**for each** $q = g(z, S_+, k) \in Q$ **and** $q' = g(za, S_+, k) \in Q$, $a \in \Sigma_T$ **do**
$\quad \delta(q, a) := q'$;

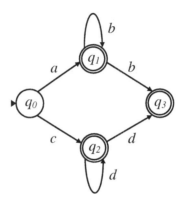

Fig. 5.1　The automaton $A(S_+, 1)$ inferred with the $k$-tail-method.

The automaton $A(S_+, 1) = (Q, \Sigma_T, \delta, q_0, F)$ for our sample $S_+$ is defined according to the Induction Scheme 5.2 in the following way (cf. Fig. 5.1):
$Q = \{q_0, q_1, q_2, q_3\}$, $\Sigma_T = \{a, b, c, d\}$, $q_0 = g(\lambda, S_+, 1)$, $F = \{q_1, q_2, q_3\}$.
The transition function $\delta$ is defined as follows:

$$\delta(q_0, a) = q_1 \quad \delta(q_1, b) = q_1 \quad \delta(q_1, b) = q_3$$

$$\delta(q_0, c) = q_2 \quad \delta(q_2, d) = q_2 \quad \delta(q_2, d) = q_3$$

The adjusting of the parameter $k$ is a crucial issue of the method. If $k = 0$, then we receive an automaton which is too generalized. If $k \geq \max_{x \in S_+} \{| \ x \ |\}$ then $L(A(S_+, k)) = S_+$, i.e., an automaton is not generalized at all.

As we will see further on, the notion of $k$-tails is used in other grammatical inference methods as well.

---

[5]We assume that the transition function $\delta$ is in the form of a control table.

### 5.1.3 *Inference of k-Testable Languages*

The inference method for the subclass of *k-testable languages* was introduced in [García and Vidal (1990); García *et al.* (1990b)]. Let us define this subclass.

> **Definition 5.3 ($k$-Testable-Language):** Let $L$ be a regular language over $\Sigma_T$. $L$ is called a $k$-testable language, $k$-TSSL, iff for every two strings $uv, u'v \in L$, where $u, u', v \in \Sigma_T^*$, $|v| \geq k$ the following holds.
>
> $$uv \in L \iff u'v \in L$$

The so-called *k-testable machine* (in the strict sense), *k*-TSS, is defined for a sample $S_+$ in the first step of the method.

> **Definition 5.4 ($k$-Testable Machine):** Let $S_+$ be a positive sample, $k \geq 1$. A $k$-testable machine is a quintuple
>
> $$Z_k(S_+) = (\Sigma(S_+), I_k(S_+), F_k(S_+), C_k(S_+), T_k(S_+)), \text{ where}$$
>
> $\Sigma(S_+)$ is a set of the terminals which appear in $S_+$,
> $I_k(S_+) = \{u : uv \in S_+, \ |u| = k-1, \ v \in \Sigma(S_+)^*\}$ is a set of the prefixes of length $k-1$ of the strings in $S_+$,
> $F_k(S_+) = \{v : uv \in S_+, \ |v| = k-1, \ u \in \Sigma(S_+)^*\}$ is a set of the suffixes of length $k-1$ of the strings in $S_+$,
> $C_k(S_+) = \{x : |x| < k, \ x \in S_+\}$ is a set of the short strings in $S_+$,
> $T_k(S_+) = \{w : uwv \in S_+, \ |w| = k, \ u, v \in \Sigma(S_+)^*\}$ is a set of the allowed substrings of length $k$ of the strings in $S_+$.

Let the sample $S_+ = \{a, b, aa, bb, aacce, aaccce, bbdde, bbddde\}$. The 3-testable machine $Z_3(S_+) = (\Sigma(S_+), I_3(S_+), F_3(S_+), C_3(S_+), T_3(S_+))$ is defined as follows:

$\Sigma(S_+) = \{a, b, c, d, e\}$
$I_3(S_+) = \{aa, bb\}$
$F_3(S_+) = \{aa, bb, ce, de\}$
$C_3(S_+) = \{a, b, aa, bb\}$
$T_3(S_+) = \{aac, acc, cce, ccc, bbd, bdd, dde, ddd\}$

A *k-TSS-based automaton* $A = (Q, \Sigma_T, \delta, q_\lambda, F)$ is induced from a $k$-testable machine $Z_k(S_+) = (\Sigma(S_+), I_k(S_+), F_k(S_+), C_k(S_+), T_k(S_+))$ in the second step of the method according to the following scheme.

---

**Induction Scheme 5.3: $k$-TSS-Based Automaton Inference**

$\Sigma_T := \Sigma(S_+);\ \ Q := \emptyset;\ \ F := \emptyset;$
**for each** $uv \in I_k(S_+) \cup C_k(S_+),\ u, v \in \Sigma(S_+)^*$ **do**
  $Q := Q \cup \{q_u\};$
**for each** $av \in T_k(S_+),\ a \in \Sigma(S_+),\ v \in \Sigma(S_+)^*$ **do**
  $Q := Q \cup \{q_v\};$
**for each** $ua \in T_k(S_+),\ a \in \Sigma(S_+),\ u \in \Sigma(S_+)^*$ **do**
  $Q := Q \cup \{q_u\};$
**for each** $v \in \Gamma_k(S_+) \cup C_k(S_+),\ v \in \Sigma(S_+)^*$ **do**
  $F := F \cup \{q_v\};$
**for each** $uav \in I_k(S_+) \cup C_k(S_+),\ a \in \Sigma(S_+),\ u, v \in \Sigma(S_+)^*$ **do**
  $\delta(q_u, a) = q_{ua};$
**for each** $awb \in T_k(S_+),\ a, b \in \Sigma(S_+),\ w \in \Sigma(S_+)^*$ **do**
  $\delta(q_{aw}, b) = q_{wb};$

Let us define the automaton $A = (Q, \Sigma_T, \delta, q_\lambda, F)$ for our $k$-testable machine $Z_k(S_+)$ according to the Induction Scheme 5.3.

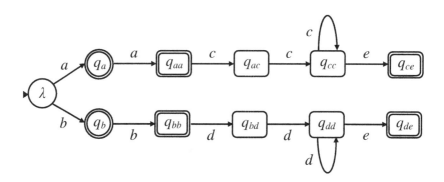

Fig. 5.2   The automaton $A$ inferred from the 3-testable machine $Z_3(S_+)$.

$\Sigma_T = \{a, b, c, d, e\}$
$Q = \{q_\lambda, q_a, q_b, q_{aa}, q_{bb}, q_{ac}, q_{cc}, q_{ce}, q_{bd}, q_{dd}, q_{de}\}$
$F = \{q_a, q_b, q_{aa}, q_{bb}, q_{ce}, q_{de}\}$
The transition function $\delta$ is defined as follows (see Fig. 5.2):

$$\delta(q_\lambda, a) = q_a \qquad \delta(q_b, b) = q_{bb} \qquad \delta(q_{ac}, c) = q_{cc} \qquad \delta(q_{dd}, d) = q_{dd}$$

$$\delta(q_\lambda, b) = q_b \qquad \delta(q_{aa}, c) = q_{ac} \qquad \delta(q_{bd}, d) = q_{dd} \qquad \delta(q_{cc}, e) = q_{ce}$$

$$\delta(q_a, a) = q_{aa} \qquad \delta(q_{bb}, d) = q_{bd} \qquad \delta(q_{cc}, c) = q_{cc} \qquad \delta(q_{dd}, e) = q_{de}$$

At the end of this section let us present the following theorem.

> **Theorem 5.1 ($k$-TSSL Inference Complexity [García *et al.* (1990b)])**
>
> *The running time of the inference algorithm for $k$-testable languages is $\mathcal{O}(\|\, S_+ \,\|)$, where $S_+$ is the sample.*

### 5.1.4 *Inference of Reversible Regular Languages*

The method which was introduced in [Angluin (1982)] infers the subclass of $k$-reversible languages. For a sample $S_+$ the *prefix tree acceptor, PTA*, is defined in the first step of the method.

Let $\mathit{Pref}(Y) = \{u \in \Sigma_T^* : \exists v \in \Sigma_T^*, uv \in Y\}$ denote the set of prefixes of $Y \subseteq \Sigma_T^*$.

> **Definition 5.5 (Prefix Tree Acceptor for $S_+$):** Let $S_+$ be a positive sample. The prefix tree acceptor for $S_+$ is a quintuple
>
> $$PTA(S_+) = (Q, \Sigma_T, \delta, Q_0, F), \text{ where}$$
>
> $Q = \mathit{Pref}(S_+)$, $\Sigma_T$ is a set of terminals which appear in $S_+$, $\delta(u, a) = ua$ whenever $u, ua \in Q$, $Q_0 = \{\lambda\}$ is the set of initial states, $F = S_+$.

Let $S_+ = \{a, b, aab, bba, aaaab, bbbba\}$. The $PTA(S_+)$ defined according to Definition 5.5 is shown in Fig. 5.3a.[6]

Now, we shall introduce the notions which are used for defining $k$-reversible automata. Let $A = (Q, \Sigma_T, \delta, Q_0, F)$ be an automaton.[7]

- The reverse of $u \in \Sigma_T^*$ is denoted $u^R$.
- We define the reverse of $\delta$, denoted $\delta^R$, as follows

$$\delta^R(q, a) = \{q' \in Q : q \in \delta(q', a)\} \quad \text{for all } a \in \Sigma_T, \ q \in Q.$$

- The *reverse of the automaton* $A$ is $A^R = (Q, \Sigma_T, \delta^R, F, Q_0)$.[8]
- $u \in \Sigma_T^*$ is a *$k$-follower* of $q \in Q$ iff $|\,u\,| = k$ and $\delta(q, u) \neq \emptyset$. $\mathit{Foll}_k(q)$ denotes the set of all $k$-followers of q.
- $u \in \Sigma_T^*$ is a *$k$-leader* of $q \in Q$ iff $|\,u\,| = k$ and $\delta^R(q, u^R) \neq \emptyset$. $\mathit{Lead}_k(q)$ denotes the set of all the $k$-leaders of q.
- $A$ is *deterministic with a lookahead $k$* iff for any $q', q'' \in Q$, $q' \neq q''$ such that $q', q'' \in Q_0$ or $q', q'' \in \delta(q, a), q \in Q, a \in \Sigma_T$: $\mathit{Foll}_k(q') \cap \mathit{Foll}_k(q'') = \emptyset$.

---

[6]The states of $PTA(S_+)$ are denoted with prefixes.

[7]Let us note that we define a set of initial states $Q_0$ instead of one initial state $q_0$.

[8]That is, we interchange the initial and final states and we reverse every transition.

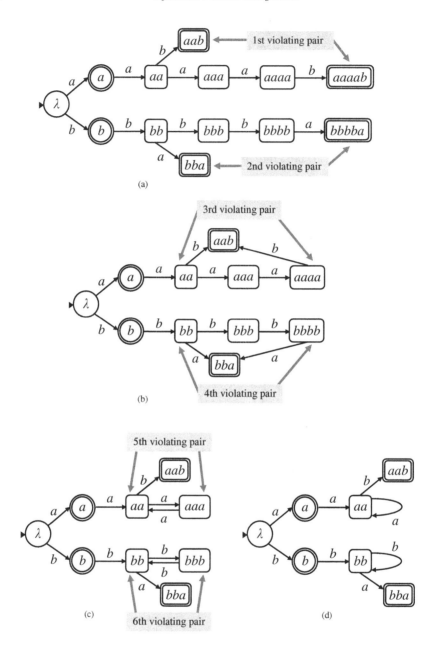

Fig. 5.3   Inferring the 2-reversible automaton $A$ *via* merging violating pairs of states.

We say that $A = (Q, \Sigma_T, \delta, Q_0, F)$ is $k$-reversible if and only if $A$ is deterministic and $A^R$ is deterministic with a lookahead $k$.[9] We can define it formally as follows:

---

[9]A language $L$ is $k$-reversible if and only if there exists a $k$-reversible automaton $A$ such that $L = L(A)$.

**Definition 5.6 ($k$-Reversible Automaton):** An automaton $A$ is $k$-reversible iff the following conditions hold.

(1) The determinism condition: $\delta : Q \times \Sigma_T \longrightarrow Q$.
(2) The look-ahead condition:

  (a) $q', q'' \in F, q' \neq q'' \implies Lead_k(q') \cap Lead_k(q'') = \emptyset$  and
  (b) $\delta(q', a) = \delta(q'', a), q' \neq q'' \implies Lead_k(q') \cap Lead_k(q'') = \emptyset$ .

The $k$-reversible automaton is constructed on the basis of $PTA$ in the second step of the method. This is made *via* merging (repeatedly) any pairs of states which violate the conditions of Definition 5.6. Let us define the notion of a violating pair of states in order to construct the $k$-reversible language inference algorithm.

A pair of states $(q', q'')$, $q', q'' \in Q$, $q' \neq q''$ is called a *violating pair* iff

(1) $\exists q \in Q : q', q'' \in \delta(q, a), a \in \Sigma_T$, or
(2) $q', q'' \in F \ \wedge \ Lead_k(q') \cap Lead_k(q'') \neq \emptyset$, or
  $\delta(q', a) = \delta(q'', a) \ \wedge \ Lead_k(q') \cap Lead_k(q'') \neq \emptyset$.

*Merging* of states $q', q''$ into $q'$ consists of the following simple operations.

- $\forall q \in Q \ \forall a \in \Sigma_T$ if $q'' \in \delta(q, a)$ then $\delta(q, a) := \delta(q, a) \cup \{q'\}$,
- $\forall q \in Q \ \forall a \in \Sigma_T$ if $q \in \delta(q'', a)$ then $\delta(q', a) := \delta(q', a) \cup \{q\}$,
- if $q'' \in Q_0$ then $Q_0 := Q_0 \setminus \{q''\} \cup \{q'\}$,
- if $q'' \in F$ then $F := F \setminus \{q''\} \cup \{q'\}$,
- $Q := Q \setminus \{q''\}$.

Let us come back to our $PTA(S_+)$ as shown in Fig. 5.3a. Let us assume that $k = 2$. The succeeding pairs of violating states are identified and merged repeatedly as it is depicted in Figs. 5.3 a-c. For example, the first[10] violating pair of states is $(aab, aaaab)$ because $aab, aaaab \in F$ and $Lead_2(aab) \cap Lead_2(aaaab) = \{ab\}$. The 2-reversible automaton $A$ inferred is shown in Fig. 5.3d.

The algorithm of $k$-reversible automaton inference uses the function *merge_violating_pair_of_states*$(A)$ which finds and merges a violating pair of states of $A$. If there is not any violating pair in $A$, the function returns *false*.

---

**Induction Scheme 5.4: $k$-Reversible Automaton Inference**

$A := PTA(S_+)$;
*violating_pair_found* := *false*;
**repeat**
  *violating_pair_found* := *merge_violating_pair_of_states*$(A)$;
**until not** *violating_pair_found*;

---

[10]The order in which violating pairs are merged does not matter.

At the end of this section let us present the following theorem.

**Theorem 5.2 ($k$-Reversible Inference Complexity [Angluin (1982)])**

*The running time of the inference algorithm for $k$-reversible languages is $\mathcal{O}(k \cdot \| S_+ \|^3)$, where $S_+$ is the sample.*

## 5.2 Informed Learning Methods for Regular Languages

Two well-known methods of inference using positive and negative samples, Gold-Trakhtenbrot-Bārzdiņš scheme and RPNI, are presented in this section.

### 5.2.1 *Gold-Trakhtenbrot-Bārzdiņš Model*

The idea of the inference scheme presented in this section was developed independently in [Trakhtenbrot and Barzdin' (1970)] and [Gold (1978)]. We present it on the basis of Gold's state characterization matrix which is built for $(S_+, S_-)$ in the first phase of the method. As in the previous section, we will assume that automaton states are denoted with the prefixes of sample words. Before we define the matrix, let us introduce the following notions:

- A set $Y \subseteq \Sigma_T^*$ is *prefix-complete* iff $uw \in Y \implies u \in Y$.
- A set $Y \subseteq \Sigma_T^*$ is *suffix-complete* iff $uw \in Y \implies w \in Y$.
- $Suff(Y) = \{v \in \Sigma_T^* : \exists u \in \Sigma_T^*, uv \in Y\}$ is the set of suffixes of $Y \subseteq \Sigma_T^*$.

**Definition 5.7 (State Characterization Matrix):** A state characterization matrix for $(S_+, S_-)$, in which $\Sigma_T$ is a set of terminals which appear in $S_+$ and $S_-$, is a triple

$$(ST, EX, M), \text{ where}$$

$ST = T \cup X(T)$ is a set of *states*, in which $T = \{u : u \in \Sigma_T^*\}$ is a set of *test states* and $X(T) = \{wv : w \in T, v \in \Sigma_T, wv \notin T\}$ is a set of *transition states*, $EX = \{e : e \in \Sigma_T^*\}$ is a set of suffixes of $S_+ \cup S_-$, called a set of *experiments*, $M : T \times EX \longrightarrow \{0, 1, \uparrow\}$ is a matrix with rows labelled with elements of $ST$ and columns labelled with elements of $EX$ such that

$$M[u, e] = \begin{cases} 1, & \text{if } ue \in S_+, \\ 0, & \text{if } ue \in S_-, \\ \uparrow, & \text{otherwise (not known); then a pair } (u, e) \text{ is called a } hole. \end{cases}$$

We require $ST$ to be prefix-complete and $EX$ to be suffix-complete in order to receive the resulting automaton which is consistent with $(S_+, S_-)$.

Table 5.1  M initialized.

|   | $\lambda$ | $a$ | $b$ | $aa$ | $ab$ | $ba$ | $bb$ | $aba$ | $abb$ | $bab$ |
|---|---|---|---|---|---|---|---|---|---|---|
| $\lambda$ |   | 1 | 1 | 0 | 1 | 0 | 0 | 0 | 1 | 0 |
| $a$ | 1 | 0 | 1 |   |   | 0 | 1 |   |   |   |
| $b$ | 1 | 0 | 0 |   | 0 |   |   |   |   |   |

An identification of the states of an automaton to be constructed is the primary task of the procedure of constructing a state characterization matrix. *Test states*[11] $T$ correspond to states which have been already identified as states of the resulting automaton $A$, whereas *transition states* $X(T)$ are candidates for automaton states. In order to define this procedure, let us introduce the following auxiliary notions. Let $M[u, \cdot]$ denote the row labelled with $u$, where $u$ is (a label of) a state.[12]

- Rows $M[u, \cdot]$ and $M[v, \cdot]$ (states $u$ and $v$) are *obviously different* iff $\exists e \in E$ such that $M[u, e], M[v, e] \in \{0, 1\}$ and $M[u, e] \neq M[v, e]$.
- A matrix $(ST, EX, M)$ is *complete* iff it has no holes (no entry is equal to $\uparrow$).
- Rows $M[u, \cdot]$ and $M[v, \cdot]$ (states $u$ and $v$) are *compatible*, denoted $M[u, \cdot] \simeq M[v, \cdot]$ ($u \simeq v$) iff $\nexists e \in E$ such that $(M[u, e] = 0$ and $M[v, e] = 1)$ or $(M[u, e] = 1$ and $M[v, e] = 0)$.
- A matrix $(ST, EX, M)$ is *closed* iff $\forall v \in X(T)$ $\exists u \in T$ such that $M[v, \cdot] = M[u, \cdot]$.

The procedure of constructing a state characterization matrix at each step moves one *transition state*, which is obviously different from every *test state*, from $X(T)$ to $T$. Then, $X(T)$ is updated and the procedure repeats itself until no obviously different transition state is found. Finally, the procedure fills the holes of the matrix, on the basis of row compatibility, in order to obtain a complete matrix. Once the matrix is complete and closed, it can be used for constructing the automaton. Let us present the stages of the procedure of constructing a matrix $(ST, EX, M)$.

(1) The matrix is *initialized* by setting $T := \{\lambda\}$, $EX := \text{Suff}(S_+ \cup S_-)$. Then, according to Definition 5.7, $X(T) := \{a : a \in \Sigma_T\}$. Finally, the entries of the matrix are filled according to the definition.

For example, let there be given $(S_+, S_-)$, $S_+ = \{a, b, ab, abb\}$, $S_- = \{aa, ba, bb, aba, bab\}$. The matrix $M$ after initialization is shown in Table 5.1. The states $ST$ correspond to rows[13] and the experiments $EX$ correspond to columns. Instead of $\uparrow$s we employ empty entries.

(2) The transition states are *promoted* until there is no obviously different transition state in the matrix.

---

[11] Sometimes test states are called *Red states* and transition states are called *Blue states*.
[12] Rows and states will be equated further on.
[13] *Test states* $T$ are separated from *transition states* $X(T)$.

Table 5.2   M after promoting $a$.

|      | λ | a | b | aa | ab | ba | bb | aba | abb | bab |
|------|---|---|---|----|----|----|----|-----|-----|-----|
| λ    |   | 1 | 1 | 0  | 1  | 0  | 0  | 0   | 1   | 0   |
| a    | 1 | 0 | 1 |    |    | 0  | 1  |     |     |     |
| b    | 1 | 0 | 0 |    | 0  |    |    |     |     |     |
| aa   | 0 |   |   |    |    |    |    |     |     |     |
| ab   | 1 | 0 | 1 |    |    |    |    |     |     |     |

Table 5.3   M after promoting $b$.

|      | λ | a | b | aa | ab | ba | bb | aba | abb | bab |
|------|---|---|---|----|----|----|----|-----|-----|-----|
| λ    |   | 1 | 1 | 0  | 1  | 0  | 0  | 0   | 1   | 0   |
| a    | 1 | 0 | 1 |    |    | 0  | 1  |     |     |     |
| b    | 1 | 0 | 0 |    | 0  |    |    |     |     |     |
| aa   | 0 |   |   |    |    |    |    |     |     |     |
| ab   | 1 | 0 | 1 |    |    |    |    |     |     |     |
| ba   | 0 |   | 0 |    |    |    |    |     |     |     |
| bb   | 0 |   |   |    |    |    |    |     |     |     |

Table 5.4   M after promoting $ba$.

|      | λ | a | b | aa | ab | ba | bb | aba | abb | bab |
|------|---|---|---|----|----|----|----|-----|-----|-----|
| λ    |   | 1 | 1 | 0  | 1  | 0  | 0  | 0   | 1   | 0   |
| a    | 1 | 0 | 1 |    |    | 0  | 1  |     |     |     |
| b    | 1 | 0 | 0 |    | 0  |    |    |     |     |     |
| ba   | 0 |   | 0 |    |    |    |    |     |     |     |
| aa   | 0 |   |   |    |    |    |    |     |     |     |
| ab   | 1 | 0 | 1 |    |    |    |    |     |     |     |
| bb   | 0 |   |   |    |    |    |    |     |     |     |
| baa  |   |   |   |    |    |    |    |     |     |     |
| bab  | 0 |   |   |    |    |    |    |     |     |     |

The iterative step of the promotion stage consists of the following operations.

- Find a transition state $u \in X(T)$ which is *obviously different* from every test state.
- Move $u$ from $X(T)$ to $T$.
- For each $a \in \Sigma_T$ add a state $ua$ to $X(T)$.
- Fill the entries corresponding to the new states according to Definition 5.7.

Let us come back to our example. As we can see in Table 5.1, the transition state $a$ (the row $M[a, \cdot]$) is obviously different from the test state $\lambda$ (the row $M[\lambda, \cdot]$). So

Table 5.5  M after filling the holes of the test state rows.

|      | λ | a | b | aa | ab | ba | bb | aba | abb | bab |
|------|---|---|---|----|----|----|----|-----|-----|-----|
| λ    | 0 | 1 | 1 | 0  | 1  | 0  | 0  | 0   | 1   | 0   |
| a    | 1 | 0 | 1 |    |    | 0  | 1  |     |     |     |
| b    | 1 | 0 | 0 |    | 0  |    |    |     |     |     |
| ba   | 0 |   | 0 |    |    |    |    |     |     |     |
| aa   | 0 |   |   |    |    |    |    |     |     |     |
| ab   | 1 | 0 | 1 |    |    |    |    |     |     |     |
| bb   | 0 |   |   |    |    |    |    |     |     |     |
| baa  |   |   |   |    |    |    |    |     |     |     |
| bab  | 0 |   |   |    |    |    |    |     |     |     |

Table 5.6  M after completing the test state rows with 1s.

|      | λ | a | b | aa | ab | ba | bb | aba | abb | bab |
|------|---|---|---|----|----|----|----|-----|-----|-----|
| λ    | 0 | 1 | 1 | 0  | 1  | 0  | 0  | 0   | 1   | 0   |
| a    | 1 | 0 | 1 | 1  | 1  | 0  | 1  | 1   | 1   | 1   |
| b    | 1 | 0 | 0 | 1  | 0  | 1  | 1  | 1   | 1   | 1   |
| ba   | 0 | 1 | 0 | 1  | 1  | 1  | 1  | 1   | 1   | 1   |
| aa   | 0 |   |   |    |    |    |    |     |     |     |
| ab   | 1 | 0 | 1 |    |    |    |    |     |     |     |
| bb   | 0 |   |   |    |    |    |    |     |     |     |
| baa  |   |   |   |    |    |    |    |     |     |     |
| bab  | 0 |   |   |    |    |    |    |     |     |     |

it is promoted, i.e., it is moved to $T$, and the transition states $aa$ and $ab$ (the rows $M[aa, \cdot]$ and $M[ab, \cdot]$) are added to $X(T)$ (cf. Table 5.2). Then, the entries of new rows are filled according to Definition 5.7. In the next iteration of the promotion stage the transition state $b$ is identified as being obviously different (from both test states: $\lambda$ and $a$) and it is promoted, as it is shown in Table 5.3. After promoting the state $ba$ (obviously different from the test states: $\lambda$, $a$ and $b$), none of the transition states is obviously different from the test states (see Table 5.4).

(3) The holes are filled in order to obtain the complete matrix.

The *filling holes* stage consists of the following steps:

(3a) *Filling holes of test state rows on the basis of transition state rows.*

For each transition state $u \in X(T)$ find a test state $v \in T$ which is compatible ($u \simeq v$) and $M[v, e] := M[u, e]$ for every $e \in EX$ such that $M[u, e] \neq \uparrow$ .

(3b) *Completing test state rows with 1s.*

Table 5.7    M after filling the holes of the transition state rows.

|     | $\lambda$ | $a$ | $b$ | $aa$ | $ab$ | $ba$ | $bb$ | $aba$ | $abb$ | $bab$ |
|-----|-----------|-----|-----|------|------|------|------|-------|-------|-------|
| $\lambda$ | 0 | 1 | 1 | 0 | 1 | 0 | 0 | 0 | 1 | 0 |
| $a$ | 1 | 0 | 1 | 1 | 1 | 0 | 1 | 1 | 1 | 1 |
| $b$ | 1 | 0 | 0 | 1 | 0 | 1 | 1 | 1 | 1 | 1 |
| $ba$ | 0 | 1 | 0 | 1 | 1 | 1 | 1 | 1 | 1 | 1 |
| $aa$ | 0 | 1 | 1 | 0 | 1 | 0 | 0 | 0 | 1 | 0 |
| $ab$ | 1 | 0 | 1 | 1 | 1 | 0 | 1 | 1 | 1 | 1 |
| $bb$ | 0 | 1 | 1 | 0 | 1 | 0 | 0 | 0 | 1 | 0 |
| $baa$ | 0 | 1 | 1 | 0 | 1 | 0 | 0 | 0 | 1 | 0 |
| $bab$ | 0 | 1 | 1 | 0 | 1 | 0 | 0 | 0 | 1 | 0 |

Complete the remaining entries of the test state rows with 1s.

(3c) *Filling holes of transition state rows on the basis of test state rows.*
For each transition state $u \in X(T)$ find a test state $v \in T$ which is compatible $(u \simeq v)$ and $M[u, e] := M[v, e]$ for every $e \in EX$ such that $M[u, e] = \uparrow$.

Let us come back to our example again. In Table 5.4, in order to fill the holes of the test state rows (point 3a) for the state $aa \in X(T)$ we identify the state $\lambda \in T$ such that $aa \simeq \lambda$. Therefore we can set $M[\lambda, \lambda] := M[aa, \lambda] = 0$. This is the only operation we can conduct in this step. We obtain Table 5.5. In the second step (3b), the entries of test state rows which contain holes are filled with 1s, giving Table 5.6 as a result. In the third step (3c), the following pairs of compatible states are identified: $aa \simeq \lambda$, $ab \simeq a$, $bb \simeq \lambda$, $baa \simeq \lambda$ and $bab \simeq \lambda$. After filling the holes of the transition state rows on the basis of the compatible pairs we obtain Table 5.7. Let us note that the matrix is complete and closed.

An automaton is inferred according to the following definition:

**Definition 5.8 (Automaton for State Characterization Matrix):** Let $(ST, EX, M)$, $ST = T \cup X(T)$ be a complete and closed state characterization matrix for $(S_+, S_-)$. The finite-state automaton for $(ST, EX, M)$ is a quintuple

$$A(ST, EX, M) = (Q, \Sigma_T, \delta, q_0, F), \text{ where}$$

$Q = T$, $\Sigma_T$ is a set of terminals which appear in $S_+$ and $S_-$,
$\delta(u, a) = v$ whenever $v \in T$ and $M[ua, \cdot] = M[v, \cdot]$,
$q_0 = \lambda$,
$F = (F_A, F_R)$ such that
$F_A = \{ue \in T : M[u, e] = 1\}$,
$F_R = \{ue \in T : M[u, e] = 0\}$.

In the example considered we have received $(ST, EX, M)$, shown in Table 5.7, which is complete and closed. We infer the automaton $A(ST, EX, M) =$

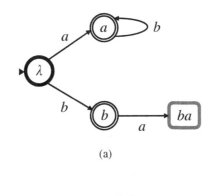

(a)

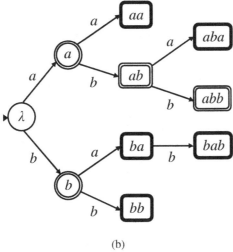

(b)

Fig. 5.4 (a) The automaton inferred for $(S_+, S_-)$. (b) The prefix tree acceptor for $(S_+, S_-)$.

$(Q, \Sigma_T, \delta, q_0, F)$ according to Definition 5.8 as follows.
$Q = \{\lambda, a, b, ba\}$, $\Sigma_T = \{a, b\}$, $q_0 = \lambda$,
$\delta(\lambda, a) = a$ since $M[\lambda a, \cdot] = M[a, \cdot]$,
$\delta(\lambda, b) = b$ since $M[\lambda b, \cdot] = M[b, \cdot]$,
$\delta(a, b) = a$ since $M[ab, \cdot] = M[a, \cdot]$,
$\delta(b, a) = ba$ since $M[ba, \cdot] = M[ba, \cdot]$,
$F_A = \{a, b\}$ since $M[\lambda, a] = 1$ and $M[\lambda, b] = 1$,
$F_R = \{\lambda, ba\}$ since $M[\lambda, \lambda] = 0$ and $M[b, a] = 0$.

The automaton $A(ST, EX, M)$ is shown in Fig. 5.4a. (A rejecting state of $F_R$ is marked with a thick border.) This is consistent with our sample. If the method cannot generate $(ST, EX, M)$ which is complete and closed or the automaton $A(ST, EX, M)$ is not consistent with $(S_+, S_-)$ then $\text{PTA}(S_+, S_-)$ is returned. The exemplary PTA for our sample is shown in Fig. 5.4b.

The Gold-Trakhtenbrot-Bārzdiņš induction scheme uses the following functions.

- *initialize_state_char_matrix*$(M, S_+, S_-)$ - the function initializes $M$ according to point (1) presented above,
- *promote*$(u)$ - the function promotes $u \in X(T)$ according to point (2) presented above,
- *complete_matrix*$(M)$ - the function fills holes in order to complete $M$ according to point (3) presented above; if generating $M$ which is complete and closed is not possible then *false* is returned,
- *construct_automaton*$(M)$ - the function constructs an automaton according to Definition 5.8,
- *consistent*$(A, S_+, S_-)$ - the function checks whether $A$ is consistent with $(S_+, S_-)$.

---

**Induction Scheme 5.5: Gold-Trakhtenbrot-Bārzdiņš Inference**

*initialize_state_char_matrix*$(M, S_+, S_-)$;
**while** $\exists u \in X(T):$ *u is obviously different in M* **do** *promote*$(u)$;
*matrix_completed* := *complete_matrix*$(M)$;
**if** *matrix_completed* **then**
   **begin**
      $A$ := *construct_automaton*$(M)$;
      **if not** *consistent*$(A, S_+, S_-)$ **then** $A := PTA(S_+, S_-)$;
   **end**;
**else** $A := PTA(S_+, S_-)$;

---

At the end of this section let us present the following theorem.

**Theorem 5.3 (G-T-B Inference Complexity [Gold (1978)])**

*The running time of the Gold-Trakhtenbrot-Bārzdiņš inference algorithm is $\mathcal{O}(n^2 \cdot \| (S_+ \cup S_-) \|)$, where $(S_+, S_-)$ is the sample, $| Q | = n$, $Q$ is the set of states of the automaton.*

### 5.2.2  *Algorithm RPNI*

The idea of the inference scheme presented in this section was developed independently in [Oncina and García (1992)] and [Lang (1992)]. We present it with the help of the RPNI algorithm [Oncina and García (1992)]. After constructing the automaton of the form of PTA for $(S_+, S_-)$ the algorithm repeatedly tries to merge pairs of the states if merging does not violate the consistency of the *deterministic* automaton with the sample.

Analogously to the Gold-Trakhtenbrot-Bārzdiņš inference algorithm, a set of states is divided into three subsets: the *Red states* $(R)$ which have been already analyzed and approved, the *Blue states* ($B$) which are candidates for merging at a given iteration of the algorithm and the remaining states. At each iteration merging of a Red state with a Blue state is considered. Let us present the stages of the algorithm.

(A) *Initialization.* The automaton $A = (Q, \Sigma_T, \delta, q_0, F)$ is initialized by setting $A := PTA(S_+, S_-)$. Then, the sets of the states are initialized: $R := \{q_0\}$, $B := \{q \in Q : \delta(q_0, a) = q\}$.

For example, let there be given $(S_+, S_-)$, $S_+ = \{aaa, bba, aaba\}$, $S_- = \{a\}$. The automaton $A$ (PTA) is shown[14] in Fig. 5.5a. The Red states ($R = \{q_0\}$) are marked with dark grey and the blue states ($B = \{q_1, q_2\}$) are marked with light grey.

(B) *Merging.* As long as there are Blue states the algorithm tries to merge the succeeding Blue state with one of the Red states. This phase consists of the following steps.

(B.1) *Extracting the succeeding Blue state*[15] $q_B$ from $B$.

In our example $q_B = q_1$ in the first iteration.

(B.2) *Checking whether merging is possible.* Having the Blue state $q_B$ chosen, the algorithm tries to merge it with any Red state and checks whether merging does not violate the consistency of the automaton with the sample. This stage consists of the following operations:

(B.2.1) *Choosing the succeeding Red state to be merged with the Blue state.*

In our example $q_R = q_0$ in the first iteration (cf. Fig. 5.5a).

(B.2.2) *Recursive merging* for $q_B$ and $q_R$ - $merge(A, q_B, q_R)$.

- Change the transition to $q_B$ to the transition to $q_R$[16]. (After merging $q_B$ with $q_R$, the state $q_B$ disappears.)
  In our example the transition $\delta(q_0, a) = q_1$ has to be changed to the transition $\delta(q_0, a) = q_0$ (cf. Figs. 5.5a and b).
- If for some $x \in \Sigma_T$: $\delta(q_B, x)$ and $\delta(q_R, x)$ are defined in $A$, then perform *recursive merging* (B.2.2) for $\delta(q_B, x)$ and $\delta(q_R, x)$ that means calling $merge(A, \delta(q_B, x), \delta(q_R, x))$. The algorithm has to perform such a merging, because otherwise we obtain an automaton which is not deterministic.
  In our example after merging $q_1$ with $q_0$ ($q_1$ disappears), we have $\delta(q_0, a) = q_0$

---

[14]In this section we denote states of PTA with $q_0, q_1, \ldots$ (not with prefixes).

[15]We do not discuss the problem of an efficient choosing of the states here. This can be based e.g. on the lexicographic order.

[16]Let us notice that for any Blue state there is exactly one such transition.

and $\delta(q_0, a) = q_3$ (cf. Figs. 5.5a and b). So we should merge $q_3$ with $q_0$ in order to remove non-determinism, etc. At the end of recursive merging we obtain the situation shown in Fig. 5.5b.

(B.2.3) *Checking the consistency of A with* $(S_+, S_-)$ *after merging.*
Recursive merging can cause a losing of consistency of the automaton with the sample. So we have to check it.

In our example, in performing the recursive merging for $q_1$ and $q_0$ we have lost consistency, since $q_0$ has been merged with $q_1$ which is the final rejecting state $(q_1 \in F_R)$ and also $q_0$ has been merged with $q_6$ which is the final accepting state $(q_6 \in F_A)$, we cannot accept this merging (cf. Fig. 5.5b).

(B.2.4.a) *Rejecting merging and promoting* $q_B$ *in the case of losing consistency.*
If consistency has been lost then the merging for $q_B$ and $q_R$ is rejected. $q_B$ is promoted which means that it is added to $R$.
(B.2.4.b) *Accepting merging in the case of preserving consistency.*

(B.2.5) *Updating the set of Blue states B.*
$B := R\Sigma_T \setminus R$. Go to (B.1).

In our example, after rejecting the merging for $q_1$ and $q_0$ the situation comes back to Fig. 5.5a. The state $q_1$ is promoted (i.e. it becomes Red). The set of Blue states is updated, i.e. the state $q_3$ which is a successor of $q_1$ becomes Blue (according to B.2.5).
In the next iteration we try to merge $q_2$ and $q_0$ unsuccessfully because of losing consistency. After this attempt $R = \{q_0, q_1, q_2\}$ and $B = \{q_3, q_4\}$.
The merges: $merge(A, q_3, q_0)$ and $merge(A, q_3, q_1)$ are rejected as well.
$merge(A, q_3, q_2)$ is accepted. The situation is shown in Fig. 5.5c. After merging $R = \{q_0, q_1, q_2\}$ and $B = \{q_4, q_6\}$.
$merge(A, q_4, q_0)$ is rejected. $merge(A, q_4, q_1)$ is accepted which is shown in Fig. 5.5d.
$merge(A, q_6, q_0)$ is accepted which is shown in Fig. 5.5e. The set of Blue states $B$ is empty and the algorithm finishes.

Let us present the RPNI algorithm. It uses the following functions.

- *initialize_R_B_sets*$(A)$ - the function initializes sets of Red and Blue states according to point (A) presented above,
- *nonempty*$(B)$ - the Boolean function which checks whether set B is not empty,
- *extract_from_set*$(B)$ - the functions extracts the element from set $B$,
- *merge*$(A, q_B, q_R)$ - the function merges states $q_B$ and $q_R$ according to point (B.2.2) presented above,
- *promote*$(R, q_B)$ - the function adds state $q_B$ to set $R$,
- *update_B_set*() - the function updates set $B$ according to point (B.2.5).

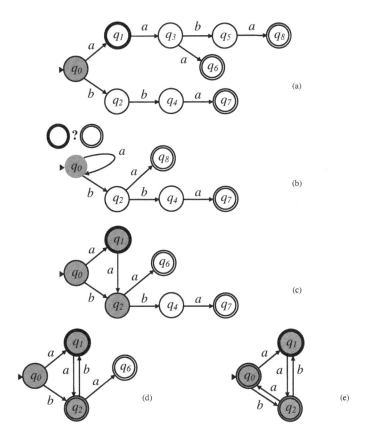

Fig. 5.5 (a) PTA for $(S_+, S_-)$. (b) The situation after merging $q_1$ with $q_0$. (c) The situation after merging $q_3$ with $q_2$. (d) The situation after merging $q_4$ with $q_1$. (e) The situation after merging $q_6$ with $q_0$.

### Induction Scheme 5.6: RPNI

$A := PTA(S_+, S_-)$;
$initialize\_R\_B\_sets(A)$;
**while** $nonempty(B)$ **do**
   **begin**
      $q_B := extract\_from\_set(B)$;
      **if** $\exists q_R \in R :$ *merging $q_B$ and $q_R$ does not violate consistency* **then**
         $A := merge(A, q_B, q_R)$;
      **else**
         $promote(R, q_B)$;
      $update\_B\_set()$;
   **end**;

At the end of this section let us present the following theorem.

**Theorem 5.4 (RPNI Complexity [Oncina and García (1992)])**

*The running time of the RPNI algorithm is $\mathcal{O}(\| S_+ \|^2 \cdot (\| S_+ \| + \| S_- \|))$, where $(S_+, S_-)$ is the sample.*

## 5.3    Inference of Reversible CF Languages

Inference of context-free languages is more difficult than the induction of regular languages. Nevertheless, looking for some analogies in order to extend the inference models developed for regular languages seems to be a sound methodological approach. The method which is an extension of the inference method for reversible regular languages is presented in this section. The method was introduced in [Sakakibara (1990, 1992)] for inferencing automata and was further developed in [Oates *et al.* (2002)] for inducing *CF* grammars.

The method infers from a positive sample (text learning) which contains additional information in the form of the structure of a derivation tree for each string. Let us introduce the following preliminary notions:

Let $G = (\Sigma_N, \Sigma_T, P, S)$ be a $\lambda$-free *CF* grammar.[17]
A subtree $T$ of a derivation tree $DT$ such that for each node $v$ of $T$ either all children of $v$ in $DT$ belong to $T$ or none of them is called a *partial derivation tree*. Let us note that the root of a partial derivation tree can be labelled with any $X \in \Sigma_N$. (If the root is labelled with $S$ then the partial derivation tree is a derivation tree.)

A derivation tree for $\alpha \in L(G)$ in which all internal nodes are labelled with the special symbol $\sigma$ is called a *skeletal description* of $\alpha$.

Since a tree can be represented with a bracketed string, elements of a sample will be represented either with skeletal descriptions or corresponding bracketed strings. A positive sample $S_+$ which consists of skeletal descriptions (or corresponding bracketed strings) is called a *structural (positive) sample*.

Let us define the structural sample $S_+$ consisting of the following elements.
$s^1 = \sigma(a\sigma(ba)b)$,
$s^2 = \sigma(a\sigma(cd)b)$,
$s^3 = \sigma(b\sigma(ab)a)$,
$s^4 = \sigma(b\sigma(b\sigma(ab)a))$.
Skeletal descriptions for elements $s^1 - s^4$ are shown in Figs. 5.6a – d.

Having a structural sample $S_+ = \{s^1, s^2, \ldots, s^m\}$, we can re-label the internal nodes (labelled with $\sigma$) of the skeletal descriptions in the following way: let $s^j \in S_+$, $j = 1, \ldots, m$. The root of $s^j$ is labelled with $N_0$. We traverse the tree $s^j$

---

[17]For applications in syntactic pattern recognition we can consider grammars which are $\lambda$-free, cf. Definition A.5 in Appendix A.1.

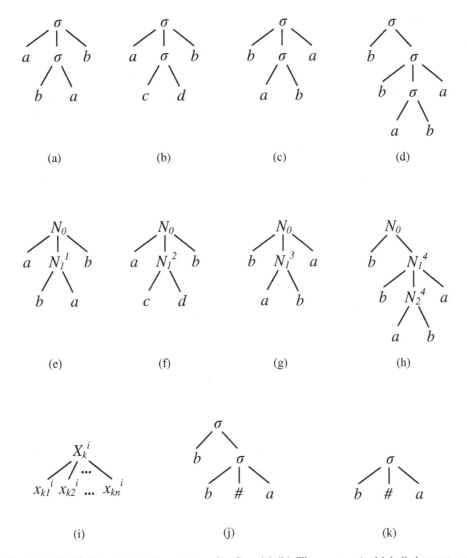

Fig. 5.6  (a)-(d) The skeletal descriptions for $S_+$. (e)-(h) The nonterminal-labelled structural sample for $S_+$. (i) A pattern for defining a production. (j) *2-context*$(s^4, N_2^4)$. (k) *1-context*$(s^4, N_2^4)$.

with a breadth-first search (BFS)[18] and we label the succeeding internal nodes with $N_1^j, N_2^j, N_3^j, \ldots$. The skeletal description $s^j$ with internal nodes labelled in such a way is called a *nonterminal-labelled skeletal description*. The structural sample $S_+$ which consists of nonterminal-labelled skeletal descriptions is called a *nonterminal-labelled structural sample*, denoted $NLS_+$.

The nonterminal-labelled structural sample for our example is shown in Figs. 5.6e $-$ h.

---

[18]We can use any traversal method.

The *initial (context-free) grammar* $G = (\Sigma_N, \Sigma_T, P, S)$ which generates a nonterminal-labelled structural sample $NLS_+$ is defined as follows. $\Sigma_N$ consists of labels defined for the internal nodes of nonterminal-labelled skeletal descriptions of $NLS_+$, $\Sigma_T$ consists of labels defined for the leaf nodes of nonterminal-labelled skeletal descriptions of $NLS_+$, $S = N_0$. The set of productions $P$ is constructed in the following way: for each subtree $X_k^i(x_{k1}^i x_{k2}^i \dots x_{kn}^i)$, $X_k^i \in \Sigma_N$, $x_{kr}^i \in (\Sigma_N \cup \Sigma_T)$, $r = 1, 2, \dots, n$, of every $s^i \in S_+$ (cf. Fig. 5.6i) the production $X_k^i \to x_{k1}^i x_{k2}^i \dots x_{kn}^i$ is added to $P$.

The initial grammar $G = (\Sigma_N, \Sigma_T, P, N_0)$, $\Sigma_N = \{N_0, N_1^1, N_1^2, N_1^3, N_1^4, N_2^4\}$, $\Sigma_T = \{a, b, c, d\}$ which generates $NLS_+$ in our example consists of the following productions:

(1) $N_0 \to aN_1^1 b$    (4) $N_0 \to bN_1^4$    (7) $N_1^3 \to ab$

(2) $N_0 \to aN_1^2 b$    (5) $N_1^1 \to ba$    (8) $N_1^4 \to bN_2^4 a$

(3) $N_0 \to bN_1^3 a$    (6) $N_1^2 \to cd$    (9) $N_2^4 \to ab$

Let $X, Y \in \Sigma_N$ be labels of a nonterminal-labelled skeletal description, $k \geq 0$. $X$ is a *k-ancestor* of $Y$ iff there exists a k-step (partial) derivation

$$X \Longrightarrow \dots \Longrightarrow \theta Y \gamma .$$

For example, $N_1^4$ is a 1-ancestor of $N_2^4$, $N_0$ is a 2-ancestor of $N_2^4$ and $N_2^4$ is a 0-ancestor for itself in Fig. 5.6h.

Now, we can introduce the following definition.

**Definition 5.9 (*k*-Context):** Let $G = (\Sigma_N, \Sigma_T, P, S)$ be a $\lambda$-free *CF* grammar, $\alpha \in L(G)$ be a skeletal description, a derivation tree $T_\alpha$ of $\alpha$ be of the form of a nonterminal-labelled skeletal description.
Let $X$ be a $k$-ancestor of $Y$ in $T_\alpha$ such that $X \xrightarrow{*} \beta$, $\beta \in \Sigma_T^+$ and $T_\beta$ $(T_\beta \subset T_\alpha)$ is a partial derivation tree for $\beta$.
A *k-context* of $Y$ in $\alpha$, denoted $k\text{-}context(\alpha, Y)$, is the tree $T$ obtained from $T_\beta$ by:
(a) removing all the descendant nodes of $Y$,
(b) re-labelling $Y$ with # and
(c) re-labelling all other nonterminals with $\sigma$.

The set of $k$-contexts of $Y$ in $L(G)$ is the set

$$k\text{-}Contexts(L(G), Y) = \{k\text{-}context(\alpha, Y) : \alpha \in L(G)\} .$$

If $L(G)$ is the initial grammar which generates $NLS_+$, i.e. $L(G) = NLS_+$, we can write $k\text{-}Contexts(NLS_+, Y)$.

Let us come back to our example. The nonterminal-labelled skeletal description of $s^4$ is shown in Fig. 5.6h. Then, $2\text{-}context(s^4, N_2^4)$ is shown in Fig. 5.6j and

$1$-$context(s^4, N_2^4)$ is shown in Fig. 5.6k.

Now, we can define $k$-reversible CF grammars.

**Definition 5.10 ($k$-Reversible *CF* Grammar):** Let $G = (\Sigma_N, \Sigma_T, P, S)$ be a $\lambda$-free CF grammar. $G$ is called a $k$-reversible context-free grammar iff the following conditions hold:

(1) The reset-free condition. If there exist two productions $Z \to \alpha X \beta$ and $Z \to \alpha Y \beta$ in $P$ then $X = Y$.
(2) The invertibility condition. If there exist two productions $X \to \alpha$ and $Y \to \alpha$ in $P$ and $k$-*Contexts*$(L(G), X) \cap k$-*Contexts*$(L(G), Y) \neq \emptyset$ then $X = Y$.

The initial (context-free) grammar is used for constructing a $k$-reversible context-free grammar. This is achieved *via* merging (repeatedly) any pairs of non-terminals which violate the conditions of Definition 5.10. Let us define the notion of a violating pair of nonterminals.

A pair of nonterminals $(X, Y)$, $X, Y \in \Sigma_N$ is called a *violating pair* iff

(1) There exist two productions $Z \to \alpha X \beta$ and $Z \to \alpha Y \beta$ in $P$ and $X \neq Y$ or
(2) there exist two productions $X \to \alpha$ and $Y \to \alpha$ in $P$ and $k$-*Contexts*$(L(G), X) \cap k$-*Contexts*$(L(G), Y) \neq \emptyset$ and $X \neq Y$.

*Merging* of nonterminals $X, Y$ into $X$ consists in replacing all the occurrences of $Y$ in all the productions of $P$ with $X$. Then, the redundant productions are removed.

Let us come back to our exemplary initial grammar $G$. Let us set the parameter $k = 1$. Firstly, one can easily notice that productions: (1) $N_0 \to a N_1^1 b$ and (2) $N_0 \to a N_1^2 b$ violate the reset-free condition, i.e. the pair of nonterminals $N_1^1$ and $N_1^2$ is violating. So, we merge them into $N_1^1$. Secondly, we see that productions: (7) $N_1^3 \to ab$ and (9) $N_2^4 \to ab$ violate the invertibility condition because

$$1\text{-}Contexts(L(G), N_1^3) \cap 1\text{-}Contexts(L(G), N_2^4) = \{\sigma(b\#a)\} \text{ (cf. Fig. 5.6)}.$$

Therefore, we merge the violating pair of nonterminals $N_1^3$ and $N_2^4$ into $N_1^3$. Now, the grammar $G$ is $1$-reversible and it contains the following productions.

(1) $N_0 \to a N_1^1 b$  (4) $N_1^1 \to ba$  (7) $N_1^4 \to b N_1^3 a$

(2) $N_0 \to b N_1^3 a$  (5) $N_1^1 \to cd$

(3) $N_0 \to b N_1^4$  (6) $N_1^3 \to ab$

The algorithm of $k$-reversible CF grammar inference uses: the function *initial_grammar*$(S_+)$ which constructs the initial grammar on the basis of a structural positive sample $S_+$ and the function *merge_violating_pair_of_nonterminals*$(G)$

which finds and merges the violating pair of nonterminals of $G$. If there is no violating pair in $G$, then the function returns *false*.

---

**Induction Scheme 5.7: $k$-Reversible $CF$ Inference**

$G := initial\_grammar(S_+)$;
$violating\_pair\_found := false$;
**repeat**
$\qquad violating\_pair\_found := merge\_violating\_pair\_of\_nonterminals(G)$;
**until not** $violating\_pair\_found$;

---

At the end of this section let us present the following theorem.

---

**Theorem 5.5 ($k$-Reversible $CF$ Inference Time [Sakakibara (1990)])**

*The running time of the inference algorithm for $k$-reversible context-free languages is polynomial with respect to the size of the structural positive sample.*

---

## 5.4 Baum-Welch Learning of HMMs

In the previous sections we have presented algorithms which learn the structure of an automaton. In the case of probabilistic automata/systems we have to estimate the probabilities as well. We present this issue for hidden Markov models introduced in Sec. 3.3.4. We assume that the set of states $Q$ of a *HMM* (cf. Scheme 3.8) and an emitted (observed) string $x = x_1 x_2 \dots x_T$ are given. We have to estimate the state-transition probability distribution $\Pi$ and the state-based symbol emission probability distribution $E$.[19]

The *Baum-Welch algorithm* [Baum et al. (1970)] is a standard method of estimating $\Pi$ and $E$. This is based on the *expectation maximization (EM) algorithm* scheme [Dempster et al. (1977)]. The *EM* algorithm is used for finding the maximum likelihood estimates of statistical model parameters, if the model depends on hidden variables. The sequence of two steps is performed iteratively. During the *expectation (E) step* the hidden variables are estimated with the help of observed variables and the current estimate of the parameters. During the *maximization (M) step* the likelihood function is maximized assuming that the hidden variables are known.[20]

In order to present the algorithm we have to introduce the notion of backward probability which is analogous to the forward probability defined in Sec. 3.3.4. Let $x = x_1 x_2 \dots x_T$ be an emitted (observed) string and $z = (z_1, z_2, \dots, z_T)$ be a valid sequence of states. Let $b_t(i)$ be the probability of observing the part

---

[19]The reader is advised to recall the notions and algorithms introduced in Sec. 3.3.4.
[20]The hidden variables estimate obtained at *E step* is used instead of the actual hidden variables.

$x_{(t+1)}x_{(t+2)}\dots x_T$ of the string $x$ assuming that state $z_t = q_i$, called a partial backward probability, i.e.,

$$b_t(i) = p(x_{(t+1)}x_{(t+2)}\dots x_T \mid z_t = q_i) \, .$$

The *backward probability algorithm* [Baum *et al.* (1970); Rabiner (1989)] computes the probabilities $b_t(i)$ in the following inductive way (compare *forward probability algorithm* in Sec. 3.3.4.):

(1) Initialize backward probability:

$$b_T(i) := 1, \ i = 1, \dots, N \, .$$

(2) Compute partial backward probabilities:

$$b_t(i) := \sum_{j=1}^{N} b_{(t+1)}(j)\pi_{ij}e_j(x_{(t+1)}), \ t = (T-1), (T-2), \dots, 1 \, , \ i = 1, \dots, N \, .$$

The running time of the backward probability algorithm is $\mathcal{O}(N^2 \cdot T)$.

During the expectation step of the Baum-Welch algorithm we define two functions with the help of forward and backward probabilities.

(E.1) The (expected) probability of visiting state $q_i$ at time $t$ assuming that the string $x$ has been observed is given by the following formula:

$$\gamma_t(j) = p(z_t = q_j \mid x) = \frac{f_t(j)b_t(j)}{p(x)}$$

(E.2) The (expected) probability of the transition from state $q_i$ at time $t$ to state $q_j$ (at time $(t+1)$) assuming that the string $x$ has been observed is given by the following formula;

$$\xi_t(i,j) = p(z_t = q_i, z_{(t+1)} = q_j \mid x) = \frac{f_t(i)\pi_{ij}e_j(x_{(t+1)})b_{(t+1)}(j)}{p(x)}$$

During the maximization step the algorithm estimates the parameters of *HMM*.

(M.1) The state-transition probability distribution $\hat{\Pi}(q_i, q_j) = \hat{\pi}_{ij}$ is estimated as follows:

$$\hat{\pi}_{ij} = \frac{\sum_{t=1}^{T-1} \xi_t(i,j)}{\sum_{t=1}^{T-1} \gamma_t(j)}$$

(M.2) The state-based symbol emission probability distribution $\hat{E}(q_j, a_m) = \hat{e}_j(a_m)$ is estimated in the following way:

$$\hat{e}_j(a_m) = \frac{\sum_{t=1}^{T} 1_{x_t=a_m} \cdot \gamma_t(j)}{\sum_{t=1}^{T} \gamma_t(j)} \, ,$$

where

$$1_{x_t=a_m} = \begin{cases} 1, & \text{if } x_t = a_m \text{ ,} \\ 0, & \text{otherwise} \end{cases}$$

is an indicator function.

Let us present the Baum-Welch algorithm. It employs the following functions:

- *initialize* - the function sets random initial parameters ($\Pi$ and $E$),
- *compute_expected_state_visiting_probabilities* - the function computes $\gamma_t(j)$, $t = 1, \ldots, T$, $j = 1, \ldots, N$ according to point (E.1),
- *compute_expected_state_transition_probabilities* - the function computes $\xi_t(i,j)$, $t = 1, \ldots, (T-1)$, $i = 1, \ldots, N$, $j = 1, \ldots, N$ according to point (E.2),
- *estimate_transition_probability_distribution* - the function estimates $\hat{\pi}_{ij}$, $i = 1, \ldots, N$, $j = 1, \ldots, N$ according to point (M.1),
- *estimate_emission_probability_distribution* - the function estimates $\hat{e}_j(a_m)$, $j = 1, \ldots, N$, $m = 1, \ldots, M$ according to point (M.2).

---

**Induction Scheme 5.8: Baum-Welch Algorithm**

*initialize*;
**repeat**
　/\* Expectation Step \*/
　　*compute_expected_state_visiting_probabilities*;
　　*compute_expected_state_transition_probabilities*;
　/\* Maximization Step \*/
　　*estimate_transition_probability_distribution*;
　　*estimate_emission_probability_distribution*;
**until** *convergence*;

---

Let us note that the Baum-Welch algorithm converges to a local maximum.

At the end of this section let us present the following theorem [Baum *et al.* (1970)].

---

**Theorem 5.6 (Baum-Welch Algorithm Complexity)**

*The running time of the Baum-Welch algorithm is $\mathcal{O}(N^2 \cdot T)$, where $N$ is the number of states of HMM, $T$ is the input length.*

---

## 5.5   Remarks on the Inference of String Languages

For the induction algorithms presented in this chapter, we have assumed that the automata inferred are (symmetrically) structurally complete with respect to the

corresponding samples.[21] We say that the automaton $A$ is (symmetrically) structurally complete with respect to the sample $S_+$ (the sample $(S_+, S_-)$) [Higuera de
la (2010)] iff

- $\forall q \in F_A \; \exists x \in S_+ : \; \delta(q_0, x) = q$ (and $\forall q \in F_R \; \exists x \in S_- : \; \delta(q_0, x) = q$),
- $\forall x \in S_+ : \; x \in L_{F_A}(A)$ (and $\forall x \in S_- : \; x \in L_{F_R}(A)$),
- $\forall q \in Q \; \forall a \in \Sigma_T$ such that $\delta(q, a)$ is defined, $\exists x \in S_+ : x = uav$ and $\delta(q_0, u) = q$
  ($\forall q \in Q \; \forall a \in \Sigma_T$ such that $\delta(q, a)$ is defined, $\exists x \in S_+ \cup S_- : x = uav$ and
  $\delta(q_0, u) = q$).

The (symmetrical) structural completeness of a grammar is defined in an analogous way.

Many grammatical inference methods are constructed according to the following
scheme. Firstly, a *canonical grammar/automaton* is defined. Secondly, it is modified iteratively and the series of *derived grammars/automata* is obtained. Let us
introduce the following notions [Hartmanis (1960); Hartmanis and Stearns (1964,
1966); Fu and Booth (1975a)].

Let $L$ be a language, $u \in \Sigma_T^*$. The left quotient of $L$ by $u$ is defined as follows:

$$L_u = \{v \in \Sigma_T^* : uv \in L\}.$$

Let $L$ be a regular language. The *canonical automaton* for $L$, $A_C = (Q, \Sigma_T, \delta, q_0, F)$ is defined in the following way:

- $Q := \{L_u : u \in \mathit{Pref}(L)\}$,
- $q_0 := \{L_\lambda\}$,
- $F := \{L_w : w \in L\}$,
- $\delta(L_u, a) := L_{ua}, \; u, ua \in \mathit{Pref}(L), \; a \in \Sigma_T$.

An automaton $A$ is called *canonical* iff $A$ is isomorphic to the canonical automaton for $L(A)$.

A *canonical grammar* has been defined in Sec. 3.1 (Scheme 3.1).

Let $X$ be a set. A *partition $\pi$* of $X$ is a set of pairwise disjoint nonempty subsets
of $X$ whose union is $X$. For any $x \in X$ there is a unique element of $\pi$, called
the *block* of $\pi$, which contains $x$. For any equivalence relation on $X$, the set of its
equivalence classes constitutes a partition of $X$.

Let $G_C$ be a canonical grammar for a sample $S_+$. A *derived grammar $G_D$* is
obtained by the *partitioning* of the set of the nonterminals of $G_C$ into equivalence
classes. Each nonterminal of $G_D$ corresponds to one block of the partition.

Let $A_C$ be a canonical automaton for the sample $S_+$. A *derived automaton $A_D$*
is obtained by the *partitioning* of the set of the states of $A_C$ into equivalence classes.
Each state of $A_D$ corresponds to one block of the partition.

---

[21]In the case of text learning we talk about structural completeness, whereas in the case of informed
learning we talk about symmetrical structural completeness.

Selected basic algorithms of the inference of string languages have been presented in this chapter. The text learning methods for regular languages which are also important for syntactic pattern recognition include: the tail-clustering method [Miclet (1980)], the pattern languages [Angluin (1980a)], the recursive merging method [Itoga (1981)], the successor method [Richetin and Vernadet (1984)], the skeleton-based method [Radhakrishnan and Nagaraja (1987)], the partial similarities method [Kudo and Shimbo (1988)], the morphic generator method [García *et al.* (1987, 1990a)], function-distinguishable languages [Fernau (2003)]. In the case of the informed learning of regular languages the following methods are also of importance for the field: the hill-climbing-based method [Tomita (1982)], the genetic-search-based method [Dupont (1994)], the combined symbolic-neural network active method [Sanfeliu and Alquézar (1995a)], the incremental method [Sanfeliu and Alquézar (1995b)], the Evidence-Driven State Merging (EDSM) algorithm [Lang *et al.* (1998)][22], the Residual Finite State Automata (RFSA) inference [Denis *et al.* (2004)], the evolutionary-algorithm-based method [Lucas and Reynolds (2005)], the neural-network-based method [Delgado and Pegalajar (2005)], the heuristic-search-based method [Bugalho and Oliveira (2005)].

Learning context-free languages is more difficult than in the case of regular languages. Therefore, a few grammatical inference methods have been developed for such subclasses of CFGs these include: precedence grammars [Crespi-Reghizzi (1970); Crespi-Reghizzi *et al.* (1973)], even linear grammars [Takada (1988); Koshiba *et al.* (1997); Sempere and García (1994)], extended regular expression-based induction [Yokomori (1988); Sempere (2000)] (the first extensions of regular expressions for CFLs were defined in [Gruska (1971)]), deterministic linear languages [Higuera de la and Oncina (2002)], very simple grammars [Yokomori (2003)], substitutable grammars [Clark and Eyraud (2007)], distributional-based multiple grammars [Clark and Yoshinaka (2014)]. The CYK-parsing-based methods were proposed in [Sakakibara (2005b); Nakamura and Matsumoto (2005)]. The inference of context-free programmed grammars was studied in [Tai and Fu (1982); Lu and Fu (1984a,b)]. Learning transducers were presented in [Oncina *et al.* (1993); Casacuberta *et al.* (2005)].

The induction methods for stochastic regular languages were published in [Maryanski and Booth (1977); Mude Van Der and Walker (1978); Carrasco and Oncina (1999); Higuera de la and Thollard (2000); Clark and Thollard (2004); Dupont *et al.* (2005); Casacuberta and Vidal (2007)] and for stochastic context-free languages in [Filipski (1980); Humenik and Pinkham (1990); Banerjee and Rosenfeld (1992); Casacuberta (1995); Sánchez and Benedí (1997); Keller and Lutz (2005); Corazza and Satta (2007); Zhu *et al.* (2009)]. Learning fuzzy languages was investigated in [Tamura and Tanaka (1973); Majumdar and Roy (1983); Peeva (1991); Watrous and Kuhn (1992); Zeng *et al.* (1994); Omlin and Giles (1996); Blanco *et al.* (2001)].

---

[22]The *Red-* and *Blue*-states terminology was introduced in this paper.

Fundamental monographs on grammatical inference include [Higuera de la (2010); Heinz and Sempere (2016); Wieczorek (2017)] with surveys being published in [Fu and Booth (1975a,b, 1986a,b); Sakakibara (1997); Higuera de la (2005)]. The seminal papers in the field of grammatical inference [Gold (1967); Feldman (1967); Horning (1969); Trakhtenbrot and Barzdin' (1970); Feldman (1972); Gold (1978); Angluin (1978, 1980b, 1987); Valiant (1984); Takada (1995); Higuera de la (1997)] equally contain theoretical foundations.

# Chapter 6

# Applications of String Methods

The methods based on string grammars and automata have a variety of applications. We shall present these methods in the succeeding sections dividing them into the following main application areas: shape and picture analysis, optical character recognition (OCR), structure analysis in bioinformatics, analysis of medical signals and images, speech recognition and natural language processing (NLP), analysis of visual events and activities (including sign language recognition and anomaly detection), signal analysis for process monitoring and control, analysis of architectural objects, feature recognition for computer aided design and manufacturing (CAD/CAM), structure analysis in chemistry, radar signal analysis, pattern recognition in seismology, pattern recognition in geology, fingerprint recognition, analysis of financial and economics time series, and image processing. A summary of these application in the tabular form is included in the last section.

## 6.1 Shape and Picture Analysis

The fundamental generic models for shape and picture analysis were introduced in the seminal papers [Freeman (1961); Kirsch (1964); Narasimhan (1964); Feder (1968); Shaw (1969); Pavlidis (1968); Chang (1970); Pavlidis (1972b); Pavlidis and Ali (1979); Shaw (1970); Milgram and Rosenfeld (1971); Stiny and Gips (1972); Siromoney *et al.* (1972, 1973); Rosenfeld (1973, 1979); Shapiro (1980); Maurer *et al.* (1982); Alquézar and Sanfeliu (1997)].

Recognition of distorted shapes was investigated by K. S. Fu and his collaborators in the 1970s. Stochastic grammars and stochastic programmed grammars were proposed for this purpose in [Fu (1973)] and [Swain and Fu (1972)], respectively. Subsequently, attribute grammars were defined in [You and Fu (1979)]. Attributes were used to describe primitives and connection relations. An inference algorithm was also presented. A method based on attributed grammars and error-correcting techniques was defined in [You and Fu (1980)].

Hierarchical grammar models, which allow for the defining of syntactic and semantic contextual constraints between primitives, were proposed in [Henderson and Davis (1981)]. The models were applied for airplane shape recognition. Shape grammar compilers were, then, defined within this approach [Henderson and Samal (1986)]. The parsers were a generalization of *LR* parsing.

Extended error-correcting Earley parsing of multi-valued strings was presented in [Bunke and Pasche (1990)].

Augmented Regular Expressions (AREs) [Alquézar and Sanfeliu (1997)] were applied by A. Sanfeliu and his collaborators for shape analysis in the 1990s. Learning the model and its use for recognizing traffic signs was presented in [Sanfeliu and Sainz (1996); Sainz and Alquezar (1996)]. The problem of inferring the model and the use of the learned recognizer for analysis of contours of frontal views of 3D solids obtained by their rotation was investigated in [Sanfeliu and Alquézar (1996); Alquézar and Sanfeliu (1996)]. The model was strong enough to be used for recognizing planar shapes with symmetries belonging to a nontrivial class of context-sensitive languages.

A system for the structural analysis of drawings *Mirabelle* was presented in [Masini and Mohr (1983)]. The application of inference of even linear grammars for picture description languages (PDL) was described in [Radhakrishnan and Nagaraja (1988)]. Finite-state automata were used for recognition of dimensions in engineering machine drawings in [Dori and Pnueli (1988); Dori (1989)]. Efficient error-correcting Viterbi parsing was defined for shape recognition in [Amengual and Vidal (1998)]. The extended CYK parser for Siromoney's array languages was defined in [Crespi-Reghizzi and Pradella (2008)]. Adjacency Grammars were used for interpretation of sketched diagrams in [Mas *et al.* (2010)]. A comprehensive overview of syntactic methods in line drawing analysis can be found in [Tombre (1996)].

The Cocke-Younger-Kasami parser was adapted to solve the starting point problem in the chain-code-based description efficiently in [Oncina (1996)].

## 6.2   Optical Character Recognition

Optical character recognition (OCR) is one of the earliest applications of syntactic pattern recognition. R. A. Kirsch considered the OCR problem in [Kirsch (1963)]. R. N. Narasimhan investigated the problem of recognition of handwritten (English) letters in [Narasimhan (1964, 1966)]. Labelling schemata and the syntax-directed interpretation method were proposed for this purpose. The research was continued and its results were published in [Narasimhan and Reddy (1971)].

Picture processing grammars were introduced for analyzing hand-written numerals, mathematical expressions and line drawings in [Chang (1971)]. Fractionally fuzzy grammars were used for handwritten English script recognition in [DePalma and Yau (1975)]. Handwritten capital letters were recognized based on fuzzy set theory and formal grammars in [Kickert and Koppelaar (1976)]. The method presented in [Stringa (1990)] makes use of hierarchical re-description of images of unconstrained alphanumeric characters in order to identify significant elements only.

Cursive script recognition was investigated by R. Parizeau, M. Plamondon and collaborators in the 1990s. A handwriting model for the recognition of cursive scripts is applied for extracting primitives used in shape grammars. These grammars model allographs and their adjacency rules [Parizeau and Plamondon (1992)]. In [Parizeau *et al.* (1992)] the parsing process is used for allograph segmentation and fuzzy logic is applied for evaluating the likelihood of possible ways of segmentation. The method of developing a writer-independent recognition system which uses fuzzy-shape grammars is presented [Parizeau and Plamondon (1995)].

Off-line handwritten sentence recognition with hidden Markov models was studied by H. Bunke and the collaborators in [Bunke *et al.* (1995); Marti and Bunke (2001); Vinciarelli *et al.* (2004); Zimmermann *et al.* (2006); Bertolami and Bunke (2008)]. Array grammars and automata were used for recognizing handwritten characters in [Wang (1984); Fernau and Freund (1996); Fernau *et al.* (1998)]. The issue of recognizing strings with substitutions, insertions, deletions and generalized transpositions was studied in [Oommen and Loke (1997)]. The method of comparing the legal and courtesy amount in bank checks with a syntax-directed translation scheme was proposed in [Kaufmann and Bunke (1998)]. Fuzzy languages and an *LR*-type parser were applied for on-line handwriting analysis in [Malaviya and Peters (2000)]. Stochastic error-correcting parsing was applied for handwritten OCR system in [Perez-Cortes *et al.* (2000)]. The hybrid *HMM/ANN* model was proposed in [España Boquera *et al.* (2011)].

Printed and hand-printed character recognition was also investigated in syntactic pattern recognition. Finite-state automata were used for the on-line recognition of hand-printed characters drawn on a graphic tablet in [Berthod and Maroy (1979)]. Context-free languages were applied in an omni-font character recognition system in [Wolberg (1987)]. The error-correcting grammatical inference was used for a printed digit recognition task in [Vidal *et al.* (1992)].

Chinese and Korean character recognition has been studied in syntactic pattern recognition as well. Grammars were used for the analysis of hand-printed Chinese and Korean characters in [Agui and Nagahashi (1979); Nagahashi and Kakatsuyama (1986); Zhao (1990)]. For recognizing Korean characters attribute-dependent programmed grammars were applied in [Lee *et al.* (1992)]. The hybrid method based on self-organizing feature maps and stochastic regular grammars was used for recognizing on-line handwritten Chinese characters in [Kuroda *et al.* (1997, 1999)].

The first results of research into the syntactic pattern recognition of mathematical expressions were published in [Anderson (1968); Chang (1970)]. The system for recognizing two-dimensional mathematic formulas written on a graphic tablet was presented in [Belaid and Haton (1984)]. Constrained attribute grammars were used in [Pagallo (1998)]. The *LR* parsing for positional grammars was applied in [Costagliola and Chang (1999)]. The method of analysis of on-line handwritten mathematical expressions with definite clause grammars was proposed in [Chan and Yeung (2000)] and its error-correcting version in [Chan and Yeung (2001)].

The syntactic pattern recognition method for processing mathematical expressions in printed documents was presented in [Garain and Chaudhuri (2000)]. Stochastic context-free grammars and hidden Markov models were used for recognizing on-line handwritten mathematical expressions in [Álvaro *et al.* (2014, 2016)]. The hybrid method based on a probabilistic SVM classifier and the CYK-type parsing for stochastic context-free grammars was presented in [Simistira *et al.* (2015)].

## 6.3   Structure Analysis in Bioinformatics

Chromosome analysis was the first application area of syntactic pattern recognition in bioinformatics. In the 1960s R. S. Ledley and his collaborators developed the FIDAC system which scanned the photomicrographs of chromosomes in order to perform karyotype analysis [Ledley (1964); Ledley *et al.* (1965); Golab *et al.* (1971)]. R. A. Kirsch investigated the problem of biological images in [Kirsch (1971)]. Research into the analysis of photomicrographs of chromosomes was led by K. S. Fu and his collaborators in the 1970s. Stochastic *CF* programmed grammars [Fu and Huang (1972); Huang and Fu (1972)] and precedence parsing were used [Lee and Fu (1972)]. The error-correcting recognition system was presented in [Thomason and Gonzales (1975)]. The direct parsing method was defined in [Tanaka *et al.* (1986)].

The possibilities for the use of formal languages, grammars and automata in molecular biology and genetics were studied in the 1980s and early 1990s in [Brendel and Busse (1984); Head (1987); Collado-Vides (1989, 1992); Searls (1992, 1993); Dong and Searls (1994); Bralley (1996)]. Stochastic context-free grammars (*CFGs*) were used for tRNA modelling in [Sakakibara *et al.* (1994)]. String variable grammars, being an extension of definite clause grammars, were applied for parsing DNA sequences in [Searls (1995)]. Multi-tape S-attribute grammars were proposed for multiple sequence alignment in [Lefebvre (1996)]. The identification of regulatory sites was performed with syntactic pattern recognition-based techniques in [Rosenblueth *et al.* (1996)]. The modelling of RNA pseudoknot structures was performed with the help of stochastic *CFGs* in [Brown and Wilson (1996)]. A method for the inference of strictly locally testable languages for DNA sequence analysis was developed in [Yokomori and Kobayashi (1998)].

A method based on stochastic *CFGs* was used for constructing small subunit ribosomal RNA multiple alignments in [Brown (2000)]. The problem of predicting RNA secondary structures containing pseudoknots was discussed in [Lyngso and Pedersen (2000)] and it was proved to be NP complete. An augmented *CFG* which generates pseudoknotted structures and allows the constructing of a polynomial time parser was proposed in [Rivas and Eddy (2000)]. Pair stochastic *CFGs* were used for ncRNA gene detection in [Rivas and Eddy (2001)]. Basic gene grammars suitable for processing DNA sequences were defined in [Leung *et al.* (2001)]. The method of grammatical inference for the recognition of human neuropeptide precursors was presented in [Muggleton *et al.* (2001)]. The method of pairwise RNA structure comparison with stochastic *CFGs* was proposed in [Holmes and Rubin (2002)]. Parallel communicating grammars for modelling RNA pseudoknotted structures were defined in [Cai *et al.* (2003)]. The use of stochastic *CFGs* for RNA secondary structure prediction was investigated in [Knudsen and Heyn (1999, 2003); Dowell and Eddy (2004); Chuong *et al.* (2006); Anderson *et al.* (2012); Ding *et al.* (2014)]. The inference of even linear grammars for predicting transmembrane domains in proteins was proposed in [Peris *et al.* (2008)]. Stochastic multiple *CFGs* were applied for RNA-RNA interaction prediction in [Kato *et al.* (2009)]. Stochastic *CFGs* were used for the analysis of protein sequences in [Dyrka and Nebel (2009); Dyrka *et al.* (2013)]. The method of inference of regular grammars for larger-than-gene structures was presented in [Tsafnat *et al.* (2011)]. A grammatical inference method for classification of amyloidogenic hexapeptides was proposed in [Wieczorek and Unold (2016)].

Fundamental research into the formal linguistics foundations of bioinformatics was made as well. A comprehensive overview of research into the use of formal languages in bioinformatics and its future directions can be found in [Searls (1997, 2001, 2002)]. The possible existence of protein grammar generating folding patterns in protein domains was considered in [Przytycka *et al.* (2002)]. The issue of the application of NLP methods in genomics was studied in [Yandell and Majoros (2002)]. The issue of learning stochastic grammars from biological sequences was discussed in [Sakakibara (2005a)]. The use of computational linguistics for exploring biopolymer structures was investigated in [Dill *et al.* (2007)].

Hidden Markov models are also used in bioinformatics. They were used[1] for sequence alignment [Baldi *et al.* (1994); Pachter *et al.* (2002)], gene prediction [Krogh *et al.* (1994b); Reese *et al.* (2000); Munch and Krogh (2006)], modelling sequencing errors [Lottaz *et al.* (2003)], base calling [Liang *et al.* (2007); Shen and Vikalo (2012)], ncRNA identification [Zhang *et al.* (2006); Singh *et al.* (2009)], ncRNA annotation [Weinberg and Ruzzo (2006); Brejová *et al.* (2007)], RNA folding and alignment [Harmanci *et al.* (2007)], predicting protein secondary structures [Won *et al.* (2007)] and ncRNA structural alignment [Yoon and Vaidyanathan (2008)].

A variety of modifications of hidden Markov models was introduced in the area of bioinformatics. *Profile hidden Markov models* [Krogh *et al.* (1994a); Eddy (1998); Karplus *et al.* (1998); Ahola *et al.* (2003); Wistrand and Sonnhammer (2004); Bernardes *et al.* (2007); Srivastava *et al.* (2007)] are specific *HMMs* which are suitable for representing and analyzing sequence profiles. *Pair hidden Markov models* [Durbin *et al.* (2002); Pachter *et al.* (2002); Knudsen and Miyamoto (2003); Do *et al.* (2005); Wang *et al.* (2006b)] are extensions of *HMMs* which are used for finding sequence alignments by emitting two (aligned) strings. *Generalized hidden Markov models* [Kulp *et al.* (1996); Reese *et al.* (2000); Majoros *et al.* (2005)], used for gene prediction, can emit a string at a state (instead of one symbol). *Evolutionary hidden Markov models* [Pedersen and Hein (2003)] combine *HMMs*, which model the

---

[1]Here we shall provide only a few examples. There are hundreds of publications on the use of *HMMs* in bioinformatics. A bibliography can be found in the monographs presented below.

structures of biological sequences, with continuous Markov chains, which - in turn - model the evolution of these structures. In the so-called *context-sensitive hidden Markov models* [Yoon and Vaidyanathan (2008); Agarwal *et al.* (2010)], previously emitted substrings can be used for determining the probabilities of future states. Thus, they can be used for describing correlations between subsequences.

An overview of the applications of hidden Markov models in bioinformatics can be found in [Gollery (2008); Yoon (2009)]. The applications of formal grammars/automata and hidden Markov models are presented in the monographs on bioinformatics [Durbin *et al.* (2002); Baldi and Brunak (2001)].

## 6.4   Medical Image/Signal Analysis

Syntactic pattern recognition is extensively used for the analysis of *ECGs* (*electrocardiograms*). Context-free grammars were used for peak detection in electrocardiograms in [Horowitz (1975, 1977)]. Electrocardiogram interpretation was performed with stochastic finite-state automata in [Albus (1977)]. Linear grammars were applied for the detection of QRS complexes in [Belforte *et al.* (1979)]. Context-free languages were used for representing patterns of ventricular arrhythmias in [Udupa and Murthy (1980)]. A hybrid learning algorithm of QRS morphologies using syntactic patterns was proposed in [Birman (1982)]. Attribute grammars were applied for detection of QRS complexes in [Papakonstantinou *et al.* (1986)]. A review of syntactic pattern recognition for ECG analysis was presented in [Skordalakis (1986)]. A syntactic-semantic approach was proposed for the recognition of QRS patterns in [Trahanias *et al.* (1989)] and for the recognition of all ECG patterns in [Trahanias and Skordalakis (1990)]. Analysis of ECG arrhythmias was performed with the help of attribute context-free grammars and Earley parsing in [Luo and Zhou (1992)]. Attributed finite-state automata were used for the syntactic recognition of ECG signals in [Koski *et al.* (1995)] and a preprocessing method of primitive extraction was proposed in [Koski (1996)]. Hidden Markov models were proposed for ECG signal analysis in [Koski (1998)]. The possibility of the use of fuzzy automata for ECG signal classification was studied in [Pedrycz (1990); Pedrycz and Gacek (2001)]. Hierarchical fuzzy finite-state automata were applied for the diagnosis of the ECG in [Tümer *et al.* (2003)].

Context-free grammars were proposed for the analysis of *EEGs* (*electroencephalograms*) in [Giese *et al.* (1979)]. Attributed grammars were used for classifying and validating intermittent EEG patterns in [Ferber (1986)]. A model consisting of a derivative-based inference of regular grammars and a minimum-distance error-correcting parser was applied for the recognition of EEG patterns at sleep stage I and stage REM in [Gath and Schwartz (1989)].

A top-down parsing system was used for the recognition of *carotid pulse waves* in [Stockman *et al.* (1976)]. The WAPSYS system based on a hybrid approach for the analysis of carotid pulse waves was proposed in [Stockman and Kanal (1983)].

Syntactic pattern recognition is used not only for medical signal analysis, but

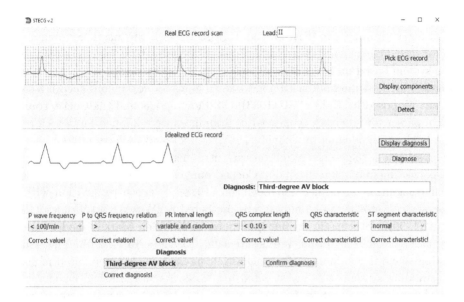

Fig. 6.1 STECG - System for Teaching ElectroCardioGraphy verifies ECG diagnoses with dynamically programmed attributed finite-state automata (Flasiński, M., Flasiński, P., and Konduracka, E. (2013). On the use of programmed automata for a verification of ECG diagnoses, *Advances in Intelligent Systems and Computing* **226**, pp. 593–601).

also for the analysis of *medical images*. The identification of skeletal bone maturity from X-rays of the hand and wrist was achieved with the help of context-free grammars in [Pathak *et al.* (1984)] and with the help of fuzzy grammars in [Pathak and Pal (1986)]. Attributed grammars and *LR* parsing were used for the analysis of pancreatic ducts for the diagnosing of pathologic changes such as chronic pancreatitis and pancreas carcinoma in [Ogiela and Tadeusiewicz (1999)]. A model for the analysis of coronary artery images based on the *LALR* parsing for the diagnosing of ischemic cardiovascular diseases was proposed in [Ogiela and Tadeusiewicz (2002, 2003)]. The *LALR* parsing was applied for the analysis of morphological lesions in the urinary tract in [Tadeusiewicz and Ogiela (2004)]. Shape feature languages [Jakubowski (1985, 1986, 1990)] were used for detecting erosions and osteophytes from hand radiographs in [Bielecka *et al.* (2011); Zieliński *et al.* (2015)].

The *LR* parser was used in the analysis of saccadic eye movements in [Juhola (1986)]. Stochastic grammars were applied for hypnogram analysis in [Fred and Leitao (1992)].

## 6.5 Speech Recognition and NLP

The first syntactic pattern recognition method of automatic *speech recognition* was published in [Mori De (1972)]. Recognizing pulses of glottal chord vibrations through stochastic finite-state automata analyzing speech waveforms was performed in [Mori De *et al.* (1977)]. Isolated words spoken in Italian were recognized with the help of fuzzy grammars in [Rivoira and Torasso (1978)]. Stochastic automata were used for recognizing spoken words and phrases in [Kashyap (1979)]. A speech recognition system based on transition network grammars was presented in [Rivoira and Torasso (1982)]. A method based on Markov models for continuous speech recognition was proposed in [Bahl *et al.* (1983)]. Markov models and the Cocke-Younger-Kasami parser for stochastic context-free grammars were applied for speech recognition language modelling in [Jelinek (1985); Jelinek and Lafferty (1991)]. A fuzzy parsing scheme for speech recognition was introduced in [Vidal *et al.* (1985)]. The error-correcting maximum-likelihood Cocke-Younger-Kasami parser was applied for speech recognition in [Miller and Levinson (1988)]. Speech recognition with the *LR* parsing for stochastic grammars was presented in [Wright and Wrigley (1989); Wright (1990)]. Stochastic regular grammars and hidden Markov models used in automatic speech recognition were studied in [Casacuberta (1990)]. The issue of adapting island-driven parsers for stochastic context-free grammars used in speech understanding systems was investigated in [Corazza *et al.* (1991)]. Dynamic programming parsing of context-free languages was used for continuous speech recognition in [Ney (1991)]. A semi-continuous extension of the morphic generator grammatical inference method [García *et al.* (1990a)] was proposed for acoustic-phonetic decoding and semantic-constrained continuous speech recognition in [Segarra *et al.* (1992)]. Context-free grammars and probabilistic network structures were applied to construct the TINA speech understanding system in [Seneff (1992)]. The induction of finite-state transducers for phonological rules was presented in [Gildea and Jurafsky (1995)]. A model based on stochastic context-free grammars for speech recognition was proposed in [Jurafsky *et al.* (1995)]. A time-synchronous continuous speech recognizer was developed with the help of the *LR* parsing and hidden Markov models in [Shimizu *et al.* (1995)]. Error-correcting parsing, finite-state automata and the Viterbi algorithm were studied for speech processing in [Amengual and Vidal (1996)]. A hybrid method based on grammatical inference and artificial neural networks for continuous speech recognition was proposed in [Castro and Casacuberta (1996)]. Weighted finite-state transducers for speech processing were presented in [Mohri *et al.* (1996); Mohri (1997)]. The issue of estimating probabilities for stochastic context-free grammars with the help of the Inside-Outside algorithm and the Viterbi algorithm for speech recognition was studied in [Sánchez *et al.* (1996)]. k-Testable in the Strict Sense, k-TSS, languages (the subclass of regular languages) and stochastic finite-state automata were used for continuous speech recognition in [Varona and Torres (2000)]. An improved method of probabilistic *FSAs* inference was used for speech recognition in [Kermorvant *et al.* (2004)]. The further results of research into the use of weighted finite-state transducers for speech recognition were presented in [Mohri *et al.* (2008)].

Syntactic pattern recognition methods are extensively used in the area of *natural language processing* (*NLP*) as well. The generalized LR (GLR) parser for NLP was presented in [Tomita (1985, 1987)]. A method based on probabilistic context-free grammars in CNF, the Baum-Welch algorithm, the Viterbi algorithm, and the Cocke-Younger-Kasami parser for sentence disambiguation was presented in [Fujisaki *et al.* (1989)]. The issue of generating grammars for statistical training in natural language applications was studied in [Sharman *et al.* (1990)]. The probabilistic *LR* parsing of natural language (corpora) was presented in [Briscoe and Carroll (1993)]. A method based on stochastic context-free grammars for driving interpretations of sentences in natural language processing was described in [Corazza *et al.* (1994)]. An Earley-based parser suitable for stochastic context-free grammars which is suitable for natural language processing was defined in [Stolcke (1995)]. Stochastic *FSAs* were used for NLP in [Sproat *et al.* (1996); Sánchez *et al.* (2018)]. The problem of the estimation of probabilistic context-free grammars was investigated in [Chi and Geman (1998)]. An efficient method of statistical induction of stochastic context free grammars from bracketed corpora was proposed in [Hogenhout and Matsumoto (1998)]. Stochastic grammars for natural language processing were studied in [Samuelsson (2000); Verdú-Mas *et al.* (2002)]. Finite automata as a tool for the compact representation of tuple dictionaries were presented in [Daciuk and Noord van (2004)]. The issue of distances between distributions for comparing language models was investigated in [Murgue and Higuera de la (2004)]. The probabilistic model of the unsupervised learning of hierarchical natural language grammar was presented in [Klein and Manning (2005)]. The space-efficient finite-state automata representation for natural language dictionaries was proposed in [Daciuk and Weiss (2012)].

Studies into the use of syntactic pattern recognition into *machine translation* began in the 1990s. Pattern-based context-free grammars for machine translation were defined in [Takeda (1996)]. Stochastic inversion transduction grammars and the bilingual parsing of parallel corpora were presented in [Wu (1997)]. Finite-state head transducers were used for translation from English into Spanish and Japanese in [Alshawi *et al.* (2000)]. The issue of computer-assisted translation with the help of finite-state transducers was considered in [Civera *et al.* (2004)]. The method of constructing inference algorithms for generation finite-state transducers from parallel corpora was proposed in [Picó *et al.* (2004)]. A model of inference of finite-state transducers from regular languages for machine translation was presented in [Casacuberta *et al.* (2005)]. Synchronous context-free grammars for machine translation were defined in [Chiang (2007)]. Two-pass methods of machine translation with the help of synchronous context-free grammars were presented in [Venugopal *et al.* (2007)].

An overview of the applications of weighted automata in natural language processing can be found in [Knight and May (2009)]. The issues of access and disambiguation in natural language processing were discussed in [Jurafsky (1996)].

The models used in speech processing and natural language processing were presented in the monographs [Jurafsky and Martin (2008); Clark *et al.* (2010)].

## 6.6 Analysis of Visual Events and Activities

Syntactic pattern recognition methods have been used for the analysis of visual events and activities since the 1990s. The recognition of human actions with *HMMs* was presented in [Yamato *et al.* (1992)]. Behavioral events were recognized by parsing for attributed grammars in [Clark (1994)]. *HMMs* were used for constructing a gesture input system in [Schlenzig *et al.* (1994)]. Dutch Sign Language was recognized with *HMMs* in [Grobel and Assan (1997)]. A method of learning visual behavior for gesture recognition based on *HMM* approach was proposed in [Wilson and Bobick (1995); Bobick and Wilson (1997)]. *HMMs* were applied for real-time American Sign Language (ASL) recognition in [Starner *et al.* (1998)]. The issue of human motion analysis was considered in [Aggarwal and Cai (1999)].

Stochastic context-free grammar parsing was used for gesture recognition and video surveillance in [Ivanov and Bobick (2000)]. A method based on finite-state automata for gesture recognition was presented in [Hong *et al.* (2000)]. Parallel hidden Markov models were proposed for recognizing ASL in [Vogler and Metaxas (2001)]. Hand gesture recognition was performed with hidden Markov models in [Yoon *et al.* (2001)]. German Sign Language was recognized with *HMMs* in [Bauer and Kraiss (2002)]. Stochastic grammars and the Earley-Stolcke parser [Stolcke (1995)] were applied for recognizing multi-tasked activities [Moore and Essa (20032)] and for the prediction of temporally extended activities in [Minnen *et al.* (2003)]. Hidden Markov models and the Kalman filter were used for recognizing dynamic hand gestures in [Ramamoorthy *et al.* (2003)]. The method of recognizing human actions through the inference of stochastic regular grammars was presented in [Cho *et al.* (2004)]. Chinese Sign Language was recognized with *HMMs* in [Gao *et al.* (2004)]. Learning and recognizing activities from movement trajectories were performed with the help of hierarchical Hidden Markov models in [Nguyen *et al.* (2005)]. Context-free grammars were applied for the recognition of activities in [Ryoo and Aggarwal (2006); Wang *et al.* (2010)]. Attributed context-free grammars and the Earley parsing were used for the detection of abnormal events in [Joo and Chellappa (2006a)] and for the recognition of multi-object events in [Joo and Chellappa (2006b)]. Multi-dimensional *HMMs* were applied for recognizing American Sign Language in [Wang *et al.* (2006a)]. Large-vocabulary recognition of continuous Chinese Sign Languages was performed with hidden Markov models in [Fang *et al.* (2007)]. Real-time hand gesture recognition was performed with stochastic context-free grammars in [Chen *et al.* (2008)]. The hybrid *HMM/PAC* model for gesture recognition was proposed in [Muñoz-Salinas *et al.* (2008)].

Temporal fuzzy automata were applied for hand gesture recognition in [Bailador and Triviño (2010)]. Continuous hand gestures were recognized with finite-state automata in [Bhuyan *et al.* (2011)]. Stochastic context-free grammars extended by Allen's temporal logic were used for recognizing complex visual events in [Zhan *et al.* (2011)]. Explaining activities was made with attribute multiset grammars and Bayesian networks in [Damen and Hogg (2012)]. Arabic Sign Language was recognized with *HMMs* in [Mohandes *et al.* (2012)]. Parsing for stochastic regular grammars was applied for the recognizing of long-term behaviors in [Sanroma *et al.* (2012)]. Fuzzy finite-state automata were used for the analysis of human body motion in [González-Villanueva *et al.* (2013)]. A feature-based stochastic context-free grammar model was proposed for the learning and recognizing of natural hand gestures in [Sadeghipour and Kopp (2014)]. Stochastic grammars and hidden Markov models were used for recognizing complex actions in [Sanroma *et al.* (2014)]. Interpreting tactic concepts in sports video was performed with latent context-free grammars in [Xu and Man (2015)]. Hidden Markov models were applied for sign language recognition in [Kumar *et al.* (2017); Guo *et al.* (2018)]. The stochastic automata-based method for discovering and tracking spatiotemporal event patterns was presented in [Zhang *et al.* (2018)].

## 6.7 Signal Analysis for Process Monitoring and Control

The fundamental assumptions for developing control systems with syntactic pattern recognition were presented in [Fu (1970)]. The inference of regular grammars and finite-state automata was used for the modelling of actual flow in chemical reactors in [Vernadat *et al.* (1982)].

A model of *dynamically programmed grammars/automata*[2] for monitoring and controlling real-time systems was introduced in [Flasiński (1994, 1995a)]. The model was used for constructing the first version of the real-time expert system ZEX to monitor, diagnose and control the software-hardware environment of a high energy physics experiment [Behrens *et al.* (1994)]. *Dynamically programmed LL(k)*, *DPLL(k)*, grammars and the *DPLL* parsing were applied for constructing the final version of the expert system ZEX [Flasiński (1995a); Flasiński and Jurek (1999)]. *DPLL(k)* grammars were generalized for the efficient controlling of industrial equipment in [Jurek (2000, 2005)]. An inference algorithm for the synthesis of *DPLL(k)* grammar-based control systems was proposed in [Jurek (2004)].

*Finite-state automata* were used for diagnosing faults in Web service processes [Yan *et al.* (2009)]. Stochastic finite-state automata were applied for state observation and the diagnosis of discrete event systems in [Lunze and Schröder (2001)]. A model based on finite-state Moore automata for fault diagnosis was proposed in [Hashtrudi Zad *et al.* (2003)]. Wind power prediction was made with stochastic (regression) finite-state automata in [Lin *et al.* (2016)]. *Hidden Markov models* were applied for accident identification in nuclear power plants [Kwon and Kim (1999)]. Tool wear condition monitoring in drilling operations was performed with *HMMs* in [Ertunc *et al.* (2001)]. The system for condition monitoring and the classification of rotating machinery with *HMMs* was presented in [Miao and Makis (2007)].

Generative grammars were used for the monitoring of fluidized catalytic cracking unit (FCCU) processes and fault diagnosis in [Rengaswamy and Venkatasubrama-

---

[2]Dynamically programmed grammars and automata have been introduced in Sec. 4.2.2.

nian (1995)]. Context-free grammars were applied for recognizing malicious system behavior in [Thompson and Flynn (2007); Luh *et al.* (2018)]. The method of inference of stochastic context-free grammars for the modelling of mobility patterns in networks was proposed in [Geyik *et al.* (2013)]. The learning of context-free grammars for time series anomaly detection (ECG, power demand data) was presented in [Senin *et al.* (2015)]. Context-free grammars were applied for recognizing driver behavior to improve safety in [Husen *et al.* (2017)].

Timed [Alur and Dill (1994)] and *real-time automata* [Dima (2001)][3] were also used in the area presented in this section. Fault diagnosis of discrete event systems was performed with timed automata in [Lunze and Supavatanakul (2002); Tripakis (2002); Bouyer *et al.* (2005); Supavatanakul *et al.* (2006)]. Weighted timed automata were studied for static scheduling problems and air-traffic control problems in [Torre La *et al.* (2002)]. The issue of timed controller synthesis was investigated in [D'Souza and Madhusudan (2002); Bouyer *et al.* (2003)]. Anomaly detection in production plants was performed with timed automata in [Maier *et al.* (2011)]. Models for the driving behavior of truck drivers were learnt with stochastic real-time automata in [Verwer *et al.* (2011); Zhang *et al.* (2017)]. Timed automata were used for learning of behavior models in [Niggemann *et al.* (2012)]. Model-based anomaly detection in technical systems was performed with timed automata in [Klerx *et al.* (2014)]. ATM (Automated Teller Machine) fraud detection with timed automata was presented in [Priesterjahn *et al.* (2015)].

Finite-state automata were also used in the approach to the *supervisory control of discrete event processes/discrete event dynamic systems, DEDS*, which was introduced in [Ramadge and Wonham (1987)]. Several models were constructed on the basis of this approach. The supervisory control of discrete event processes with partial observations and the case of decentralized control were studied in [Cieslak *et al.* (1988)]. The issue of observability in discrete event dynamic systems was investigated in [Ozveren and Willsky (1990)]. Supervisory control for Rapid Thermal Multiprocessor was described in [Balemi *et al.* (1993)]. The supervised control concept, where control and supervision were separated, was proposed in [Charbonnier *et al.* (1999)]. The method of supervisor reduction for discrete-event systems was presented in [Su *et al.* (2004)]. The model for the coordination control of discrete-event systems was described in [Komenda *et al.* (2012, 2015)].

*Pushdown automata* were applied for reducing an operational supervisory control problem in [Schneider *et al.* (2014)]. Supervisory controller synthesis was extended to pushdown automata in [Schmuck *et al.* (2014, 2016)].

The model for the failure diagnosis of discrete event systems presented in [Sampath *et al.* (1995, 1996)] was equally based on finite-state automata.

The use of finite-state automata for discrete event processes was presented in [Raisch (2013)]. A survey of timed automata for constructing real-time systems

---

[3]Some authors of the papers herein presented, in using real-time automata, refer to them as "timed automata".

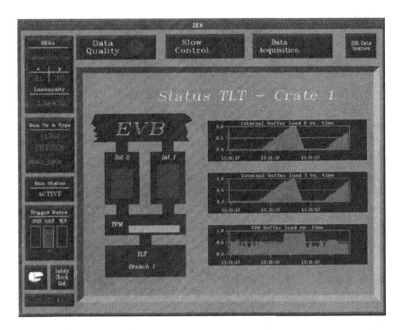

Fig. 6.2 ZEX - ZEUS Expert System for monitoring and controlling a high energy physics experiment by recognizing waveforms with the $DPLL(k)$ parsing [Flasiński and Jurek (1999)].

was conducted in [Waez *et al.* (2013)]. Discrete event systems are presented in the monograph [Cassandras and Lafortune (2010)].

## 6.8 Architectural Object Analysis

*Shape grammars*[4] have been used for the modelling of various architectural styles since the 1970s. A parametric shape grammar was applied to design room layouts for Palladian villa plans in [Stiny and Mitchell (1978)]. Buffalo bungalows were modelled with a parametric shape grammar in [Downing and Flemming (1981)]. Parametric shape grammars generated prairie houses according to the Frank Lloyd Wright's prairie house style in [Koning and Eizenberg (1981)]. A method for defining new design languages from existing ones was presented in [Knight (1981)]. Shape grammars which generate houses in the Queen Anne style were constructed in [Flemming (1981)]. A shape grammar for Alvaro Siza's patio houses at Malagueira was defined on the basis of the corpus of thirty five houses in [Duarte (2005)].

Research into the use of syntactic pattern recognition for the *automatic analysis and modelling* of architectural objects started in the first decade of the 21st century. The novel methodology based on *split grammars*, an extension of shape grammars, was proposed for this purpose in [Wonka *et al.* (2003)]. Then, the variety of methods was developed especially for *urban reconstruction*. Syntactic pattern recognition

---

[4]The shape grammars and split grammars considered in this section are introduced in Sec. 4.5.4.

methods in this area can be divided into two groups.

The first one concerns the important issue of *façade parsing* which is the reconstruction of a building façade by dividing it into its structural elements (e.g., windows, balconies) on the basis of *a priori* knowledge on its valid structure and semantics. In the case of syntactic pattern recognition methods, this knowledge is in the form of formal grammar. An approach for the semantic interpretation of building façades based on stochastic attributed context-free grammars was proposed in [Alegre and Dellaert (2004)]. Shape grammars were used for the image-based procedural modelling of façades in [Müller *et al.* (2007)]. Façade reconstruction was performed by means of a derivation in a split grammar controlled by the Markov Chain Monte Carlo method in [Ripperda and Brenner (2007)]. Context-sensitive grammars were used for façade reconstruction from mobile LiDAR mapping [Becker and Haala (2009)]. A method based on shape grammars and Markov Random Fields for single view reconstruction was presented in [Koutsourakis *et al.* (2009)]. A method using split grammars and the Cocke-Younger-Kasami parsing-based algorithm for generic façade reconstruction was proposed in [Riemenschneider *et al.* (2012)]. A 3D reconstruction of buildings from ground-level sequences was conducted with the help of shape grammars and an evolutionary algorithm in [Simon *et al.* (2012)]. An efficient façade parsing with the rank-one approximation method was presented in [Yang *et al.* (2012)]. Constrained attributed grammars were used for semantizing 3D architectural objects in [Boulch *et al.* (2013)]. Binary split grammars and reinforcement learning were applied to façade parsing in [Teboul *et al.* (2013)]. A model of learning generic split grammars from annotated images for façade parsing was proposed in [Gadde *et al.* (2016)].

The second group of methods concerns the key issue of *reconstructing whole buildings from various sources* (e.g., photographs, LiDAR data). In *inverse procedural modelling* (*ILP*) grammars are not only used for generating building (something that has been presented at the beginning of this section), but also for reconstructing existing buildings. Shape grammars coded with Generative Modeling Language (GML) were used for reconstructing buildings in [Hohmann *et al.* (2010)]. A generative grammar and a parsing algorithm were defined for building detection from 3D point clouds in [Toshev *et al.* (2010)]. A method of reconstructing 3D building models with the help of Manhattan-World grammars was presented in [Vanegas *et al.* (2010)]. Shape grammars were used for 3D building reconstruction in [Mathias *et al.* (2011)]. Attributed stochastic context-free grammars and the Earley parsing-based algorithm were used as models of inverse procedural modelling in [Martinović and Gool Van (2013)]. A shape grammar-based model for inferring grammar rules, separating façades and finding the style of a façade was presented in [Weissenberg (2014)]. An inference algorithm for split grammars used for urban reconstruction and large-scale urban modelling was proposed in [Wu *et al.* (2014)]. Stochastic attribute grammars and their parsing suitable for both interior design and architectural object analysis were proposed in [Liu *et al.* (2014)].

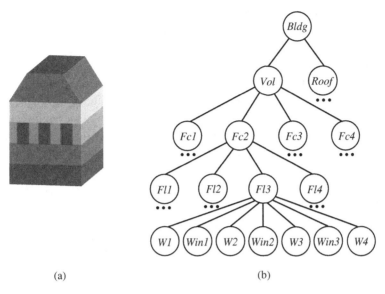

(a)                        (b)

Fig. 6.3 An exemplary architectural object model and the part of its derivation tree after shape/split grammar parsing.

An overview of the issue of urban reconstruction can be found in [Musialski *et al.* (2013)].

## 6.9 Feature Recognition for CAD/CAM

The first syntactic pattern recognition methods for computer-aided design and manufacturing were developed by R. Jakubowski[5] and his collaborators in the late 1970s and early 1980s. A method based on String Adjunct Grammars[6] for the recognition of rotary machined parts was presented in [Jakubowski and Kasprzak (1977)]. The *LR* parsing was used in this model in [Jakubowski (1982)]. A generalized shape feature language for describing machined parts modelled by the rotational or translational sweeping was proposed in [Jakubowski (1985)]. The model was completed by introducing a multi-level language translation for grouping similar machined parts into subclasses [Jakubowski (1986, 1990)] and using parsable *ETPL(k)* graph grammars at the highest level of machined part representation [Jakubowski and Flasiński (1992)].

In the Kyprianou model [Kyprianou (1980)], feature grammars were defined for feature recognition based on the concavity/smoothness/convexity concept. This model influenced the development of other syntactic pattern recognition methods for CAD/CAM feature recognition.

The Earley parsing was used for feature recognition in [Staley *et al.* (1983)]. A

---

[5]The Jakubowski model is presented in Sec. 4.5.5.
[6]String Adjunct Grammars are introduced in Sec. 4.1.

syntactic pattern recognition method for the identification of machined surfaces was proposed in [Choi *et al.* (1984)]. The issue of the extraction of manufacturing details from CAD models with syntactic methods was studied in [Srinivasan *et al.* (1985)]. Feature extraction for process planning with finite-state automata was considered in [Joshi and Chang (1990)]. Attributed grammars for engineering design were studied in [Mullins and Rinderle (1991); Rinderle (1991)]. Lindenmayer systems were used in a CAD system in [Mandorli *et al.* (1993)]. Shape grammars for engineering design were investigated in [Brown *et al.* (1995)]. The syntactic pattern recognition system for the extraction of 3D part features was presented in [Kulkarni and Pande (1995)]. The system extracting generic classes of manufacturing features from engineering drawings was proposed in [Prabhu (1999)]. A feature recognition module which applies B-rep data for the syntactic pattern recognition of manufacturing features in prismatic parts was presented in [Arivazhagan *et al.* (2008)]. Grammar rules were used for generating objects for layered manufacturing machines from initial shapes in CAD in [Sass (2008)].

## 6.10 Structure Analysis in Chemistry

Structure analysis in chemistry is one of the earliest applications of syntactic pattern recognition. Syntax analysis of linear structural formulas was presented in [Fehder and Barnett (1965)]. Topological grammars for representing the connectivity of the chemical structure diagrams and geometric grammars describing the arrangement of the diagrams in a plane were defined in [Tauber and Rankin (1972)]. A formal linguistic approach to the representation of generic chemical formulae in chemical patents was proposed in [Krishnamurthy and Lynch (1981)]. Context-sensitive grammars were used for representing and searching generic chemical (Markush) formulas, which are typical in chemical patents, in [Lynch *et al.* (1981); Barnard *et al.* (1981); Welford *et al.* (1981); Barnard *et al.* (1984)].

A formal linguistic approach was used for defining languages for describing molecular patterns, i.e. molecular descriptors. Linear notations, such as WLN, SMILES, SLN and InChI, are especially suitable because they are efficiently parsable by chemoinformatics applications. WLN (Wiswesser Line Notation) was described in [Smith and Baker (1975); Wiswesser (1982)]. SMILES (Simplified Molecule Input Line Entry System) was presented in [Weininger (1988, 2003)]. SLN (SYBYL Line Notation) was defined in [Ash *et al.* (1997); Homer *et al.* (2008)]. InChI (the IUPAC International Chemical Identifier) was described in [Heller *et al.* (2015)].

Context-free grammars were used for defining Molecular Query Language (MQL) in [Proschak *et al.* (2007)]. Grammatical inference was applied for the prediction of chemical activity in [Sidorova and Anisimova (2014)]. The problem of chemical toxicity prediction was modelled with attributed grammars in [Sidorova and Garcia (2015)]. The syntax-based translator for SMILES from strings to feature vectors was presented in [Sagar and Sidorova (2016)].

## 6.11 Radar Signal Analysis

Finite-state automata were used for detecting airborne objects in maritime infra-red images in [Barnard (1989)]. Syntactic pattern recognition of radar measurements of commercial aircraft was made with *FSAs* in [Sands and Garber (1990)]. The error-correcting parsing for high range resolution (HRR) target recognition was presented in [Bhatnagar *et al.* (2000)]. A syntactic pattern recognition-based system for target detection using HRR signatures was presented in [Turnbaugh *et al.* (2008)].

Syntactic-stochastic pattern recognition models for radar signal analysis were developed by V. Krishnamurthy and his collaborators in the 21st century. Stochastic context-free grammars were applied for surveillance and tracking with multifunction radars (MFRs) in [Visnevski *et al.* (2007)]. A method for the signal interpretation of multifunction radars with stochastic *CFGs* was proposed in [Wang and Krishnamurthy (2008)]. Stochastic context-free grammars were used for identifying suspicious spatial trajectories tracking with ground moving target indicator (GMTI) radar in [Wang *et al.* (2011)]. Detection of anomalous trajectory patterns with stochastic context-free grammars was presented in [Fanaswala and Krishnamurthy (2013)]. Stochastic context-free grammars and Earley-Stolcke parsing were applied for trajectory constrained track-before-detect in [Fanaswala and Krishnamurthy (2014)].

## 6.12 Pattern Recognition in Seismology

The syntactic recognition of seismic patterns was investigated by K. S. Fu and his collaborators in the 1980s. The method for inferring regular grammars from earthquake/explosion data was presented in [Liu and Fu (1982, 1983)]. Syntactic pattern recognition techniques were used for the classification of Ricket wavelets and the detection of bright spots in [Huang and Fu (1984, 1985a,b)].

This research was continued by K. Y. Huang and his collaborators. The extended minimum-distance error-correcting Earley parsing was constructed for seismic signal analysis in [Huang and Leu (1992)]. The application of *Picture Description Languages* for the recognition of seismic patterns was presented in [Huang (1992)]. Error-correcting finite-state automata were applied for the recognition of Ricker wavelets in [Huang and Leu (1995)]. A comprehensive syntactic pattern recognition model for seismic oil exploration, including error-correcting finite-state automata, attributed grammars, error-correcting Earley parsing, and tree automata (SPECTA and GECTA),[7] was presented in the monograph [Huang (2002)]. A method of analysis of seismic waveforms based on augmented transition network grammars was proposed in [Anderson (1982)].

---

[7]These automata are introduced in the next chapter.

## 6.13   Pattern Recognition in Geology

A method based on the grammar of unit associations and the parsing of logderived lithology units for interpretation of sedimentary environments from wireline logs was presented in [Griffiths (1990)]. Stochastic context-free grammars were used for the simulation of 1D sedimentary sequences in a coal bearing succession in [Duan et al. (1996)]. The conditional simulation of 2D parasequences in shallow marine depositional sequences was performed with attributed controlled grammars in [Duan et al. (1999)].

Sections from a sedimentary succession were simulated with stochastic attributed grammars in [Hill and Griffiths (2007)]. A method for describing data collected from field studies based on context-free grammars was proposed in [Hill and Griffiths (2008)]. Attributed regular grammars and their parsing were applied for generating facies models for reservoir characterization in [Hill and Griffiths (2009)].

## 6.14   Fingerprint Recognition

A method for the recognition of fingerprint patterns based on context-free grammars was presented in [Moayer and Fu (1975)]. Stochastic context-free grammars were used for analysis of fingerprints in [Moayer and Fu (1976a)]. Type classification of fingerprints was performed with programmed context-free grammars in [Rao and Balck (1980)]. Nondeterministic finite-state automata were applied for fingerprint classification in [Chang and Fan (2002)].

A survey of fingerprint analysis methods can be found in [Yager and Amin (2004)].

## 6.15   Financial/Economics Time Series Analysis

A syntactic pattern recognition model for technical analysis in portfolio trading was presented in [Pau (1991)]. Context-free grammars and error-correcting parsing were studied for financial trading with a technical analysis of price curves in [Gianotti (1993)]. The use of syntactic pattern recognition for the NASDAQ structural time-series patterns are considered in [Batyrshin et al. (2007)]. Hidden Markov models were used for predicting the sign of local financial trends in [Bicego et al. (2008)].

## 6.16   Image Processing

Syntactic pattern recognition methods were used for the segmentation and labelling of digitized pages of technical documents in [Krishnamoorthy et al. (1993)]. Stochastic automata were applied for relaxation labelling in [Sastry and Thathachar (1994)]. Image segmentation and hierarchical representation modelling were performed with augmented context-free grammars in [Siskind et al. (2007)].

## 6.17  Summary

A summary of the applications of string syntactic pattern recognition methods described in the previous sections is presented in Table 6.1.

Table 6.1   The applications of string-based methods.

| Applications | Models | References |
|---|---|---|
| Shape and picture analysis | Error-correcting finite-state automata, stochastic grammars, programmed grammars, shape grammars, *LR* parsing, CYK parsing, Earley parsing, Augmented Regular Expressions, Picture Description Languages, Siromoney array grammars | [Freeman (1961)], [Narasimhan (1964)], [Feder (1968)], [Shaw (1968, 1969, 1970)], [Milgram and Rosenfeld (1971)], [Stiny and Gips (1972)], [Rosenfeld (1973)], [Swain and Fu (1972)], [Fu (1973)], [Siromoney *et al.* (1972)], [Siromoney *et al.* (1973)], [Rosenfeld (1976, 1979)], [You and Fu (1979)], [You and Fu (1980)] [Henderson and Davis (1981)], [Maurer *et al.* (1982, 1983)], [Masini and Mohr (1983)], [Henderson and Samal (1986)], [Radhakrishnan and Nagaraja (1988)], [Dori and Pnueli (1988; Dori (1989)], [Bunke and Pasche (1990)], [Oncina (1996)], [Alquézar and Sanfeliu (1996)], [Sanfeliu and Alquézar (1996)], [Sainz and Alquezar (1996)] [Sanfeliu and Sainz (1996)], [Tombre (1996)], [Alquézar and Sanfeliu (1997)], [Amengual and Vidal (1998)], [Crespi-Reghizzi and Pradella (2008)], [Mas *et al.* (2010)] |
| Optical character recognition | Regular grammars, finite-state automata, hidden Markov models, context-free grammars, *LR* parsing, precedence grammars, programmed grammars, fuzzy grammars, stochastic grammars, CYK parsing, two-dimensional automata, constraint multiset grammars, positional grammars, adjacency grammars | [Kirsch (1963)], [Narasimhan (1964)], [Narasimhan (1966)], [Narasimhan and Reddy (1971)], [Anderson (1968)], [Chang (1970)], [Chang (1971)], [DePalma and Yau (1975)], [Kickert and Koppelaar (1976)], [Agui and Nagahashi (1979)], [Berthod and Maroy (1979)], [Belaid and Haton (1984)], [Wang (1984)], [Nagahashi and Kakatsuyama (1986)], [Wolberg (1987)], [Stringa (1990)], [Zhao (1990)], [Lee *et al.* (1992)], [Vidal *et al.* (1992)], [Parizeau and Plamondon (1992)], [Parizeau *et al.* (1992)], [Parizeau and Plamondon (1995)], [Bunke *et al.* (1995)], [Fernau and Freund (1996)], [Kuroda *et al.* (1997)], [Oommen and Loke (1997)], [Fernau *et al.* (1998)], [Kaufmann and Bunke (1998)], [Pagallo (1998)], [Kuroda *et al.* (1999)], [Garain and Chaudhuri (2000)], [Malaviya and Peters (2000)], [Chan and Yeung (2000)], [Perez-Cortes *et al.* (2000)], [Chan and Yeung (2001)], [Marti and Bunke (2001)], [Vinciarelli *et al.* (2004)], [Zimmermann *et al.* (2006)], [Bertolami and Bunke (2008)], [España Boquera *et al.* (2011)], [Álvaro *et al.* (2014)], [Simistira *et al.* (2015)], [Álvaro *et al.* (2016)] |

Table 6.1 *(Continued)*

| Applications | Models | References |
|---|---|---|
| Structure analysis in bioinformatics | Regular grammars, stochastic context-free grammars, programmed context-free grammars, attributed grammars, hidden Markov models, precedence parsing, CYK parsing | [Ledley (1964)], [Ledley *et al.* (1965)], [Golab *et al.* (1971)], [Kirsch (1971)], [Fu and Huang (1972)], [Lee and Fu (1972)], [Thomason and Gonzales (1975)], [Brendel and Busse (1984)], [Tanaka *et al.* (1986)], [Head (1987)], [Collado-Vides (1989, 1992)], [Searls (1992, 1993, 1995, 1997, 2001, 2002)], [Dong and Searls (1994)], [Krogh *et al.* (1994a,b)], [Sakakibara *et al.* (1994)], [Bralley (1996)], [Brown and Wilson (1996)], [Kulp *et al.* (1996)], [Lefebvre (1996)], [Rosenblueth *et al.* (1996)], [Eddy (1998)], [Karplus *et al.* (1998)], [Yokomori and Kobayashi (1998)], [Knudsen and Heyn (1999)], [Brown (2000)], [Lyngso and Pedersen (2000)], [Reese *et al.* (2000)], [Rivas and Eddy (2000, 2001)], [Leung *et al.* (2001)], [Muggleton *et al.* (2001)], [Holmes and Rubin (2002)], [Pachter *et al.* (2002)], [Przytycka *et al.* (2002)], [Yandell and Majoros (2002)], [Ahola *et al.* (2003)], [Cai *et al.* (2003)], [Knudsen and Heyn (2003)], [Knudsen and Miyamoto (2003)], [Lottaz *et al.* (2003)], [Pedersen and Hein (2003)], [Dowell and Eddy (2004)], [Wistrand and Sonnhammer (2004)], [Do *et al.* (2005)], [Majoros *et al.* (2005)], [Sakakibara (2005a)], [Chuong *et al.* (2006)], [Munch and Krogh (2006)], [Wang *et al.* (2006b)], [Weinberg and Ruzzo (2006)], [Zhang *et al.* (2006)], [Bernardes *et al.* (2007)], [Brejová *et al.* (2007)], [Dill *et al.* (2007)], [Harmanci *et al.* (2007)], [Liang *et al.* (2007)], [Srivastava *et al.* (2007)], [Won *et al.* (2007)], [Peris *et al.* (2008)], [Yoon and Vaidyanathan (2008)], [Dyrka and Nebel (2009)], [Kato *et al.* (2009)], [Singh *et al.* (2009)], [Yoon (2009)], [Agarwal *et al.* (2010)], [Tsafnat *et al.* (2011)], [Anderson *et al.* (2012)], [Shen and Vikalo (2012)], [Dyrka *et al.* (2013)], [Ding *et al.* (2014)], [Wieczorek and Unold (2016)] |

Table 6.1 (*Continued*)

| Applications | Models | References |
|---|---|---|
| Medical image and signal analysis | Finite-state automata, context-free grammars, Shape Feature Languages, attributed automata, stochastic automata, fuzzy automata, *LR* parsing, Earley parsing, minimum-distance parsing | [Horowitz (1975, 1977)], [Stockman *et al.* (1976)], [Albus (1977)], [Belforte *et al.* (1979)], [Giese *et al.* (1979)], [Udupa and Murthy (1980)], [Birman (1982)], [Stockman and Kanal (1983)], [Pathak *et al.* (1984)], [Pathak and Pal (1986)], [Ferber (1986)], [Papakonstantinou *et al.* (1986)], [Skordalakis (1986)], [Juhola (1986)], [Trahanias *et al.* (1989)], [Gath and Schwartz (1989)], [Trahanias and Skordalakis (1990)], [Pedrycz (1990)], [Fred and Leitao (1992)], [Luo and Zhou (1992)], [Koski *et al.* (1995)], [Koski (1996, 1998)], [Pedrycz and Gacek (2001)], [Ogiela and Tadeusiewicz (1999, 2002, 2003)], [Tümer *et al.* (2003)], [Tadeusiewicz and Ogiela (2004)], [Bielecka *et al.* (2011)], [Zieliński *et al.* (2015)] |
| Speech recognition and natural language processing (NLP) | Regular grammars, stochastic finite-state automata, fuzzy finite-state automata, hidden Markov models, finite-state transducers, context-free grammars, stochastic grammars, Earley-Stolcke parsing, CYK parsing, *LR* parsing, error-correcting parsing | [Mori De (1972)], [Mori De *et al.* (1977)], [Rivoira and Torasso (1978, 1982)], [Kashyap (1979)], [Bahl *et al.* (1983)], [Jelinek (1985)], [Vidal *et al.* (1985)], [Tomita (1985, 1987)], [Miller and Levinson (1988)], [Fujisaki *et al.* (1989)], [Wright and Wrigley (1989)], [Casacuberta (1990)], [García *et al.* (1990a)], [Sharman *et al.* (1990)], [Wright (1990)], [Corazza *et al.* (1991)], [Jelinek and Lafferty (1991)], [Ney (1991)], [Segarra *et al.* (1992)], [Seneff (1992)], [Briscoe and Carroll (1993)], [Corazza *et al.* (1994)], [Gildea and Jurafsky (1995)], [Jurafsky *et al.* (1995)], [Shimizu *et al.* (1995)], [Stolcke (1995)], [Amengual and Vidal (1996)], [Castro and Casacuberta (1996)], [Jurafsky (1996)], [Mohri *et al.* (1996)], [Sánchez *et al.* (1996)], [Sproat *et al.* (1996)], [Takeda (1996)], [Mohri (1997)], [Wu (1997)], [Chi and Geman (1998)], [Hogenhout and Matsumoto (1998)], [Alshawi *et al.* (2000)], [Samuelsson (2000)], [Verdú-Mas *et al.* (2002)], [Varona and Torres (2000)], [Civera *et al.* (2004)], [Daciuk and Noord van (2004)], [Kermorvant *et al.* (2004)], [Murgue and Higuera de la (2004)], [Picó *et al.* (2004)], [Casacuberta *et al.* (2005)], [Klein and Manning (2005)], [Chiang (2007)], [Venugopal *et al.* (2007)], [Mohri *et al.* (2008)], [Knight and May (2009)], [Daciuk and Weiss (2012)], [Sánchez *et al.* (2018)] |

Table 6.1 *(Continued)*

| Applications | Models | References |
|---|---|---|
| Analysis of visual events and activities | Regular grammars, finite-state automata, context-free grammars, attributed grammars, stochastic grammars, attributed multiset grammars, hidden Markov models, stochastic automata, fuzzy automata, Earley parsing, Earley-Stolcke parsing | [Yamato *et al.* (1992)], [Clark (1994)], [Schlenzig *et al.* (1994)], [Wilson and Bobick (1995)], [Bobick and Wilson (1997)], [Grobel and Assan (1997)], [Starner *et al.* (1998)], [Aggarwal and Cai (1999)], [Ivanov and Bobick (2000)], [Hong *et al.* (2000)], [Vogler and Metaxas (2001)], [Yoon *et al.* (2001)], [Bauer and Kraiss (2002)], [Moore and Essa (20032)], [Minnen *et al.* (2003)], [Ramamoorthy *et al.* (2003)], [Cho *et al.* (2004)], [Gao *et al.* (2004)], [Nguyen *et al.* (2005)], [Ryoo and Aggarwal (2006)], [Joo and Chellappa (2006a)], [Joo and Chellappa (2006b)], [Wang *et al.* (2006a)], [Chen *et al.* (2008)], [Fang *et al.* (2007)], [Muñoz-Salinas *et al.* (2008)], [Bailador and Triviño (2010)], [Wang *et al.* (2010)], [Bhuyan *et al.* (2011)] [Zhan *et al.* (2011)], [Damen and Hogg (2012)], [Mohandes *et al.* (2012)], [Sanroma *et al.* (2012)], [González-Villanueva *et al.* (2013)], [Sadeghipour and Kopp (2014)], [Sanroma *et al.* (2014)], [Xu and Man (2015)], [Kumar *et al.* (2017)], [Guo *et al.* (2018)], [Zhang *et al.* (2018)] |
| Signal analysis for process monitoring and control | Finite-state automata, pushdown automata, dynamically programmed grammars and automata, *DPLL* parsing, hidden Markov models, context-free grammars, stochastic grammars, timed automata, real-time automata | [Fu (1970)], [Vernadat *et al.* (1982)], [Ramadge and Wonham (1987)], [Cieslak *et al.* (1988)], [Ozveren and Willsky (1990)], [Balemi *et al.* (1993)], [Behrens *et al.* (1994)], [Flasiński (1994, 1995a)], [Rengaswamy and Venkatasubramanian (1995)], [Sampath *et al.* (1995)], [Sampath *et al.* (1996)], [Kwon and Kim (1999)], [Flasiński and Jurek (1999)], [Charbonnier *et al.* (1999)], [Jurek (2000, 2004, 2005)], [Ertunc *et al.* (2001)], [Lunze and Schröder (2001)], [Lunze and Supavatanakul (2002)], [D'Souza and Madhusudan (2002)], [Torre La *et al.* (2002)], [Tripakis (2002)], [Bouyer *et al.* (2003)], [Hashtrudi Zad *et al.* (2003)], [Su *et al.* (2004)], [Bouyer *et al.* (2005)], [Supavatanakul *et al.* (2006)], [Miao and Makis (2007)], [Thompson and Flynn (2007)], [Yan *et al.* (2009)], [Cassandras and Lafortune (2010)], [Maier *et al.* (2011)], [Verwer *et al.* (2011)], [Komenda *et al.* (2012)], [Niggemann *et al.* (2012)], [Geyik *et al.* (2013)], [Raisch (2013)], [Waez *et al.* (2013)], [Klerx *et al.* (2014)], [Schmuck *et al.* (2014)], [Schneider *et al.* (2014)], [Komenda *et al.* (2015)], [Priesterjahn *et al.* (2015)], [Senin *et al.* (2015)], [Lin *et al.* (2016)], [Schmuck *et al.* (2016)], [Husen *et al.* (2017)], [Zhang *et al.* (2017)], [Luh *et al.* (2018)] |

Table 6.1 (*Continued*)

| Applications | Models | References |
|---|---|---|
| Architectural object analysis | Context-free grammars, attributed grammars, stochastic grammars, shape grammars, split grammars, constraint multiset grammars, CYK parsing, Earley parsing | [Stiny and Mitchell (1978)], [Downing and Flemming (1981)], [Koning and Eizenberg (1981)], [Knight (1981)], [Flemming (1981)], [Wonka *et al.* (2003)], [Alegre and Dellaert (2004)], [Duarte (2005)], [Müller *et al.* (2007)], [Ripperda and Brenner (2007)], [Becker and Haala (2009)], [Koutsourakis *et al.* (2009)], [Hohmann *et al.* (2010)], [Toshev *et al.* (2010)], [Vanegas *et al.* (2010)], [Mathias *et al.* (2011)], [Riemenschneider *et al.* (2012)], [Simon *et al.* (2012)], [Yang *et al.* (2012)], [Boulch *et al.* (2013)], [Martinović and Gool Van (2013)], [Musialski *et al.* (2013)], [Teboul *et al.* (2013)], [Liu *et al.* (2014)], [Weissenberg (2014)], [Wu *et al.* (2014)], [Gadde *et al.* (2016)] |
| Feature recognition for computer aided design and manufacturing | Finite-state automata, context-free grammars, Shape Feature Languages, attributed grammars, *LR* parsing, Earley parsing | [Jakubowski and Kasprzak (1977)], [Jakubowski (1982, 1985, 1986, 1990)], [Jakubowski and Flasiński (1992)], [Kyprianou (1980)], [Staley *et al.* (1983)], [Choi *et al.* (1984)], [Srinivasan *et al.* (1985)], [Joshi and Chang (1990)], [Mullins and Rinderle (1991)], [Rinderle (1991)], [Mandorli *et al.* (1993)], [Brown *et al.* (1995)], [Kulkarni and Pande (1995)], [Prabhu (1999)], [Arivazhagan *et al.* (2008)], [Sass (2008)] |
| Structure analysis in chemistry | Context-free grammars, attributed grammars, context-sensitive grammars | [Fehder and Barnett (1965)], [Tauber and Rankin (1972)], [Smith and Baker (1975)], [Barnard *et al.* (1981)], [Lynch *et al.* (1981)], [Krishnamurthy and Lynch (1981)], [Welford *et al.* (1981)], [Wiswesser (1982)], [Barnard *et al.* (1984)], [Weininger (1988)], [Ash *et al.* (1997)], [Weininger (2003)], [Homer *et al.* (2008)], [Sidorova and Anisimova (2014)], [Sidorova and Garcia (2015)], [Heller *et al.* (2015)], [Sagar and Sidorova (2016)] |
| Radar signal analysis | Finite-state automata, context-free grammars, stochastic grammars, error-correcting parsing, Earley-Stolcke parsing | [Barnard (1989)], [Sands and Garber (1990)], [Bhatnagar *et al.* (2000)], [Visnevski *et al.* (2007)], [Turnbaugh *et al.* (2008)], [Wang and Krishnamurthy (2008)], [Wang *et al.* (2011)], [Fanaswala and Krishnamurthy (2013)], [Fanaswala and Krishnamurthy (2014)] |

Table 6.1 (*Continued*)

| Applications | Models | References |
|---|---|---|
| Pattern recognition in seismology | Regular grammars, attributed grammars, stochastic grammars, finite-state automata, error-correcting parsing, Earley parsing | [Liu and Fu (1982)], [Anderson (1982)], [Liu and Fu (1983)], [Huang and Fu (1985a)], [Huang and Fu (1985b)], [Huang and Leu (1992)], [Huang (1992)], [Huang and Leu (1995)], [Huang (2002)] |
| Structure analysis in geology | Regular grammars, context-free grammars, stochastic grammars, attributed grammars, finite-state automata | [Griffiths (1990)], [Duan et al. (1996)], [Duan et al. (1999)], [Hill and Griffiths (2007)], [Hill and Griffiths (2008)], [Hill and Griffiths (2009)] |
| Fingerprint recognition | Finite-state automata, context-free grammars, stochastic grammars, programmed grammars | [Moayer and Fu (1975)], [Moayer and Fu (1976a)], [Rao and Balck (1980)], [Chang and Fan (2002)], [Yager and Amin (2004)] |
| Financial and economics time series analysis | Context-free grammars, context-sensitive grammars, hidden Markov models | [Pau (1991)] , [Gianotti (1993)], [Batyrshin et al. (2007)] , [Bicego et al. (2008)] |
| Image processing | Context-free grammars, stochastic automata | [Krishnamoorthy et al. (1993)], [Sastry and Thathachar (1994)], [Siskind et al. (2007)] |

# PART 3
# TREE-BASED MODELS

# Chapter 7

# Pattern Recognition Based on Tree Languages

Whereas the theory of string languages has been developed mainly for applications in the areas of programming languages and compiler design, tree grammars and automata were introduced in the mid 1960s for solving decidability problems within second order logic [Doner (1965); Thatcher and Wright (1968)]. A tree grammar is generalization of a string grammar, i.e. its left- and right-hand sides are trees. *Regular tree grammars* were introduced in [Brainerd (1969)][1] Their left-hand sides consist of one-node trees labelled with nonterminal symbols.

*Finite-state tree automata* are defined for these grammars. They differ from finite-state (string) automata in that they walk along tree paths, somehow, in parallel. So, they are in "more than one state at a given moment." In other words, we can say a tree is parsed with more than one reading head. There are two basic classes of finite-state tree automata. A *frontier-to-root automaton* (*bottom-up tree automaton*) [Doner (1965); Thatcher and Wright (1968)] parses a tree starting from the leaves upward to the root. A *root-to-frontier automaton* (*top-down tree automaton*) [Rabin (1969)] performs parsing in the opposite direction.[2]

*Context-free tree grammars* were defined in [Rounds (1970)]. Their left-hand sides are in the form of two-level trees. Two types of context-free tree languages are distinguished according to a way the trees are derived [Engelfriet and Schmidt (1977, 1978)]. For *OI-tree languages* (*outside-in*) a production is applied to a node $v$ such that none of the ancestors of $v$ is nonterminal node. For *IO-tree languages* (*inside-out*) a production is applied to a node $v$ such that none of the descendants of $v$ is a nonterminal node. For CF tree languages, top-down pushdown tree automata [Guessarian (1983)] and bottom-up tree pushdown automata [Schimpf (1982); Schimpf and Gallier (1985)], which are analogous to string $LL$ and $LR$ syntax analyzers (respectively), were defined. *Tree transducers* were introduced in [Rounds (1968); Thatcher (1970)] and investigated in [Baker (1978, 1979)].

Although the theory of tree languages has been developed intensively for the last

---

[1]The notion of Brainerd's *regular tree systems* differs from the definition of *regular tree grammars* assumed nowadays.

[2]There are also classes of tree automata using other strategies of parsing, e.g., two-way automata, tree-walking automata.

179

few decades and delivering important results [Gécseg and Steinby (1984); Comon *et al.* (2007)], research has focused on theoretical issues rather than on the practical applications. Therefore, although the predominance of tree syntax analyzers over string ones had been noticed in syntactic pattern recognition already in the early 1970s [Fu and Bhargava (1973); Fu (1976b)], novel models had to be developed, mainly by K. S. Fu and his collaborators, in order to solve problems in this area.

Tree models allow one to express various inter-primitive relations contrary to string models which use only the concatenation relation. This results in a greater complexity of tree automata which have to parse structures with a partial ordering only, contrary to the linearly-ordered structures analyzed by string automata. However, as it turned out already in the 1970s, this is not the crucial problem in the case of pattern recognition. The main effort was concentrated on carrying out research into the recognition of distorted patterns. Therefore, tree models which are analogous to the string ones presented in Sec. 3.3 were developed. These models were worked out on the basis of finite-state tree automata because of their computational efficiency. The first *stochastic finite tree automaton* was defined in 1980 [Fu (1980a)]. Two basic types of *error-correcting finite tree automata*, namely the structure-preserved ones (*SPECTA*) which do not encompass modifications of tree structure and the generalized ones (*GECTA*) allowing for structural modifications, were defined in [Lu and Fu (1976)] and [Lu and Fu (1978)], respectively. Fuzzy tree automata were presented in [Lee (1982)]. In [López *et al.* (2000)] a novel approach for the constructing error-correcting tree automata was proposed.

*Tree Adjoining Languages* introduced in [Joshi *et al.* (1975); Joshi (1985)] are also an important class of languages in syntactic pattern recognition, which is mainly used in NLP, image analysis and bioinformatics.

Before we present tree automata we shall introduce the notions concerning tree structures [Gorn (1967); Brainerd (1969); Fu (1982); Gécseg and Steinby (1984)].

Let $\mathcal{U} = (\mathbb{N}_+, \bullet, \lambda)$, where $\mathbb{N}_+$ is the set of positive integers, $\bullet$ is the operation, $\lambda$ is the identity, be the free monoid. Let us introduce the partial ordering $\leq$ on $\mathcal{U}$ in the following way. $x \leq y$, $x, y \in \mathcal{U}$ iff there exists $z \in \mathcal{U}$ such that $x \bullet z = y$. $x$ and $y$ are incomparable iff $x \nleq y$ and $y \nleq x$. $\mathcal{U}$ is called the *Gorn universal tree domain* and it is shown in Fig. 7.1a.

A subset $D \subset \mathcal{U}$ is a *tree domain* iff for all $x, y \in \mathcal{U}$ and all $i, j \in \mathbb{N}_+$ the following conditions are satisfied: (1) if $x \bullet y \in D$ then $x \in D$ and (2) if $x \bullet j \in D$ and $i \leq j$ then $x \bullet i \in D$. The *root* is represented by $\lambda$. The *leaves* are the nodes which are maximal with respect to $\leq$. The example of a tree domain is shown in Fig. 7.1b.

Let $\mathbb{N}$ be the set of nonnegative integers, $A$ be a finite subset of $\mathbb{N}$. A *ranked alphabet* is a pair $(\Sigma, r)$, where $\Sigma$ is a finite alphabet, $r : \Sigma \to 2^A$ is a rank multi-valued mapping. $n \in r(a), a \in \Sigma$ is called the rank of $a$. We denote $\Sigma_n = \{a : n \in r(a)\}$. (If we are considering the alphabet of terminal symbols $\Sigma_T$, we write $\Sigma_{T,n}$.)

A *tree* over $(\Sigma, r)$ is a function $t : D \to \Sigma$, $D$ is a tree domain, such that: (1) $t(x) \in \Sigma_0$, if $x$ is a leaf in $D$ and (2) $t(x) \in \Sigma_n$, where $n = max\{i \in \mathbb{N}_+ : x \bullet i \in D\}$,

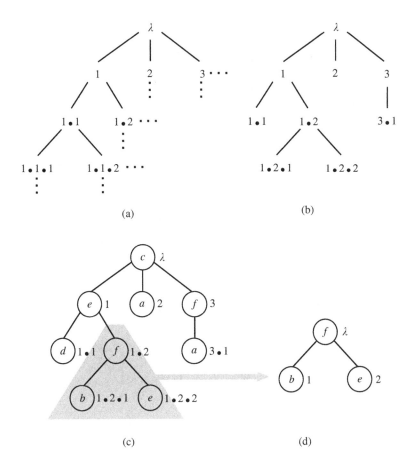

Fig. 7.1 (a) The Gorn universal tree domain. (b) Example of a tree domain. (c) Example of a tree. (d) Example of a subtree.

otherwise. The domain of a tree $t$ is denoted by $D_t$. The set of all finite trees over $\Sigma$ is denoted by $T_\Sigma$. A *node* is a pair $(x, a) \in D \times \Sigma$, where $x$ is called an *address*. A node $(x, a)$ is called a *parent* of a node $(x \bullet i, b)$, $i \in \mathbb{N}_+$. A node $(x \bullet i, b)$ is called a *child* of a node $(x, a)$. The example of a tree (for a domain depicted in Fig. 7.1b) is shown in Fig. 7.1c. The *frontier* of $t$ is the sequence of its leaves.

Let $t \in T_\Sigma$ and $x \in D_t$. The subtree of $t$ at $x$, denoted $t/x$, is defined by the function which is the set of pairs $\{(y, a) : (x \bullet y, a) \in t, \ a \in \Sigma\}$. For example, if a tree shown in Fig. 7.1c is denoted with $t$ then its subtree at $1 \bullet 2$, denoted $t/1 \bullet 2$, is shown in Fig. 7.1d. (Let us notice that the addresses of this subtree are created by removing the prefix $1 \bullet 2$.)

In most further examples addresses will not be presented for trees in figures. For a notational convenience we will use the bracketed Polish prefix notation. For example, the tree shown in Fig. 7.1c will be represented as $c(e(df(be))af(a))$.

In the area of syntactic pattern recognition tree-based models have been used,

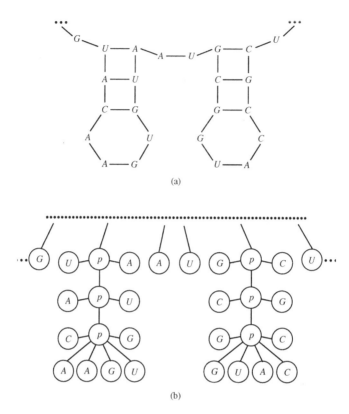

(a)

(b)

Fig. 7.2   (a) Example of a part of an RNA-like structure. (b) Its tree representation.

among others, for circuit verification, image understanding, texture analysis, optical character recognition, satellite data interpretation, tissue analysis in histopathology, RNA structure analysis (see Fig. 7.2 in which the example of the *extended RNA forest representation* [Höchsmann *et al.* (2003)] is shown), chemical structure recognition, fingerprint identification, protein structure prediction, seismic pattern recognition, urban architecture analysis and reconstruction. These applications will be presented in Chap. 9.

The classic methods of syntactic pattern recognition which are based on tree languages are presented in the following sections. Bottom-up finite tree automata for expansive tree languages are introduced in Sec. 7.1. Two types of structure-preserved error-correcting tree automata (SPECTA), i.e., minimum-distance SPECTA and maximum-likelihood SPECTA, are defined in Sections 7.2 and 7.3, respectively. Generalized error-correcting tree automata (GECTA) are presented in Sec. 7.4. Tree Adjoining Grammars (TAGs) are introduced in Sec. 7.5. The last section contains remarks on tree automata.

## 7.1 Recognition of Expansive Tree Languages

Let us define regular tree grammars [Brainerd (1969); Gécseg and Steinby (1984)].

**Definition 7.1 (Regular Tree Grammar):** A regular tree grammar over $(\Sigma_T, r)$ is a quintuple

$$G = (\Sigma_N, \Sigma_T, r, P, S), \text{ where}$$

$\Sigma_N$ is a finite set of nonterminal symbols,
$(\Sigma_T, r)$ is a ranked alphabet of terminal symbols, $\Sigma_N \cap \Sigma_T = \emptyset$, $\Sigma = \Sigma_N \cup \Sigma_T$,
$P$ is a set of productions of the form: $X \to t$, $X \in \Sigma_N$ and $t \in T_\Sigma$ is such that
nonterminal symbols may appear at the leaves only,
$S \in \Sigma_N$ is the start symbol.

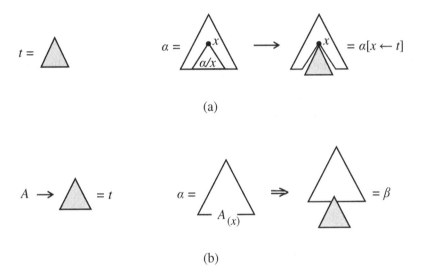

(a)

(b)

Fig. 7.3 (a) Replacement of a subtree and (b) derivation in regular tree grammar.

Let us note that for every tree belonging to a derivation in a regular tree grammar nonterminal symbols may appear at the leaves only according to Definition 7.1.

We will introduce the notion of a derivation step as a kind of more general notion of subtree replacement. (Subtree replacements will be used for defining error transformations on trees in Sec. 7.4.) Let $\alpha, t \in T_\Sigma$ and $x \in D_\alpha$. The *replacement* of the subtree $\alpha/x$ by $t$, denoted $\alpha[x \leftarrow t]$, is the tree defined by the function which is the set of pairs (see Fig. 7.3a)

$$\{(y, \alpha(y)) : y \in D_\alpha \, , \; x \text{ is not a prefix of } y\} \cup \{(x \bullet z, t(z)) : z \in D_t\} \, .$$

Let $\alpha, \beta \in T_\Sigma$ and $x \in D_\alpha$. We say that $\alpha$ directly derives $\beta$ in a regular tree grammar $G$, denoted $\alpha \underset{G}{\Longrightarrow} \beta$, iff there exists $A \to t \in P$ such that $\alpha(x) = A$ and

$\beta = \alpha[x \leftarrow t]$ (see Fig. 7.3b).

The reflexive and transitive closure of the relation $\underset{G}{\Longrightarrow}$, denoted $\underset{G}{\overset{*}{\Longrightarrow}}$, is called a derivation in $G$. The tree language generated by the grammar $G$ is the set

$$L(G) = \{\phi \in T_{\Sigma_T} : S \underset{G}{\overset{*}{\Longrightarrow}} \phi\}.$$

Now, we shall define expansive tree grammars [Brainerd (1969)] which were used for constructing models of fingerprint recognition [Moayer and Fu (1976b)], satellite data interpretation [Li and Fu (1976)] and optical character recognition [Fu and Bhargava (1973)].

**Definition 7.2 (Expansive Tree Grammar):** Let $G = (\Sigma_N, \Sigma_T, r, P, S)$ be a regular tree grammar. $G$ is called an expansive tree grammar (a tree grammar in normal form) iff each production is of the form:

$$X_0 \rightarrow a(X_1 X_2 \ldots X_n) \text{ or } X_0 \rightarrow a,$$

where $a \in \Sigma_{T,n}$, $X_0, X_1, X_2, \ldots, X_n \in \Sigma_N$.

The requirement introduced by Definition 7.2 is not restrictive because of the following theorem.

**Theorem 7.1 (Regular and Expansive Grammars [Brainerd (1969)])**

*For each regular tree grammar $G$, an expansive tree grammar $\bar{G}$ such that $L(G) = L(\bar{G})$ can be effectively constructed.*

For example, we define the following expansive tree grammar.
$G = (\Sigma_N, \Sigma_T, r, P, S)$, where:
$\Sigma_N = \{S, A, B, C\}$,
$\Sigma_T = \{a, b, c\}$, $r(a) = \{0, 2\}$, $r(b) = \{0, 1\}$, $r(c) = \{0, 1, 2\}$,
$P$ consists of the following productions (see Fig. 7.4a):

    (1) $S \rightarrow c(AB)$    (3) $B \rightarrow b(B)$    (5) $A \rightarrow a$    (7) $C \rightarrow c$

    (2) $A \rightarrow a(AC)$    (4) $C \rightarrow c(C)$    (6) $B \rightarrow b$

Let us derive the tree $t = c(a(ac(c))b(b))$ in the grammar $G$ as it is shown in Fig. 7.4b. (The following sequence of productions is applied: 1, 2, 3, 5, 4, 6, 7.)

$S \Rightarrow c(AB) \Rightarrow c(a(AC)B) \Rightarrow c(a(AC)b(B)) \Rightarrow c(a(aC)b(B)) \Rightarrow$
$\Rightarrow c(a(ac(C))b(B)) \Rightarrow c(a(ac(C))b(b)) \Rightarrow c(a(ac(c))b(b))$

Patterns represented with trees generated by expansive tree grammars can be analyzed with the help of frontier-to-root (bottom-up) finite tree automata [Brainerd (1968)] which are defined in the following way:

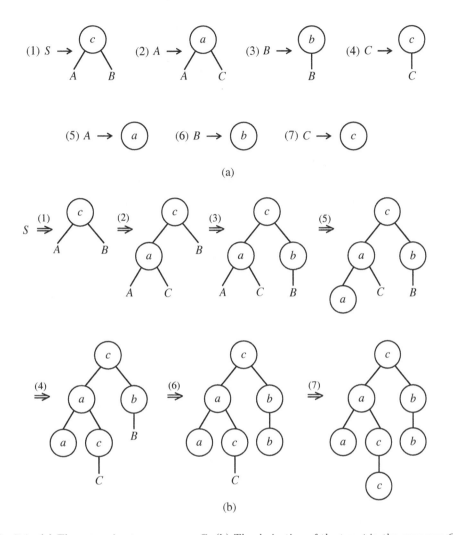

Fig. 7.4 (a) The expansive tree grammar $G$. (b) The derivation of the tree $t$ in the grammar $G$.

## Parsing Scheme 7.1: Frontier-to-Root Finite Tree Automaton

A frontier-to-root (bottom-up) deterministic finite tree automaton is a quintuple

$$A = (Q, \Sigma_T, r, \delta, Q_F), \text{ where}$$

$Q$ is a finite set of states,
$(\Sigma_T, r)$ is a ranked alphabet of input symbols,
$\delta$ is a family $\{\delta_a^n : a \in \Sigma_{T,n}, \ n \in \mathbb{N}\}$ of transition functions

$$\delta_a^n : Q^n \longrightarrow Q ,$$

$Q_F \subset Q$ is the set of final states.

If $n$ is obvious from the context, we write $\delta_a$ instead of $\delta_a^n$.

In order to represent the analyzing of trees by frontier-to-root automata let us define the *response mapping* $\varrho : T_\Sigma \longrightarrow Q$ in the following way:

(1) If $a \in \Sigma_{T,0}$ then $\varrho(a) = \delta_a$.

(2) If $a \in \Sigma_{T,n}$ , $n > 0$ then $\varrho(a(X_1 X_2 \ldots X_n)) = \delta_a(\varrho(X_1), \varrho(X_2), \ldots, \varrho(X_n))$.

The tree language accepted by the frontier-to-root automaton $A$ is the set

$$L(A) = \{\phi \in T_{\Sigma_T} : \varrho(\phi) \in Q_F\}.$$

Now, we can define the automaton $A$ for our expansive grammar $G$ in the following way[3].

$A = (Q, \Sigma_T, r, \delta, Q_F)$, where:

$Q = \{S, A, B, C\}$,

$\Sigma_T = \{a, b, c\}$, $r(a) = \{0, 2\}$, $r(b) = \{0, 1\}$, $r(c) = \{0, 1, 2\}$,

$Q_F = \{S\}$,

$\delta$ is defined as follows:

$$\delta_c(A, B) = S \quad \delta_b(B) = B \quad \delta_a = A \quad (7)\ \delta_c = C$$

$$\delta_a(A, C) = A \quad \delta_c(C) = C \quad \delta_b = B$$

For example, let us analyze the tree $t = c(a(ac(c))b(b))$ shown in Fig. 7.4b.
$\varrho(c(a(ac(c))b(b))) = \delta_c(\varrho(a(ac(c))), \varrho(b(b))) = \delta_c(\delta_a(\varrho(a), \varrho(c(c))), \delta_b(\varrho(b))) = \delta_c(\delta_a(\delta_a, \delta_c(\varrho(c))), \delta_b(\delta_b)) = \delta_c(\delta_a(\delta_a, \delta_c(\delta_c)), \delta_b(\delta_b)) = \delta_c(\delta_a(A, \delta_c(C)), \delta_b(B)) = \delta_c(\delta_a(A, C), B) = \delta_c(A, B) = S$

$A$ is really a frontier-to-root automaton, because it starts analyzing of $t$ at leaves of $t$ (i.e. at the frontier of $t$) and processes upward until it reaches the root of $t$.

## 7.2 Minimum-Distance SPECTA Model

In Sec. 3.3 we have discussed the issue of the recognition of distorted patterns. We have presented the error-correcting parsing approach to the analysis of such patterns in Sec. 3.3.3. As we will see in this section this approach can be extended from string languages to tree languages. First of all, we introduce the preliminary notions [Lu and Fu (1976)] which are analogous to those presented in Sec. 3.3.3.

Let $T_{\Sigma_T}^D = \{\alpha : \alpha \in T_{\Sigma_T}, D_\alpha = D\}$ be the set of trees in the domain $D$, $\mathcal{F} : T_{\Sigma_T}^D \longmapsto T_{\Sigma_T}^D$ be a *tree transformation*.

Let $x \in D$, $a \in \Sigma_T$ and $\alpha, \alpha' \in T_{\Sigma_T}^D$. A tree transformation $S_{(x,a)}(\alpha) = \alpha'$ such that $\alpha'$ is the result of substituting the label $b \in \Sigma_T$ $b \neq a$ of the node $(x, b)$ of the tree $\alpha$ by the label $a$ is called a *label substitution error transformation*.

Let us introduce the notion of an expanded regular tree grammar which generates also patterns containing label substitution errors.

---

[3]Comparing the productions of $G$ with the transitions of $A$, one can easily guess the rules of constructing $A$ on the basis of $G$.

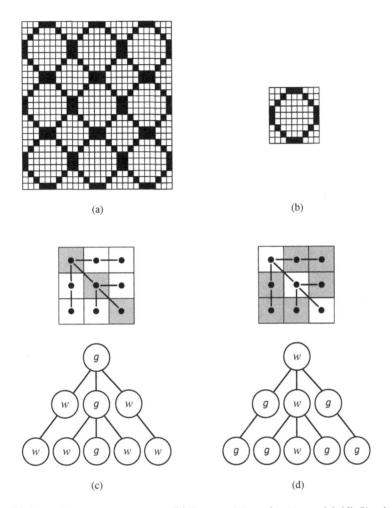

Fig. 7.5 (a) Exemplary texture pattern. (b) Its repetitive subpattern. (c)-(d) Simple texture patterns and their tree representations.

**Definition 7.3 (Expanded Tree Grammar):** Let $G = (\Sigma_N, \Sigma_T, r, P, S)$ be a (reference) expansive tree grammar. $G' = (\Sigma_N, \Sigma'_T, r', P', S)$ is called an expanded regular tree grammar for $G$ iff

$\Sigma_T \subseteq \Sigma'_T$,

$r$ is the restriction of $r'$ to $\Sigma_T$, i.e. $r'|_{\Sigma_T} = r$,

$P' = P \cup P_S$, where

$P_S = \{X_0 \rightarrow b(X_1 \ldots X_n) : X_0 \rightarrow a(X_1 \ldots X_n) \in P,\ a \in \Sigma_{T,n},\ b \in \Sigma'_{T,n},$
$a \neq b\} \cup \{X_0 \rightarrow b : X_0 \rightarrow a \in P,\ a \in \Sigma_{T,0},\ b \in \Sigma'_{T,0},\ a \neq b\}.$

The language generated by the expanded tree grammar $G'$ consists of trees which belong to the language generated by the reference grammar, $L(G)$, and their distortions resulting from label substitution errors. That is,

$$L(G') = \{\alpha' : \alpha' \in T_{\Sigma'_T} \text{ and there exists } \alpha \in L(G) \text{ such that } D_{\alpha'} = D_\alpha\}.$$

Now, we shall consider the example of applying expanded grammars for *texture analysis*. We define texture as the visual characteristics of a surface treated as a structure composed of interwoven (repetitive) elements. These elements can be considered, in turn, as variations of the visual pattern, sometimes called a *texel* (for texture element). Texture analysis is applied for materials inspection, tissue analysis, terrain classification and the like. The example of idealized texture is shown in Fig. 7.5a and its texel is shown in Fig. 7.5b.

Let us assume that we want to generate two texture elements defined with $3 \times 3$ windows and shown in Fig. 7.5 c and d. The scheme of spanning trees in pattern windows and tree representations of two elements are shown in this figure as well (the terminal label $g$ means grey, while the terminal label $w$ means white). We define the following expanded regular tree grammar $G' = (\Sigma_N, \Sigma'_T, r', P', S)$ which generates the tree language consisting of these two elements.

$\Sigma_N = \{S, C_1, C_2, D_1, D_2, G, W\}$,

$\Sigma'_T = \{g, w\}$,   $r'(g) = \{0, 1, 3\}$,   $r'(w) = \{0, 1, 3\}$,

$P' = P \cup P_S$ , where

$P$ consists of the following productions generating the texture elements (see Fig. 7.6a):

| | | |
|---|---|---|
| (1) $S \rightarrow g(C_1C_2C_1)$ | (4) $S \rightarrow w(D_1D_2D_1)$ | (7) $W \rightarrow w$ |
| (2) $C_1 \rightarrow w(W)$ | (5) $D_1 \rightarrow g(G)$ | (8) $G \rightarrow g$ |
| (3) $C_2 \rightarrow g(WGW)$ | (6) $D_2 \rightarrow w(GWG)$ | |

$P_S$ consists of the following productions generating distortions of the texture elements (see Fig. 7.6b):

| | | |
|---|---|---|
| (9) $S \rightarrow w(C_1C_2C_1)$ | (12) $S \rightarrow g(D_1D_2D_1)$ | (15) $W \rightarrow g$ |
| (10) $C_1 \rightarrow g(W)$ | (13) $D_1 \rightarrow w(G)$ | (16) $G \rightarrow w$ |
| (11) $C_2 \rightarrow w(WGW)$ | (14) $D_2 \rightarrow g(GWG)$ | |

The main idea of the minimum-distance structure-preserved error-correcting tree automaton, SPECTA, consists in finding the most similar tree $\alpha \in L(G)$ for a given tree $\alpha'$.

The distance $\rho(\alpha, \alpha')$ between the trees $\alpha, \alpha' \in T^D_{\Sigma_T}$ is defined as the smallest number of the label substitution error transformations $S$ required to obtain the tree $\alpha'$ from the tree $\alpha$. Thus, for a given tree $\alpha'$ SPECTA searches for a tree $\alpha \in L(G)$ such that

$$\rho(\alpha, \alpha') = \min_\beta\{\rho(\beta, \alpha') : \beta \in L(G), \ D_\beta = D_{\alpha'}\} \ .$$

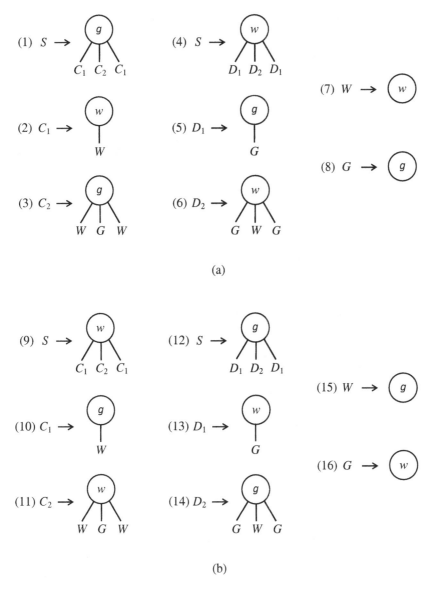

Fig. 7.6   (a) Productions generating the texture elements. (b) Productions generating distortions of the texture elements.

The tree $\alpha$ is called the minimum-distance correction of $\alpha'$ in $L(G)$. $\rho(\alpha, \alpha')$ is called the distance between $\alpha'$ and $L(G)$, denoted by $\rho(L(G), \alpha')$.

The minimum-distance SPECTA constructs the tree-like transition table $I$ for the input tree $\alpha'$. The table $I$ is constructed according to the frontier-to-root parsing of $\alpha'$. Each element $I(x)$ of the table corresponds to a node $(x, a)$ of $\alpha'$ and it contains a set of items of the form $[X, d, k]$, where $X$ is a candidate state of the node $(x, a)$, $d$ is the minimum number of label substitution errors in the subtree $\alpha'/x$ when $(x, a)$ is represented by $X$, and $k$ is the index of the production used.

Let us present the minimum-distance SPECTA algorithm. (Its functions are defined below.)

---

**Parsing Scheme 7.2: Minimum-Distance SPECTA**

/* Expanded tree grammar: $G = (\Sigma_N, \Sigma_T, r, P, S)$;  Input tree: $\alpha$  */
$error := 0$;
$accept := 0$;
**repeat**
  $(x, a) := give\_next\_node(\alpha)$;
  **if** $a$ **in** $\Sigma_T$ **then**
    **begin**
      **if** $rank(x) = 0$ **then**
        **begin**
          **for each** $(k)$ $X_0 \to a$ **in** $P$ **do** $add([X_0, 0, k], I(x))$;
          **for each** $(k)$ $X_0 \to b$ **in** $P$ **do** $add([X_0, 1, k], I(x))$;
        **end**;
      **else** /* $rank(x) > 0$  */
        **begin**
          $n := rank(x)$;
          **for each** $(k)$ $X_0 \to a(X_1 X_2 \ldots X_n)$ **in** $P$ **do**
            **if** $reduction\_possible(k, x, I)$ **then**
              **begin**
                $d := sum\_of\_children\_distances(k, x, I)$;
                $add([X_0, d, k], I(x))$;
              **end**;
          **for each** $(k)$ $X_0 \to b(X_1 X_2 \ldots X_n)$ **in** $P$ **and** $b \neq a$ **do**
            **if** $reduction\_possible(k, x, I)$ **then**
              **begin**
                $d := sum\_of\_children\_distances(k, x, I) + 1$;
                $add([X_0, d, k], I(x))$;
              **end**;
          **if** $is\_empty(I(x))$ **then** $error := 1$ **else** $delete\_redund\_items(I(x))$;
        **end**;
    **end**;
  **else** $error := 1$;
**until** $is\_root(x)$ **or** $error = 1$;
**if** $[S, u, m]$ **in** $I(\lambda)$ **then** $accept := 1$ **else** $error := 1$;  /* $\rho(L(G), \alpha) = u$ */

---

The functions of Scheme 7.2 are defined as follows.

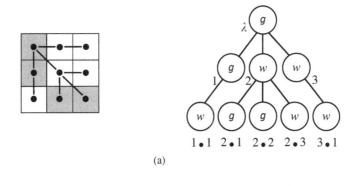

(a)

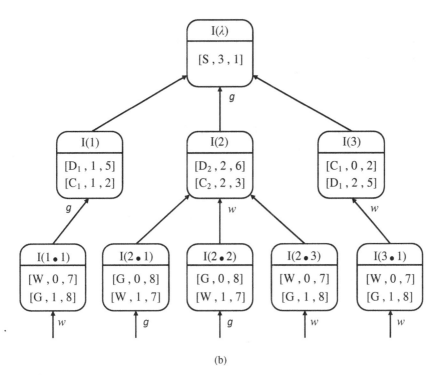

(b)

Fig. 7.7 (a) Distorted texture pattern and its tree $t$. (b) Transition table of the tree $t$.

- *give_next_node*($\alpha$) - the function gives the succeeding node of tree $\alpha$ (i.e., the next one with each succeeding call), traversing the tree in the frontier-to-root manner, specifically using the inverse breadth-first search (BFS) traversal,
- *rank*($x$) - the function gives the number of children of the node having the address $x$,
- *add*($[X, d, k], I(x)$) - the function adds item $[X, d, k]$ to element $I(x)$ of the transition table,
- *reduction_possible*($k, x, I$) - for production ($k$) $X_0 \rightarrow a(X_1 X_2 \ldots X_n)$, the

function checks whether $[X_1, d_1, k_1] \in I(x \bullet 1)$, $[X_2, d_2, k_2] \in I(x \bullet 2), \ldots,$ $[X_n, d_n, k_n] \in I(x \bullet n)$,

- *sum_of_children_distances*$(k, x, I)$ - for production $(k)$ $X_0 \rightarrow a(X_1 X_2 \ldots X_n)$ such that $[X_1, d_1, k_1] \in I(x \bullet 1)$, $[X_2, d_2, k_2] \in I(x \bullet 2), \ldots, [X_n, d_n, k_n] \in I(x \bullet n)$, the function gives the sum $d_1 + d_2 + \ldots + d_n$,
- *is_empty*$(W)$ - the Boolean function which checks whether set $W$ is empty,
- *delete_redund_items*$(I(x))$ - if element $I(x)$ contains many items with the same state $X$ (i.e., items $[X, d, k]$), the function delete items with larger numbers of errors (i.e., for each state only the item with the minimum distance is preserved),
- *is_root*$(x)$ - the Boolean function which checks whether the node having address $x$ is the root (i.e., $x = \lambda$).

For example, for the tree $t$ representing the distorted texture pattern shown in Fig. 7.7a, the algorithm generates the transition table shown in Fig. 7.7b. One can easily see *three* distortions in this tree with respect to the closest (reference) pattern which is shown in Fig. 7.5c. These errors occur for nodes having addresses: 1, 2 and $2 \bullet 1$. Therefore, the transition table contains item $[S, 3, 1]$ in $I(\lambda)$.

## 7.3   Maximum-Likelihood SPECTA Model

As we have discussed in Sec. 3.3, if statistical information for estimating the probability distribution of patterns is available, stochastic grammars can be used. In this section we introduce stochastic tree grammars and corresponding maximum-likelihood SPECTAs [Lu and Fu (1976)]. Let us introduce the following preliminary notions [Bhargava and Fu (1974a); Lu and Fu (1976); Fu (1980a, 1982)].

**Definition 7.4 (Expansive Stochastic Tree Grammar):** An expansive stochastic tree grammar over $(\Sigma_T, r)$ is a quintuple

$$G = (\Sigma_N, \Sigma_T, r, P, S), \text{ where}$$

$\Sigma_N$, $\Sigma_T$, $r$, $S$ are defined as in Definition 7.1,
$P$ is a set of productions of the form:

$$A_i \xrightarrow{p_{ij}} t_{ij}, \quad i = 1, \ldots, n, \; j = 1, \ldots, m_i,$$

in which $A_i \in \Sigma_N$ , $t_{ij} \in T_\Sigma$ is a tree which either consists of a terminal root and its nonterminal children or consists of a terminal node (i.e. $t_{ij}$ is of the form either $a(X_1 X_2 \ldots X_n)$ or $a$, $a \in \Sigma_{T,n}$, $X_1, X_2, \ldots, X_n \in \Sigma_N$), $p_{ij}$ is the probability related to the application of the production such that

$$0 < p_{ij} \leq 1 \;\; , \;\; \sum_{j=1}^{m_i} p_{ij} = 1 \; .$$

Let the tree $\theta$ be derived directly from the tree $\beta$ as the result of applying the production $A_i \xrightarrow{p_{ij}} t_{ij}$, i.e.

$$\beta \xrightarrow{p_{ij}} \theta \ .$$

We say that $\beta$ derives directly $\theta$ with the probability $p_{ij}$.

If there exists the following sequence of derivational steps

$$\alpha_k \xrightarrow{p_k} \alpha_{k+1} \ , \ k = 1, \ldots, r-1$$

then we say that $\alpha_1$ derives $\alpha_r$ with the probability $p = \prod_{k=1}^{r} p_k$, denoted $\alpha_1 \xRightarrow[*]{p} \alpha_r$.

We define the stochastic tree language generated by the grammar $G$ in the following way:

**Definition 7.5 (Stochastic Tree Language Generated):** The language generated by the expansive stochastic tree grammar $G = (\Sigma_N, \Sigma_T, r, P, S)$ is the set

$$L(G) = \{(\alpha, p(\alpha)) : \alpha \in T_{\Sigma_T}, \ S \xRightarrow[*]{p_v} \alpha, \ v = 1, \ldots, s, \ p(\alpha) = \sum_{v=1}^{s} p_v\},$$

where $s$ is the number of all the different derivations of $\alpha$ from $S$ and $p_v$ is the probability of the $v$th derivation of $\alpha$.

Now, we can introduce the idea of the maximum-likelihood model for trees [Fu (1982); Shi and Fu (1982)]. Let $T_{\Sigma_T}^{D} = \{\alpha : \alpha \in T_{\Sigma_T}, \ D_\alpha = D\}$ be the set of trees in the domain $D$. Let $\alpha = a(t_1 \ldots t_n)$, $\alpha' = a'(t_1' \ldots t_n') \in T_{\Sigma_T}^{D}$, where $t_1, \ldots, t_n$ and $t_1', \ldots, t_n' \in T_{\Sigma_T}$ are subtrees of $\alpha$ and $\alpha'$, respectively[4]. The probability of $\alpha'$ being the distorted tree of $\alpha$ is

$$p(\alpha' \mid \alpha) = p(a' \mid a) \cdot p(t_1' \mid t_1) \cdot \ldots \cdot p(t_n' \mid t_n)$$

and furthermore, for any $\alpha \in T_{\Sigma_T}^{D}$

$$\sum_{\alpha' \in T_{\Sigma_T}^{D}} p(\alpha' \mid \alpha) = 1 \ .$$

In defining the expanded stochastic tree grammar $G' = (\Sigma_N, \Sigma_T', r', P', S)$ for the expansive stochastic tree grammar $G$, we assume that the distortion probabilities $p(b \mid a)$, $a \in \Sigma_T$, $b \in \Sigma_T'$ are known.

**Definition 7.6 (Expanded Stochastic Tree Grammar):** Let $G = (\Sigma_N, \Sigma_T, r, P, S)$ be a (reference) expansive stochastic tree grammar. $G' = (\Sigma_N, \Sigma_T', r', P', S)$ is called an expanded stochastic tree grammar for $G$ iff
$\Sigma_T \subseteq \Sigma_T'$,
$r$ is the restriction of $r'$ to $\Sigma_T$, i.e. $r'|_{\Sigma_T} = r$ ,
$P' = \{X_0 \xrightarrow{p'} b(X_1 \ldots X_n) : X_0 \xrightarrow{p} a(X_1 \ldots X_n) \in P, \ a \in \Sigma_{T,n}, \ b \in \Sigma_{T,n}'\}$
$\cup \{X_0 \xrightarrow{p'} b : X_0 \xrightarrow{p} a \in P, \ a \in \Sigma_{T,0}, \ b \subset \Sigma_{T,0}'\}$, where $p' = p \cdot p(b \mid a)$.

---

[4]Each subtree can be further decomposed into its root and its subtrees, etc.

The maximum-likelihood SPECTA, for a given tree $\alpha' \in T_{\Sigma_T}^D$, searches for the tree $\alpha \in L(G)$, $\alpha \in T_{\Sigma_T}^D$ which is the highest probable distortion of $\alpha'$, i.e.

$$p(\alpha' \mid \alpha) \cdot p(\alpha) = \max_{\beta} \{p(\alpha' \mid \beta) \cdot p(\beta) : \beta \in L(G), \ \beta \in T_{\Sigma_T}^D\}.$$

The value $p(\alpha' \mid \alpha) \cdot p(\alpha)$ is called the probability of $\alpha'$ being the distorted tree of $L(G)$ and this is denoted as $p(\alpha' \mid G)$.

Now, we can present the maximum-likelihood SPECTA algorithm. (Its functions are introduced below.)

---

**Parsing Scheme 7.3: Maximum-Likelihood SPECTA**

/* Stochastic tree grammar: $G = (\Sigma_N, \Sigma_T, r, P, S)$; Input tree: $\alpha$ */
*error* := 0;
*accept* := 0;
**repeat**
    $(x, b) := give\_next\_node(\alpha)$;
    **if** $b$ in $\Sigma_T$ **then**
        **begin**
          **if** $rank(x) = 0$ **then**
            **for each** $(k)$ $X_0 \xrightarrow{p} a$ **in** $P$ **do**
                **begin**
                    $p' := p \cdot p(b \mid a)$;
                    $add([X_0, p', k], I(x))$;
                **end**;
          **else** /* $rank(x) > 0$ */
            **begin**
                $n := rank(x)$;
                **for each** $(k)$ $X_0 \xrightarrow{p} a(X_1 X_2 \ldots X_n)$ **in** $P$ **do**
                    **if** $reduction\_possible(k, x, I)$ **then**
                      **begin**
                        $p' := product\_of\_probabilities(k, x, I, b)$;
                        $add([X_0, p', k], I(x))$;
                      **end**;
                **if** $is\_empty(I(x))$ **then** *error* := 1 **else** $delete\_redund\_items(I(x))$;
            **end**;
        **end**;
    **else** *error* := 1;
  **until** $is\_root(x)$ **or** *error* = 1;
  **if** $[S, \bar{p}, m]$ **in** $I(\lambda)$ **then** *accept* := 1 **else** *error* := 1; /* $p(\alpha \mid G) = \bar{p}$ */

---

As one can see, the maximum-likelihood SPECTA constructs the tree-like transition table $I$ which was introduced for the minimum-distance SPECTA. The only difference concerning the table $I$ is that probabilities instead of distances are stored in items $[X, d, k]$. Scheme 7.3 uses functions: $give\_next\_node(\alpha)$, $rank(x)$, $reduction\_possible(k, x, I)$, $add([X, d, k], I(x))$, $is\_empty(W)$, $is\_root(x)$ which have been defined for the minimum-distance SPECTA in the previous section. Function $delete\_redund\_items(I(x))$ is modified accordingly, i.e., it deletes items with smaller probabilities (i.e., for each state only the item with the highest probability is preserved).

The new function $product\_of\_probabilities(k, x, I, b)$ is defined. This gives the product $p \cdot p(b \mid a) \cdot p'_1 \cdot p'_2 \cdot \ldots \cdot p'_n$ for production $(k)$ $X_0 \xrightarrow{p} a(X_1 X_2 \ldots X_n)$ such that $[X_1, p'_1, k_1] \in I(x \bullet 1)$, $[X_2, p'_2, k_2] \in I(x \bullet 2), \ldots, [X_n, p'_n, k_n] \in I(x \bullet n)$.

## 7.4 Generalized Error-Correcting Tree Automata (GECTA)

Three basic types of error transformations are considered in the theory of error-correcting parsing, namely: substitution, deletion and insertion. A substitution error does not modify the structure of the pattern, contrary to deletion and insertion errors. Two kinds of SPECTAs presented in the previous sections allow substitution errors only, i.e., they do not encompass modifications of tree structure. Generalized error-correcting tree automata, GECTA, [Lu and Fu (1978)] allow for structural modifications.

First of all, we discuss three basic error transformations on trees. We shall introduce them on the basis of the model presented in [Lu and Fu (1978)], specifically defining three subtypes of insertion: stretch, branch and split.[5]

The following types of errors on trees are considered.

(1) The substitution of the node by the node with another terminal symbol, denoted $S$.
(2) The insertion of an extrinsic node between a node and its parent, called a stretch and denoted $T$.
(3) The insertion of an extrinsic node to the left of all the children of a node, called a branch and denoted $B$.
(4) The insertion of an extrinsic node to the right of a node, called a split and denoted $P$.
(5) The deletion of a node, denoted $D$.

Now, we formalize our considerations. Let there be given two trees $\alpha, \alpha' \in T_{\Sigma_T}$. A transformation $\mathcal{F} : T_{\Sigma_T} \longmapsto T_{\Sigma_T}$ such that $\alpha' \in \mathcal{F}(\alpha)$ is called a *tree transformation*. We define the error tree transformations corresponding to the types of errors introduced above in the following way.[6] Let $x \in D_\alpha$ , $a \in \Sigma_T, x = y \bullet i$ , $x$ have $k$ children and $y$ have $n$ children, $\alpha[z \leftarrow t]$ denote the replacement of the subtree $\alpha/z$ by the tree $t$ in the tree $\alpha$, defined in Sec. 7.1.

---

[5]Of course, we can define other subtypes of insertion and deletion error transformations on trees than those proposed in this model.

[6]In defining tree transformations we will say *node x* instead of *the node having the address x*.

(1) The substitution of node $x$ by the node labelled with $a$[7]

$$S_{(x,a)}(\alpha) = \alpha[x \leftarrow \{(\lambda, a)\} , x \bullet 1 \leftarrow \alpha/x \bullet 1 , \ldots, x \bullet k \leftarrow \alpha/x \bullet k].$$

(2) The insertion of the node labelled with $a$ between node $x$ and its parent, as shown in Fig. 7.8a

$$T_{(x,a)}(\alpha) = \alpha[x \leftarrow \{(\lambda, a)\} , x \bullet 1 \leftarrow \alpha/x].$$

(3) The insertion of the node labelled with $a$ to the left of all the children of node $x$ (the domain is extended, i.e. $D_\alpha := D_\alpha \cup \{x \bullet (k+1)\}$), as shown in Fig. 7.8b

$$B_{(x,a)}(\alpha) = \alpha[x \leftarrow \{(\lambda, \alpha(x)), (1, a)\} , x \bullet (k+1) \leftarrow \alpha/x \bullet k , x \bullet k \leftarrow \alpha/x \bullet (k-1) , \ldots, x \bullet 2 \leftarrow \alpha/x \bullet 1].$$

(4) The insertion of the node labelled with $a$ to the right of node $x$ (the domain is extended, i.e., $D_\alpha := D_\alpha \cup \{y \bullet (n+1)\}$), as shown in Fig. 7.8c

$$P_{(x,a)}(\alpha) = \alpha[y \bullet (n+1) \leftarrow \alpha/y \bullet n , \ldots, y \bullet (i+2) \leftarrow \alpha/y \bullet (i+1) , y \bullet (i+1) \leftarrow \{(\lambda, a)\}].$$

(5) The deletion of node $x$ in the case of it having no children, $k = 0$ (the domain is reduced, i.e. $D_\alpha := D_\alpha \setminus \{y \bullet n\}$)

$$D_{(x)}(\alpha) = \alpha[y \bullet i \leftarrow \alpha/y \bullet (i+1) , \ldots, y \bullet (n-1) \leftarrow \alpha/y \bullet n].$$

(6) The deletion of node $x$ in the case it has $k$ children, $k > 0$ (the domain is extended, i.e. $D_\alpha := D_\alpha \cup \{y \bullet (n+1) , \ldots , y \bullet (n+k-1)\}$), as shown in Fig. 7.8d

$$D_{(x)}(\alpha) = \alpha[y \bullet (n+k-1) \leftarrow \alpha/y \bullet n , \ldots, y \bullet (i+k) \leftarrow \alpha/y \bullet (i+1) , y \bullet (i+k-1) \leftarrow \alpha/x \bullet k , \ldots, y \bullet i \leftarrow \alpha/x \bullet 1].$$

We write $\alpha \xmapsto{\mathcal{F}} \alpha'$, where $\mathcal{F}$ is one of the error transformations $S, T, B, P, D$, if $\alpha' \in \mathcal{F}(\alpha)$. Let $\mathcal{F}^k$ denote the composition of $\mathcal{F}$ with itself $k$ times. We write $\alpha \xmapsto{\mathcal{F}^k} \alpha'$ , $k \geq 0$, if $\alpha'$ is obtained from $\alpha$ by applying $k$ error transformations.

The distance $\rho(\alpha, \alpha')$ between trees $\alpha$ and $\alpha'$ is defined as the smallest integer $k$ for which $\alpha \xmapsto{\mathcal{F}^k} \alpha'$. For example, if $\alpha = e(b(c(a))af)$ is shown in Fig. 7.9a and $\alpha' = e(b(dc(a))a)$ is shown in Fig. 7.9b, then $\rho(\alpha, \alpha') = 2$, because $\alpha' = D_{(3)}(B_{(1,d)}(\alpha))$ and no other sequence of error transformations from $\alpha$ to $\alpha'$ is shorter than 2. Let $L$ be a tree language. If $\alpha'$ can be obtained from some tree belonging to $L$, then the distance between $\alpha'$ and $L$ is

$$\rho(L, \alpha') = \min_{\beta}\{\rho(\beta, \alpha') : \beta \in L\} .$$

In a way similar to string error transformations, we can ascribe weights $\sigma, \omega, \gamma$ to substitution, insertion and deletion tree transformations, $S$, $I = \{T, B, P\}$ and $D$, respectively. Let $M$ be a sequence of tree transformations applied to obtain the tree

---

[7]For notational convenience we will write the whole *sequence of replacements* in square brackets.

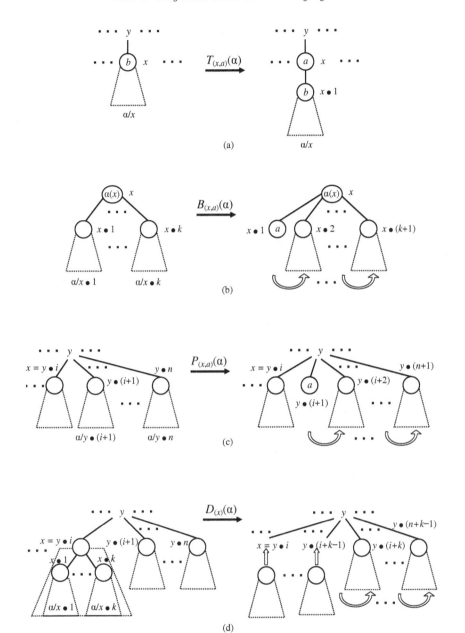

Fig. 7.8   Error transformations on $\alpha$.

$\alpha'$ from the tree $\alpha$ such that we have used $s_M$ substitution error transformations, $i_M$ insertion error transformations and $d_M$ deletion error transformations. The weighted distance $\rho_W(\alpha, \alpha')$ between trees $\alpha$ and $\alpha'$ is

$$\rho_W(\alpha, \alpha') = \min_M \{\sigma \cdot s_M + \omega \cdot i_M + \gamma \cdot d_M\} \ .$$

Generalized error-correcting tree automata are more complex than the automata presented in previous sections, since they allow for the structural modifications of trees. Therefore, in order to simplify their construction, the trees to be analyzed are normalized. The binary form of trees is introduced in [Lu and Fu (1978)]. A tree $\alpha$ is transformed to this form in the following way. If a node of $\alpha$ has zero or one child, then nothing changes. If a node $(x, a)$ has $k$ children, $k \geq 2$, then the stratification operation is performed in the following way. Let $\alpha/x = t_0 = a(t_1 t_2 \ldots t_k)$, where $t_1, t_2, \ldots, t_k$ are subtrees of $\alpha/x$. Let $*$ be a special (additional) terminal symbol. The subtree $\alpha/x$ is stratified as follows.

$$t_0 = a(t^*_{(k-1)} t_k) \ , \ t^*_{(k-1)} = *(t^*_{(k-2)} t_{(k-1)}) \ , \ \ldots, \ t^*_2 = *(t^*_1 t_2) \ , \ t^*_1 = *(t_1)$$

Thus, if a node of a tree in binary form has two children, then its left child is labelled with $*$. For example, the tree in binary form for the tree depicted in Fig. 7.9b is shown in Fig. 7.9c.

Now, we are able to introduce the binary form of regular tree grammar [Lu and Fu (1978)].

**Definition 7.7 (Binary Form of Regular Tree Grammar):** Let $G = (\Sigma_N, \Sigma_T, r, P, S)$ be a regular tree grammar. $G$ is in binary form iff
- a special symbol $*$ belongs to $\Sigma_T$ ,
- $r : \Sigma_T \to 2^{\{0,1,2\}}$ ,
- all its productions are in one of the following forms:

    (a) $X_0 \to a$       (c) $X_0 \to a(U_1 X_1)$     (e) $U_2 \to *(U_1 X_1)$

    (b) $X_0 \to a(X_1)$     (d) $U_1 \to *(X_1)$ ,

where $X_0, X_1, U_1, U_2 \in \Sigma_N$ , $a \in \Sigma_T$ , $a \neq *$.

This requirement is not restrictive because every expansive tree grammar can be easily transformed to a binary form [Lu and Fu (1978)]. If a right-hand side of a production is the one-node or two-node tree, then nothing changes. If production is of the form $X_0 \to a(X_1 X_2 \ldots X_k)$, $k \geq 2$, then it is stratified in the following way:

$$X_0 \to a(U^0_{(k-1)} X_k), \ U^0_{(k-1)} \to *(U^0_{(k-2)} X_{(k-1)}), \ \ldots, \ U^0_2 \to *(U^0_1 X_2), \ U^0_1 \to *(X_1)$$

Let $Z$ be the set of weights of the error transformations. We extend the transition function of frontier-to-root deterministic tree automaton (cf. Scheme 7.1) to the transition function with weights in the following way:

$$\delta^n_a : Q^n \longrightarrow Q \times Z \ , \ a \in \Sigma_{T,n} \ .$$

Before we introduce formally expanded tree automaton which allows for structural modifications on trees, let us consider the following example of defining its error transition functions. Let us assume that a tree grammar contains the produc-

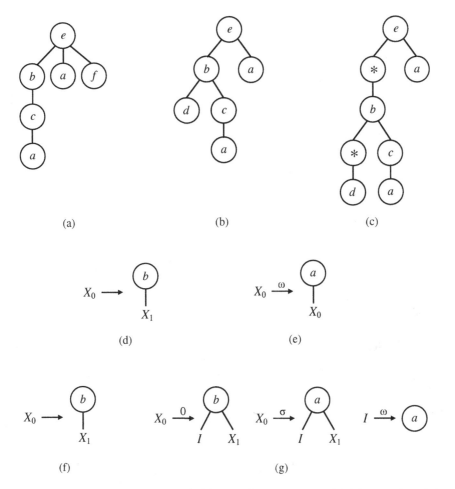

Fig. 7.9  (a) Tree α. (b) Distorted tree α′. (c) Tree α′ in binary form. (d)-(e) Example of defining productions for stretch error transformation. (f)-(g) Example of defining productions for branch error transformation.

tion shown in Fig. 7.9d[8]. If we want to model the insertion of the node labelled with any $a \in \Sigma_T$ between the node labelled with $b$ (i.e., the stretch shown in Fig. 7.8a), then we have to add productions of the form shown in Fig. 7.9e for each $a \in \Sigma_T$ ($\omega$ is the weight of insertion). This means that for the automaton transition[9]

$$\delta_b(X_1) = X_0$$

which corresponds to the production shown in Fig. 7.9d, we have to add the following insertion error transition of the expanded automaton

---

[8]Let us remember that right-hand side trees of a grammar in the binary form can have at most three nodes.

[9]In defining transition functions we omit their ranks, as these are obvious from the context.

$$\delta_a^I(X_0) = X_0, \ \omega$$

for each $a \in \Sigma_T$. ($\delta^I$ means the insertion ($I$) error transition function.)

If we want to model the insertion of the node labelled with $a$ to the left of all the children of some node (i.e., the branch shown in Fig. 7.8b) for the production shown in Fig. 7.9f, then we have to add productions of the form shown in Fig. 7.9g for each $a \in \Sigma_T$ ($\sigma$ is the weight of substitution). This means that for the automaton transition

$$\delta_b(X_1) = X_0$$

we have to add the following insertion error transitions of the expanded automaton

$$\delta_b^I(I, X_1) = X_0, \ 0 \quad , \quad \delta_a^I(I, X_1) = X_0, \ \sigma \quad , \quad \delta_a^I = I, \ \omega$$

for each $a \in \Sigma_T$. The rules of defining all the error transition functions for the model introduced in [Lu and Fu (1978)] can be found in [Lu and Fu (1978); Fu (1982)].

Now, we can define expanded finite tree automaton on the basis of the model introduced in [Lu and Fu (1978)].

---

**Parsing Scheme 7.4: Expanded Finite Tree Automaton**

Let $A = (Q, \Sigma_T, r, \delta, Q_F)$ be a (referential) deterministic frontier-to-root finite tree automaton such that $r : \Sigma_T \to 2^{\{0,1,2\}}$, $Q_F = \{q_0\}$. Let $\sigma, \omega, \gamma$ be the weights ascribed to substitution, insertion and deletion error transformations, respectively.

$A' = (Q', \Sigma_T', r', \Delta, q_0)$ is called an expanded tree automaton for $A$ iff $Q' = Q \cup \{I\}$, where $I$ is a special state used for generating insertion errors, $\Sigma_T' = \Sigma_T \cup \{*\}$, where $*$ is a special symbol introduced in Definition 7.7, $r$ is the restriction of $r'$ to $\Sigma_T$, i.e. $r'|_{\Sigma_T} = r$ ,

$\Delta = \Delta_R \cup \Delta_S \cup \Delta_I \cup \Delta_D$ , where

- $\Delta_R$ is a family $\{\delta_a^R : a \in \Sigma_T\}$ of referential transition functions with weight 0 (i.e., $\delta_a^R(\xi) = (X_0, 0)$, if $\delta_a(\xi) = X_0$ , where $\xi = \lambda$ or $\xi \in Q$ or $\xi \in Q \times Q$),
- $\Delta_S$ is a family $\{\delta_a^S : a \in \Sigma_T\}$ of substitution error transition functions with weight $\sigma$ ,
- $\Delta_I$ is a family $\{\delta_a^I : a \in \Sigma_T\}$ of insertion error transition functions with weight $\omega$ ,
- $\Delta_D$ is a family $\{\delta_a^D : a \in \Sigma_T\}$ of deletion error transition functions with weight $\gamma$ ,

$q_0$ is the final state.

---

Let $L(A)$ denote the language accepted by the expanded finite tree automaton

*A.* The minimum-distance generalized error-correcting tree automaton, GECTA, for a given tree $\alpha'$, searches for such a tree $\alpha \in L(A)$ so that the weighted distance $\rho_W(\alpha, \alpha')$ is smallest. In order to find such a tree and the corresponding weighted distance, the minimum-distance GECTA constructs the tree-like transition table $I$ in a similar way as the minimum-distance SPECTA does. The details of the algorithm are presented in [Lu and Fu (1978); Fu (1982)].

## 7.5 Tree Adjoining Grammars

The formalism of Tree Adjoining Grammars (*TAGs*) was introduced in [Joshi *et al.* (1975); Joshi (1985); Joshi and Schabes (1997)] in the context of research into the enhancement of the generative power of context-free (string) grammars.[10] However, from the point of view of the theory of abstract rewriting systems *TAGs* are tree generating systems. Therefore, we present them in this part of the book.

The notion of Tree Adjoining Grammars has evolved since its introduction in 1975.[11] We present this notion here according to [Joshi and Schabes (1997)]. Let a tree node $(x, a)$ which is not a leaf be called an *internal node*.

**Definition 7.8 (Tree Adjoining Grammar):** A Tree Adjoining Grammar, *TAG*, is a quintuple

$$G = (\Sigma_N, \Sigma_T, S, I, A), \text{ where}$$

$\Sigma_N$ is a finite set of nonterminal symbols,
$\Sigma_T$ is a finite set of terminal symbols, $\Sigma_N \cap \Sigma_T = \emptyset$, $\Sigma = \Sigma_N \cup \Sigma_T$,
$S \in \Sigma_N$ is the initial symbol,
$I$ is a finite set of *initial* trees such that for any $\alpha \in I$ the internal nodes of $\alpha$ are labelled by nonterminals and leaves are labelled by terminals or nonterminals; nonterminal leaves of $\alpha$ are marked for the *substitution* operation with a special symbol $\downarrow$,
$A$ is a finite set of *auxiliary* trees such that for any $\beta \in A$ the internal nodes of $\beta$ are labelled by nonterminals and leaves are labelled by terminals or nonterminals; nonterminal leaves of $\beta$ are marked for substitution except for one node, called the *foot node*; the foot node has the same label as the root of $\beta$; the foot node is marked for the *adjoining* operation with a special symbol $*$.

The set $I \cup A$ is called the set of *elementary trees* of $G$. A tree resulting from the application of substitution or adjoining operations is called a *derived tree*.

The substitution operation is shown schematically in Fig. 7.10a. It consists of replacing a nonterminal leaf marked $\downarrow$ (and having the address $x$) of a derived tree with some tree $s$ derived from an initial tree. The replaced node (marked $\downarrow$) should

---

[10]We have already mentioned *TAGs* when discussing this problem in Sec. 4.1.5.
[11]For example, originally, the roots of initial trees were labelled with $S$, their leaves were labelled with terminal symbols only, etc. Then, after introducing the substitution operation and other extensions these conditions were changed.

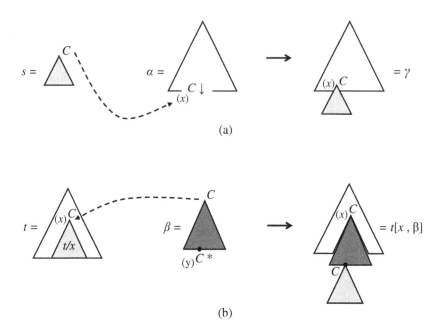

Fig. 7.10   (a) The substitution operation and (b) the adjoining operation.

have the same (nonterminal) label as the root of the tree $s$. We will not introduce formally the substitution operation since it is analogous to the direct derivation step in the regular tree grammars defined in Sec. 7.1 (cf. Fig. 7.3b).

The adjoining operation is shown schematically in Fig. 7.10b. It consists of inserting an auxiliary tree $\beta$ into an internal node having the address $x$ of a derived tree $t$. The node of $t$ having the address $x$ should have the same (nonterminal) label as the root of the tree $\beta$. The subtree $t/x$ is attached to the foot node of $\beta$ (marked with $*$). The adjoining operation can be defined formally in an analogous way to the replacing operation in Sec. 7.1 (cf. Fig. 7.3a).

Let $\beta \in T_\Sigma$ be an auxiliary tree and $y$ be the address of the foot node of $\beta$. Let $t \in T_\Sigma$. The *adjunction* of $\beta$ to $t$ at the address $x$ of $t$, denoted $t[x, \beta]$, is the tree defined by the function which is the set of pairs (see Fig. 7.10b)

$\{(z, t(z)) : z \in D_t , \ x \text{ is not a prefix of } z\} \cup$
$\cup \ \{(x \bullet u, \ \beta(u)) : u \in D_\beta\} \cup$
$\cup \ \{(x \bullet y \bullet w, \ t/x(w)) : w \in D_{t/x}\} .$

As we have mentioned in Sec. 4.1.5, Tree Adjoining Grammars can also be used for generating enhanced string context-free languages (Mildly Context-Sensitive Languages). Then, the strings defined by the terminal labels of the frontiers of the derived trees are treated as the words of these languages. In order to extract tree frontiers, let us define the *yield mapping* $Y : T_\Sigma \longrightarrow \Sigma^*_{T,0}$ in the following way.
(1) If $a \in \Sigma_{T,0}$ then $Y(a) = a$.
(2) If $a \in \Sigma_{T,n}$ , $k > 0$ and $t_1, t_2, \ldots, t_n \in T_\Sigma$ then

$$Y(a(t_1 t_2 \ldots t_n)) = Y(t_1) \cdot Y(t_2) \cdot \ldots \cdot Y(t_n)) \,,$$

where $\cdot$ is the concatenation operation.

The yield mapping gives the sequence of the labels of the frontier nodes (i.e. the leaves), writing them from left to right.

Let $\theta, \gamma \in T_\Sigma$. We say that $\theta$ directly derives $\gamma$ in a Tree Adjoining Grammar $G$, denoted $\theta \underset{G}{\Longrightarrow} \gamma$, iff either $\gamma = \theta[x, \beta]$, $x \in D_\theta$, $\beta \in A$ or $\gamma$ results from the application of a substitution operation to $\theta$.

The reflexive and transitive closure of the relation $\underset{G}{\Longrightarrow}$ is denoted with $\underset{G}{\overset{*}{\Longrightarrow}}$ . If $\theta \underset{G}{\overset{*}{\Longrightarrow}} \gamma$, then $\gamma$ is called a *derived tree of* $\theta$. The set of all derived trees of $\theta$ is denoted with $DT(\theta)$.

The tree set of $G$ is the set

$$T(G) = \{\gamma \in T_\Sigma : \gamma \in DT(\theta),\ \theta \in I,\ \theta(\lambda) = S, \text{ and } Y(\gamma) \in \Sigma_T^*\}.$$

The string language of $G$ is the set

$$L(G) = \{v : v = Y(\gamma),\ \gamma \in T(G)\}.$$

There are a variety of extensions defined for Tree Adjoining Grammars. For example, certain constraints can be imposed on the form of the adjoining operation. The *Null Adjoining* constraint imposed on some node disallows any adjunction on this node. (This is marked with the index $NA$ of the nonterminal label of the node.)

Now, let us define the following Tree Adjoining Grammar $G$ which generates the (string) context sensitive language $L = \{a^n b^n e^k c^n d^n,\ n \geq 0,\ k \geq 1\}$.
$G = (\Sigma_N, \Sigma_T, S, I, A)$, where:
$\Sigma_N = \{S, A\}$,
$\Sigma_T = \{a, b, c, d, e\}$,
$I$ consists of the following initial trees (see Figs. 7.11a, b, c):

$$\alpha_1 = S(A \downarrow) \quad \alpha_2 = A(eA \downarrow) \quad \alpha_3 = A(eA) \,,$$

$A$ consists of the following auxiliary tree (see Fig. 7.11d):

$$\beta_1 = S_{NA}(aS(bS_{NA}^* c)d) \,.$$

The derivation of the tree which has the frontier $a^2 b^2 e^2 c^2 d^2$ is shown in Figs. 7.11e - i. Firstly, the tree shown in Fig. 7.11f is obtained by substituting the node labelled $A \downarrow$ of $\alpha_1$ with $\alpha_2$. Secondly, the node labelled $A \downarrow$ is substituted with $\alpha_3$ and obtained is the tree shown in Fig. 7.11g. Finally, the adjoining operation using the auxiliary tree $\beta_1$ is applied to the node labelled $S$ (Figs. 7.11h - i).

Tree Adjoining Grammars are mainly used in natural language processing (NLP) and bioinformatics. In the case of NLP, derived trees express the hierarchical nature of natural language sentences in a convenient way. The tree shown in Fig. 1.8 in

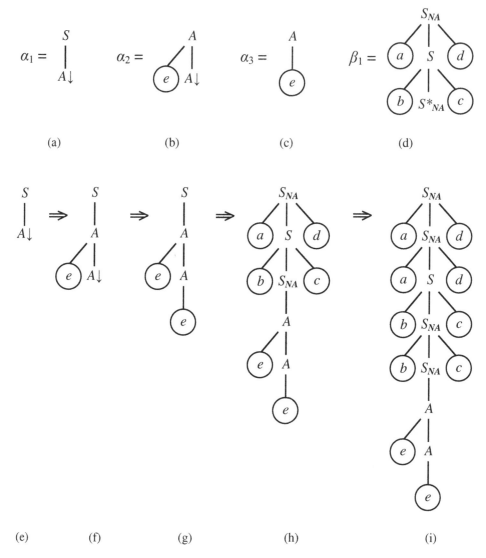

Fig. 7.11  (a)-(c) The initial trees of Tree Adjoining Grammar $G$, (d) the auxiliary tree of $G$, (e)-(i) the derivation in $G$.

Chap. 1 is a good example of a derived tree.[12] The example of the use of derived trees in bioinformatics is shown in Fig. 7.12. Three typical structures of RNA, namely: stem (a), branched structure (b) and hairpin loop (c), are represented with the (standard) *arc notation* and the correspondingly derived trees.

Parsing algorithms for Tree Adjoining Languages (*TALs*) are modifications of the parsers for context-free string languages presented in Chap. 3. The first parsing

---

[12]Of course, this tree can also be interpreted as a *derivation* tree generated by a (string) context-free grammar.

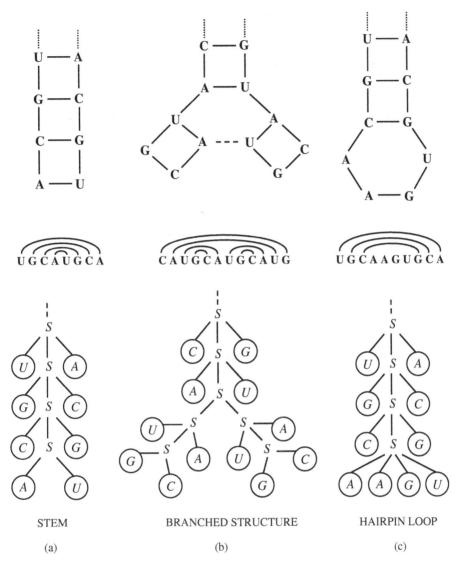

Fig. 7.12 The exemplary RNA structures, their arc representations and derived tree representations.

algorithm for TALs, a modification of the Cocke-Younger-Kasami parser, with the running time $\mathcal{O}(n^6)$, where $n$ is the number of tree frontier nodes, was presented in [Vijay-Shanker and Joshi (1985)]. Then, a number of polynomial syntax analyzers for *TALs* were proposed. The Earley parser-based algorithm was defined in [Schabes and Joshi (1988)]. An *LR* syntax analyzer was presented in [Schabes and Vijay-Shanker (1990)]. Parsing algorithms for *TALs* were also proposed in [Poller (1994); Satta (1993); Vijay-Shanker and Weir (1994b); Noord van (1994); Aizawa and Nakamura (1999a); Schabes and Waters (1995); Alonso Pardo *et al.* (2000)].

## 7.6    Remarks on Tree Languages

Frontier-to-root deterministic finite tree automata, *FR DFTA*, have been introduced
in Scheme 7.1 as a tool for syntactic pattern recognition. As stated at the beginning
of this chapter, for regular tree grammars the other three classes of finite tree
automata are defined [Doner (1965); Thatcher and Wright (1968); Rabin (1969)].
They differ from *FR DFTA*s in the form of transition functions. Let us introduce
them with the corresponding forms of transition functions (cf. Scheme 7.1).

- Root-to-frontier deterministic finite tree automata, *RF DFTA*

$$\delta_a^n : Q \longrightarrow Q^n$$

- Frontier-to-root nondeterministic finite tree automata, *FR NFTA*

$$\delta_a^n : Q^n \longrightarrow 2^Q$$

- Root-to-frontier nondeterministic finite tree automata, *RF NFTA*

$$\delta_a^n : Q \longrightarrow 2^{Q^n}$$

The relations among the classes of tree languages accepted by the classes of finite
tree automata were established in [Thatcher and Wright (1968); Doner (1970)].
These are shown in Fig. 7.13. As one can see the classes of tree languages accepted
by *FR DFTA*, *RF NFTA* and *FR NFTA* are all equal. This class is called a class of
recognizable tree languages, denoted *RECOG*. The class of languages generated by
Tree Adjoining Grammars has a greater generative power than the class *RECOG*
[Joshi and Schabes (1997)].

A. K. Joshi led the research into Harris's transformational systems[13] [Harris
(1957, 1962, 1964, 1968)] in the 1960s [Joshi (1962, 1966)]. Continuing this research, Joshi and his collaborators proposed String Adjunct Grammars in [Joshi
*et al.* (1972a,b)] which were investigated in [Levy (1973); Hart (1973, 1974); Levy
and Joshi (1978)]. Then, String Adjunct Grammars were extended to Tree Adjoining Grammars (*TAGs*) [Joshi *et al.* (1975)]. The formal properties of *TAGs* have
been studied intensively in recent decades [Joshi (1985); Kroch (1987); Shieber and
Schabes (1990); Joshi *et al.* (1991); Resnick (1992); Vijay-Shanker (1992); Joshi and
Schabes (1992); Vijay-Shanker and Weir (1994a); Joshi and Schabes (1997); Kepser
and Rogers (2011); Boullier and Sagot (2011); Kuhlmann and Satta (2012)]. The
power properties of Tree Adjoining Grammars with respect to strings grammars
have been discussed in Sec. 4.1.5.

Unranked tree languages were studied in the context of syntactic pattern recognition in [Barrero (1991b)].

As we have mentioned in the introduction to this chapter tree grammars and
automata have been introduced for solving decidability problems in mathematical
logic. In this theoretical-oriented approach trees are introduced as *terms*. Indeed,

---

[13]Harris's transformational systems do not belong to the Chomskyan paradigm.

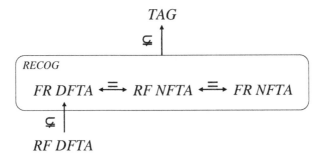

Fig. 7.13   The relations among the classes of tree regular languages.

if we consider a ranked alphabet $(\Sigma, n)$, $n \geq 0$ as a set family of $n$-ary function symbols,[14] $X$ as a set of variables, then a term $f(t_1, \ldots, t_n) \in \mathcal{T}_\Sigma(X)$, where $f \in \Sigma_n$, $n \geq 0$, $\mathcal{T}_\Sigma(X)$ is a set of terms over $\Sigma$ and $X$, $t_1, \ldots, t_n \in \mathcal{T}_\Sigma(X)$, may be viewed as a tree rooted at the node $(\lambda, f)$ and having the subtrees $t_1, \ldots, t_n$.[15]

---

[14]$\Sigma_0$ denotes here a set of 0-argument function symbols, i.e. a set of constant symbols.
[15]If $n = 0$ then the tree consists of one node.

Chapter 8

# Inference (Induction) of Tree Languages

As we have seen in Chap. 5, a variety of inference algorithms for string languages have been developed. On the other hand, only a few grammatical inference algorithms in the case of tree structures have been proposed over the last forty years. As we will see, generic schemes which have been defined for the inferring of string languages are used for the constructing of (analogous) induction algorithms for tree languages.

Inference algorithms for tree languages which have been defined for syntactic pattern recognition are presented in this chapter. The $k$-tail-based inference method for tree languages is introduced in Sec. 8.1. In Section 8.2, the algorithm of the inference of reversible tree languages is presented. The tree-derivative-based inference method is introduced in 8.3. The issue of the informed learning of tree languages is discussed in Section 8.4. Remarks on the inference of tree languages are included in the last section.

Basic notions and denotations which concern grammatical inference have been introduced at the beginning of Chap. 5.

## 8.1 k-Tail-Based Inference of Tree Languages

The preliminary version of the $k$-tail-based inference method for tree languages[1] was defined independently in [Bhargava and Fu (1974b)] and [Gonzales and Thomason (1974)]. Then, the generalized versions of this method were presented in [Brayer and Fu (1977)] and [Gonzales et al. (1976)]. We introduce this method according to [Brayer and Fu (1977)]. Since the method is based on the concept of $k$-tails, which has been already presented for string languages in Sec. 5.1.2, we will not define the general scheme of this method here. (It is analogous to the $k$-tail method for string languages.) Instead, we shall focus on the specific issues related to tree languages.

Let $S_+$ be a sample of trees over $\Sigma_T$, $dpt(\tau)$, $\tau \in T_\Sigma$, denote the depth of the tree $\tau$,[2] $\varepsilon$ denote the empty tree. We shall introduce the following notion according

---

[1]The reader is advised to recall the notions introduced in Sec. 5.1.2.
[2]The depth of a tree is the number of edges between the root $r$ and a leaf which is most distant from $r$.

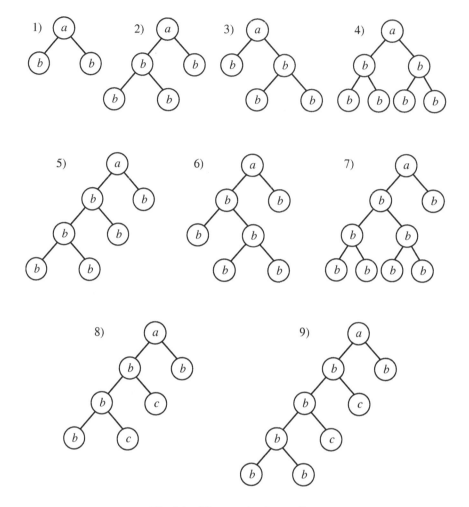

Fig. 8.1 The sample of trees $S_+$.

to the idea presented in [Brayer and Fu (1977)].

**Definition 8.1 (Set of Tree $k$-Tails):** A set

$$C_t = \{(\tau_1, \tau_2, \ldots, \tau_m) : t\tau_1\tau_2 \ldots \tau_m \in S_+ \text{ and } dpt(\tau_l) + 1 \le k,\ l = 1, 2, \ldots, m\},$$

where

$t \in T_\Sigma$ is a tree with a single special leaf; let us assume that this leaf has the address $x$,

$\tau_1, \tau_2, \ldots, \tau_m \in T_\Sigma$,

$t\tau_1\tau_2 \ldots \tau_m$ denotes the tree in which $\tau_1, \tau_2, \ldots, \tau_m$ are subtrees of $t\tau_1\tau_2 \ldots \tau_m$, such that $\tau_l = t\tau_1\tau_2 \ldots \tau_m/x \bullet l,\ l = 1, 2, \ldots, m$,

is called the set of $k$-tails with respect to the tree $t$ and the node $x$.

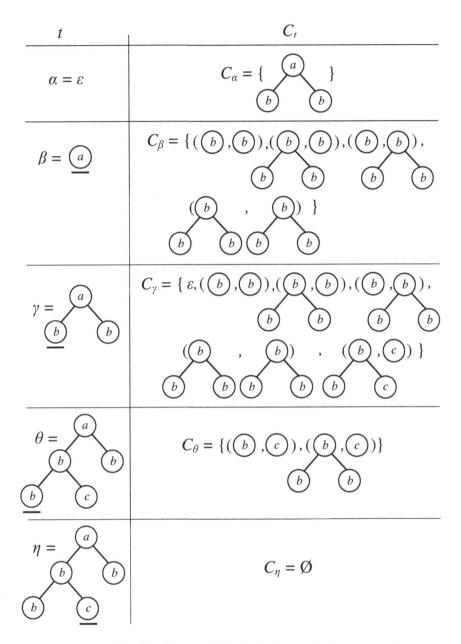

Fig. 8.2 The sets of 2-tails for the sample $S_+$.

We say that $\tau_l$ is concatenated at the $l$th position of the special leaf $x$ of the tree $t$ [Brayer and Fu (1977)].

Let us consider the following example in the case of $k = 2$. Let the sample $S_+$ contain trees shown in Fig. 8.1. The succeeding trees $t = \alpha, \beta, \gamma, \theta, \eta$ and the corresponding sets $C_\alpha, C_\beta, C_\gamma, C_\theta, C_\eta$ constructed according to Definition 8.1 are shown in Fig. 8.2. The special leaf $x$ of the tree $t$ is underlined. $C_\alpha$ is defined on the basis of sample tree 1. $C_\beta$ is defined on the basis of sample trees 1, 2, 3 and 4. $C_\gamma$ is defined on the basis of sample trees 1, 2, 5, 6, 7 and 8. $C_\theta$ is defined on the basis of sample trees 8 and 9.

In order to infer grammar productions every set of $k$-tails $C_t$ has to be decomposed into subsets such that each subset contains equinumerous tuples. This results from the fact that an $i$-tuple and an $j$-tuple, $i \neq j$, cannot be generated by the same production. Therefore, we shall introduce the following decomposition notation [Brayer and Fu (1977)].

$$C_t = C_{t0} \cup C_{t1} \cup \ldots \cup C_{tm}, \text{ where}$$

$C_{t0} = \{\varepsilon\}$, if $t \in S_+$; otherwise $C_{t0} = \emptyset$,
$C_{t1} = \{(\tau_1) : t\tau_1 \in S_+ \text{ and } dpt(\tau_1) + 1 \leq k\}$,
$C_{t2} = \{(\tau_1, \tau_2) : t\tau_1\tau_2 \in S_+ , \ dpt(\tau_1) + 1 \leq k \text{ and } dpt(\tau_2) + 1 \leq k\}$,
$C_{tm} = \{(\tau_1, \tau_2, \ldots, \tau_m) : t\tau_1\tau_2 \ldots \tau_m \in S_+ \text{ and } dpt(\tau_l) + 1 \leq k, \ l = 1, 2, \ldots, m\}$.

Let us come back to our example: the sets of $k$-tails are decomposed in the following way.
$C_\alpha = C_{\alpha 1}$
$C_\beta = C_{\beta 2}$
$C_\gamma = C_{\gamma 0} \cup C_{\gamma 2}$, where $C_{\gamma 0} = \{\varepsilon\}$ and $C_{\gamma 2} = C_\gamma \setminus \{\varepsilon\}$
$C_\theta = C_{\theta 2}$
$C_\eta = \emptyset$

Let us notice that for each node $v$ of a tree $s \in S_+$ only certain ordered combinations of the descendants of $v$ are allowed. Therefore, each decomposed set $C_{ti}$ has to be further decomposed into the subsets of $i$-tuples which represent the allowed combinations of descendants. Let us introduce the following decomposition notation [Brayer and Fu (1977)].

$$C_{ti} = C_{ti1} \cup C_{ti2} \cup \ldots \cup C_{tin}$$

where,

$$C_{tij} = \{(\tau_1, \tau_2, \ldots, \tau_i) : \tau_1 \in S_{j1} , \ \tau_2 \in S_{j2} , \ \ldots , \ \tau_i \in S_{ji}\}, j = 1, 2, \ldots, n,$$

in which $S_{jl}, l = 1, 2, \ldots, i$, is a set of trees (a tree sublanguage).

Each tree sublanguage $S_{jl}$ will be treated as a set of trees generated by the particular nonterminal symbol of the tree grammar inferred.

Let us come back to our example again. The sets of the form $C_{tij}$ are defined as follows (see also Fig. 8.3a):[3]
$C_{\alpha 1} = C_{\alpha 11} = \{(\tau_1) : \tau_1 \in S\}$, where $S$ is the sublanguage of trees, $S = \{a(bb)\}$
$C_{\beta 2} = C_{\beta 21} = \{(\tau_1, \tau_2) : \tau_1 \in B , \ \tau_2 \in B\}$, where $B = \{b , \ b(bb)\}$
$C_{\gamma 0} = C_{\gamma 01} = \{\varepsilon\}$

---

[3]Trees belonging to sets $S_{jl}$ are denoted with the help of the bracketed Polish prefix notation, which has been introduced at the beginning of the previous chapter.

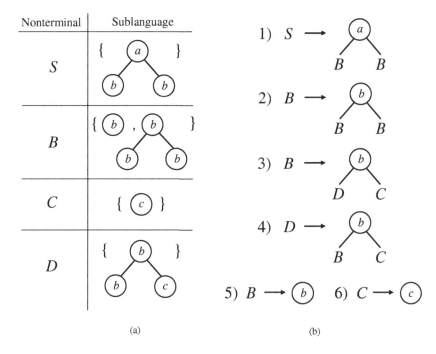

Fig. 8.3 (a) The sublanguages for the sample $S_+$ and (b) the inferred grammar $G$.

$C_{\gamma 2} = C_{\gamma 21} \cup C_{\gamma 22}$, where
$C_{\gamma 21} = \{(\tau_1, \tau_2) : \tau_1 \in B, \ \tau_2 \in B\}$
$C_{\gamma 22} = \{(\tau_1, \tau_2) : \tau_1 \in D, \ \tau_2 \in C\}$, in which $D = \{b(bc)\}$, $C = \{c\}$
$C_{\theta 2} = C_{\theta 21} = \{(\tau_1, \tau_2) : \tau_1 \in B, \ \tau_2 \in C\}$

Now, we can introduce the following rule which allows one to define tree grammar productions on the basis of the notions introduced above [Brayer and Fu (1977)].

**Rule 8.1 (Tree $k$-Tail-based Production Induction):**
A production $A_{jl} \to x(A_{n1} A_{n2} \ldots A_{nm})$ is inferred if a tree $t$ related to the set of $k$-tails $C_t$ has been defined and the following conditions hold.
1) $A_{jl}$ is the nonterminal corresponding to the sublanguage $S_{jl}$.
2) There exists a $C_{tij}$ that contains the sublanguage $S_{jl}$ in the $l$th position of its specification.
3) $tx$ is a tree with $x$ concatenated at the $l$th position of $t$.
4) There exists a $C_{txmn}$ that is specified by the sublanguages $S_{n1}, S_{n2}, \ldots, S_{nm}$.
5) $A_{n1}, A_{n2}, \ldots, A_{nm}$ are the nonterminals corresponding to the sublanguages $S_{n1}, S_{n2}, \ldots, S_{nm}$, respectively.
6) Either $x(t_1 t_2 \ldots t_m)$ is a tree in $S_{jl}$, where $t_1 \in S_{n1}, t_2 \in S_{n2}, \ldots, t_m \in S_{nm}$ or $dpt(x(t_1 t_2 \ldots t_m)) > k$.

Let us come back to our example again. The set of productions inferred for the sample $S_+$ according to Rule 8.1 is shown in Fig. 8.3b. For example, rule (4) has been inferred because the tree $\gamma$ (cf. Fig. 8.2) has been defined for $C_\gamma$ and the following conditions hold.

1) $D$ is the nonterminal corresponding to the sublanguage $\{b(bc)\}$.

2) $C_{\gamma 22}$ has $\{b(bc)\}$ concatenated at its first position.

3) $\theta = \gamma bc$ (cf. Fig. 8.2) is a tree with $b$ concatenated at the first position of $\gamma$.

4) $C_{\theta 21}$ is specified by the sublanguages $\{b , b(bb)\}$ and $\{c\}$.

5) $B$ and $C$ are the nonterminals corresponding to the sublanguages $\{b , b(bb)\}$ and $\{c\}$, respectively.

## 8.2  Inference of Reversible Tree Languages

The method of the inference of $k$-reversible tree languages was introduced in [López *et al.* (2004)]. Since we present this method using analogies to the inference method for $k$-reversible (string) languages, the reader is advised to recall the notions introduced in Sec. 5.1.4. The method of the inference of $k$-reversible tree languages allows one to generate *frontier-to-root deterministic finite tree automata* (cf. Scheme 7.1).[4] Automata of this type will be considered in this section. The *subtree automaton*, *STA*, is defined in the first step of the method. Let $S_+$ be a sample of trees over $\Sigma_T$. First of all, we shall define a *set of subtrees* [López *et al.* (2004)].

Let $t \in T_{\Sigma_T}$. The set of subtrees of $t$, denoted $Sub(t)$, is defined in the following way:

$$Sub(a) = \{a\} \text{ for each } a \in \Sigma_{T,0}$$
$$Sub(t) = \{t\} \cup \bigcup_{i=1,\ldots,n} Sub(t_i) \text{ for } t = a(t_1 \ldots t_n), \ a \in \Sigma_{T,n}, \ t_1,\ldots,t_n \in T_{\Sigma_T}$$

The set of subtrees for $S_+$ is defined as follows: $Sub(S_+) = \bigcup_{s \in S_+} Sub(s)$.

Now, we can introduce the following definition [López *et al.* (2004)]:[5]

**Definition 8.2 (Subtree Automaton for $S_+$):** The subtree automaton for $S_+$ is a quintuple

$$STA(S_+) = (Q, \Sigma_T, r, \delta, Q_F), \text{ where}$$

$Q = Sub(S_+)$ is the set of states,

$(\Sigma_T, r)$ is the ranked alphabet of input symbols which appear in $S_+$,

$\delta$ is the family $\{\delta_a^n : a \in \Sigma_{T,n}, \ n \in \mathbb{N}\}$ of transitions functions such that:

$\delta_a^0 = a$ for $a \in \Sigma_{T,0}$ ,

$\delta_a^n(t_1,\ldots,t_n) = a(t_1 \ldots t_n), a(t_1 \ldots t_n) \in Q$ for $a \in \Sigma_{T,n}$ , $n > 0$, $t_1,\ldots,t_n \in Q$,

$Q_F = S_+$ is the set of final states.

If $n$ is obvious from the context, we write $\delta_a$ instead of $\delta_a^n$.

---

[4]Trees in the form of *skeletal descriptions* (see Sec. 5.3) are considered in [López *et al.* (2004)]. We consider *common* trees in this section.

[5]A subtree automaton will be defined according to the convention of Chap. 7.

A subtree automaton *STA* is analogous to a prefix tree acceptor *PTA* defined for the inference of $k$-reversible (string) languages (cf. Definition 5.5 in Sec. 5.1.4).

Before we define $k$-reversible tree automata, we shall introduce the following notions.

Let $t \in T_\Sigma$ and $x \in D_t$, where $D_t$ is the domain of $t$. Let $dpn(x)$ denote the depth of the node $x$,[6] $dpt(t)$ denote the depth of the tree $t$ and $t(x)$ denote the label of $x$. The *$k$-root of a tree $t$*, $k \geq 0$, is defined as follows:

$$root_k(t) = \begin{cases} t, & \text{if } dpt(t) < k, \\ t' \ : \ t'(x) = t(x) \ , \ x \in D_t \ , \ dpn(x) \leq k, & \text{otherwise.} \end{cases}$$

If $T$ is a set of trees then $root_k(T) = \bigcup_{t \in T} root_k(t)$.

Let $A = (Q, \Sigma_T, r, \delta, Q_F)$ be a frontier-to-root deterministic finite tree automaton and $q \in Q$. We define $L(q) = \{t \in T_{\Sigma_T} : \delta(t) = q\}$.

Now, we can introduce the following definition [López *et al.* (2004)].[7]

**Definition 8.3 ($k$-Reversible Tree Automaton):** A tree automaton $A = (Q, \Sigma_T, r, \delta, Q_F)$ is $k$-reversible iff the following conditions hold.

(1) The determinism condition: $\delta$ is a family $\{\delta_a^n : a \in \Sigma_{T,n}, \ n \in \mathbb{N}\}$ of transition functions such that $\delta_a^n : Q^n \longrightarrow Q$.

(2) The $k$-reversibility condition:

    (a) $q', q'' \in Q_F$, $q' \neq q'' \implies root_k(L(q')) \cap root_k(L(q'')) = \emptyset$ and

    (b) $\delta_a^n(q_1, \ldots, q_{(i-1)}, q', \ldots, q_n) = \delta_a^n(q_1, \ldots, q_{(i-1)}, q'', \ldots, q_n)$, $q' \neq q'' \implies$
        $\implies root_k(L(q')) \cap root_k(L(q'')) = \emptyset$ .

The $k$-reversible tree automaton $A$ is constructed in the second step of the method in an analogous way to the construction of the $k$-reversible (string) automaton presented in Sec. 5.1.4. The automaton $A$ is defined on the basis of the subtree automaton *STA* by merging (repeatedly) any pairs of states which violate the conditions of Definition 8.3.

Both the notion of a *violating pair of states* and the concept of the *merging of states* have been presented in Sec. 5.1.4. They are defined in an analogous way for tree automata. Therefore, we will not introduce them in this section. Instead, we shall consider the example of the $k$-reversible tree automaton inference.

Let the sample $S_+ = \{a(b(db(df(gh)e)e)c(ch)) \ , \ a(b(db(db(df(gh)e)e)e)c(ch))\}$ (see Fig. 8.4). We will infer the 1-reversible tree automaton $A$ (i.e., $k = 1$).

Firstly, the subtree automaton *STA* is defined as follows (the states/subtrees of the automaton $A$ are marked in Fig. 8.4):

---

[6] The depth of a node is the number of edges between the root and this node.
[7] This definition has been reformulated in order to show it is analogous to Definition 5.6.

| | |
|---|---|
| (1) | $\delta_f(g,h) = q_1$ |
| (2) | $\delta_b(d, q_1, e) = q_2$ |
| (3) | $\delta_b(d, q_2, e) = q_3$ |
| (4) | $\delta_c(c, h) = q_4$ |
| (5) | $\delta_a(q_3, q_4) = q_5 \in Q_F$ |
| (6) | $\delta_b(d, q_3, e) = q_6$ |
| (7) | $\delta_a(q_6, q_4) = q_7 \in Q_F$ |

Now, since the final states $q_5$ and $q_7$ are violating (i.e., $root_1(L(q_5)) \cap root_1(L(q_7)) = \{a(bc)\}$ and $q_5 \neq q_7$), they are merged.[8] The following transitions are obtained:

| | |
|---|---|
| (1) | $\delta_f(g,h) = q_1$ |
| (2) | $\delta_b(d, q_1, e) = q_2$ |
| (3) | $\delta_b(d, q_2, e) = q_3$ |
| (4) | $\delta_c(c, h) = q_4$ |
| (5) | $\delta_a(q_3, q_4) = q_5 \in Q_F$ |
| (6) | $\delta_b(d, q_3, e) = q_6$ |
| (7) | $\delta_a(q_6, q_4) = q_5 \in Q_F$ |

Finally, the violating states $q_3$ and $q_6$ are identified (i.e., $\delta_a(q_3, q_4) = \delta_a(q_6, q_4)$ and $q_3 \neq q_6$ and $root_1(L(q_3)) \cap root_1(L(q_6)) = \{b(dbe)\}$) and merged. The following transitions of the 1-reversible tree automaton $A$ are obtained:

| | |
|---|---|
| (1) | $\delta_f(g,h) = q_1$ |
| (2) | $\delta_b(d, q_1, e) = q_2$ |
| (3) | $\delta_b(d, q_2, e) = q_3$ |
| (4) | $\delta_c(c, h) = q_4$ |
| (5), (7) | $\delta_a(q_3, q_4) = q_5 \in Q_F$ |
| (6) | $\delta_b(d, q_3, e) = q_3$ |

Let us notice that the automaton $A$ corresponds to our intuition concerning the language represented by the sample $S_+$. We can guess that the left subtree of trees

---

[8] The subsets of states which share a $k$-root are defined in the first step of the algorithm presented in [López *et al.* (2004)] in order to facilitate the process of state merging. We shall not define them merely because our example is simple.

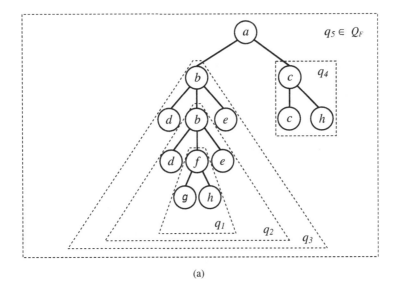

(a)

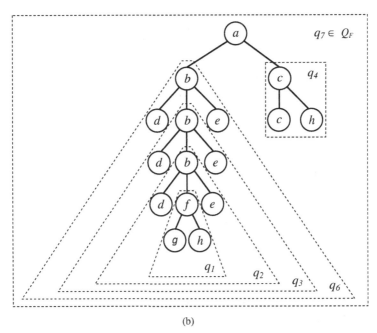

(b)

Fig. 8.4  The subtree automaton *STA*.

belonging to this language consists of sequences of $b(dbe)$ which are finished with $f(gh)$. These sequences are recognized *via* the recurrent transition (6) $\delta_b(d, q_3, c) = q_3$.

The induction scheme for $k$-reversible tree languages is analogous to the scheme for $k$-reversible regular (string) languages (Scheme 5.4) and to the scheme for $k$-reversible context-free (string) languages (Scheme 5.7).

---

**Induction Scheme 8.1: $k$-Reversible Tree Automaton Inference**

$A := STA(S_+)$;
*violating_pair_found* := *false*;
**repeat**
    *violating_pair_found* := *merge_violating_pair_of_states*$(A)$;
**until not** *violating_pair_found*;

---

At the end of this section let us present the following theorem.

**Theorem 8.1 ($k$-RTL Inference Complexity [López *et al.* (2004)])**

*The running time of the inference algorithm for $k$-reversible tree languages is $\mathcal{O}(\|\ S_+\ \|^3)$, where $S_+$ is the sample.*

## 8.3  Tree-Derivative-Based Inference

The tree-derivative-based inference method was proposed in [Levine (1981, 1982)]. Brzozowski derivatives (see Sec. 5.1.1) were extended for tree languages in the following way in [Levine (1981)].

Let $\alpha, t \in T_\Sigma$ and $x \in D_\alpha$. The *replacement* of the subtree $\alpha/x$ by $t$ is denoted by $\alpha[x \leftarrow t]$.[9]

**Definition 8.4 (Tree Derivative):** Let $Y$ be a set of trees over an alphabet $\Sigma_T$. The $m$th-order tree derivative of $Y$ with respect to the tree $t \in T_{\Sigma_T}$ is recursively defined as follows:

$$\partial_t^1(Y) = \{\alpha[x \leftarrow \$] : \alpha \in Y \text{ and } \alpha/x = t\}, \ \$ \notin \Sigma_T \text{ and}$$
$$\partial_t^{i+1}(Y) = \partial_t^1(\partial_t^i(Y)) \text{ for } i \geq 1.$$

The exemplary set $Y$ and some tree derivatives of $Y$ are shown in Fig. 8.5a.

A tree derivative can be modified in order to consider depth bounded tree derivatives in the following way. Let $dpt(u)$ denote the depth of the tree $u$. The *$k$ depth bounded tree derivative of order $m$* is defined as

$$\partial_t^{k,m}(Y) = \{u : u \in \partial_t^m(Y) \text{ and } dpt(u) \leq k\}.$$

The generating of a subtree automaton and the merging of its states is the main idea of the tree-derivative-based inference method. This merging is performed with the help of the following relation on trees [Levine (1982)]:

---

[9]The replacement of the subtree has been defined formally in Sec. 7.1.

**Definition 8.5 (Subtree-Invariant Equivalence Relation):** $R$ is a subtree-invariant equivalence relation on trees in $T_{\Sigma_T}$ iff $tRu$ implies $v[x \leftarrow t]Rv[x \leftarrow u]$ for each $x \in D_v$ and $t, u, v \in T_{\Sigma_T}$.

A *state-minimizing subtree-invariant equivalence relation* of finite index for the tree automaton $A$ is defined as follows: $tR^Au$ iff for each $v \in T_{\Sigma_T}$ and each $x \in D_v$, $v[x \leftarrow t] \in L(A)$ exactly when $v[x \leftarrow u] \in L(A)$.

The $R^A$-equivalence classes correspond to the states of the tree automaton $A$. For the determining of the minimal automaton, tree derivatives will be used. Let us introduce the following theorem [Levine (1982)]:

**Theorem 8.2 (Tree Derivatives and $\mathbf{R^A}$ [Levine (1982)])**

$$tR^Au \quad \text{iff} \quad \partial_t^{k,i}(L(A)) = \partial_u^{k,i}(L(A)), \quad k \geq 0, \ i \geq 1.$$

The inference method consists of the following two stages [Levine (1982)]:

(A) *Initialization.* The generation of the subtree automaton[10] $A$ for the sample $S_+$ and the generation of the initial subtree-invariant equivalence relation $R^A = \{t_1, \ldots, t_n\}$, where $t_1, \ldots, t_n$ are the distinct subtrees in the sample $S_+$.

For example, let the sample $S_+$ be defined as shown in Fig. 8.5b and the parameter $k = 1$. The relation $R^A = S_+ \cup \{b, d, e, g, h, c(d), f(gh)\}$. The states of $A$ correspond to the distinct subtrees in the sample $S_+$, as well. Let us ascribe symbols to the states in the following way: the symbol $S$ corresponds to the trees which belong to $S_+$. (Let us note, that we can make such an ascription because all the trees in the sample belong to the same $R^A$-equivalence class, i.e. $\partial_{t \in S_+}^{k,i}(S_+) = \{\$\}$.) The subtrees $b, d, e, g$ and $h$ correspond to the state symbols $B, D, E, G$ and $H$, respectively. The subtrees $c(d)$ and $f(gh)$ correspond to the state symbols $C$ and $F$, respectively. The transitions of the initial automaton are defined[11] as follows:

|     |                    |      |                        |
|-----|--------------------|------|------------------------|
| (1) | $\delta_b = B$     | (7)  | $\delta_f(G, H) = F$   |
| (2) | $\delta_d = D$     | (8)  | $\delta_a(B, C) = S$   |
| (3) | $\delta_e = E$     | (9)  | $\delta_a(C, E) = S$   |
| (4) | $\delta_g = G$     | (10) | $\delta_a(B, F) = S$   |
| (5) | $\delta_h = H$     | (11) | $\delta_a(F, E) = S$   |
| (6) | $\delta_c(D) = C$  |      |                        |

---

[10]The subtree automaton has been introduced in the previous section (Definition 8.2).
[11]The transitions are defined according to Definition 8.2.

(B) *Merging.* For each tree pair $(t_p, t_s)$ which is not in the same class of $R^A$ and for each values of $k$ and $i$, if:

$$\partial_{t_p}^{k,i}(S_+) = \partial_{t_s}^{k,i}(S_+) \quad \text{and} \quad \partial_{t_p}^{k,i}(S_+) \neq \emptyset \quad \text{and} \quad \partial_{t_p}^{k,i}(S_+) \neq \{\$\}$$

then merge the classes which contain $t_p$ and $t_s$.

Let us come back to our example. Since $\partial_{c(d)}^{1,1}(S_+) = \partial_{f(gh)}^{1,1}(S_+)$ as it is shown in Fig. 8.5c, the states $C$ and $F$ are merged.[12] After this merging, the following set of the transitions is obtained:

| | | | |
|---|---|---|---|
| (1) | $\delta_b = B$ | (7) | $\delta_f(G, H) = C$ |
| (2) | $\delta_d = D$ | (8), (10) | $\delta_a(B, C) = S$ |
| (3) | $\delta_e = E$ | (9), (11) | $\delta_a(C, E) = S$ |
| (4) | $\delta_g = G$ | | |
| (5) | $\delta_h = H$ | | |
| (6) | $\delta_c(D) = C$ | | |

The tree-derivative-based inference method can be presented by the following scheme.

---

**Induction Scheme 8.2: Tree-Derivative-Based Inference**

$A := STA(S_+)$;
*pair_of_equivalent_states_found* := *false*;
**repeat**
   *pair_of_equivalent_states_found* := *merge_pair_of_equivalent_states*($A$);
**until not** *pair_of_equivalent_states_found*;

---

The tree-derivative-based inference method was enhanced in [Levine (1982)] by the use of an inferential strength parameter which specifies the support required from the sample for the inference and the concept of grammatical expansion (a feedback mechanism).

## 8.4  Informed Learning of Tree Languages

The issue of an informed learning of tree languages was studied in [Barrero (1991a)]. In this section, we shall introduce the generic method of the inference of expansive tree grammars which was presented in [Barrero (1991a)]. The method is based

---

[12]Let us notice that the subtree $c(d)$ corresponds to $C$ and the subtree $f(gh)$ corresponds to $F$.

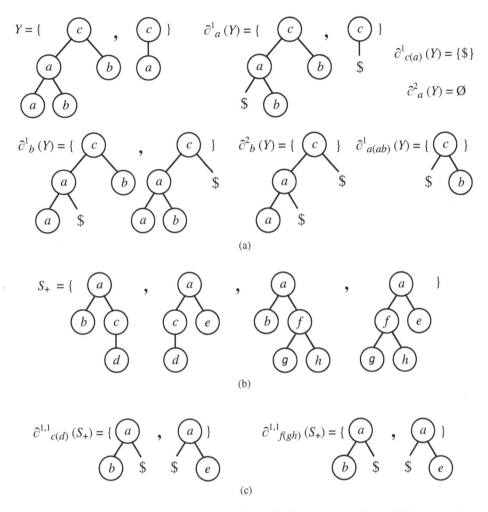

Fig. 8.5  (a) The exemplary tree derivatives for the set $Y$, (b) the sample $S_+$ and (c) two equivalent derivatives for the sample $S_+$.

on the construction of a frontier-to-root deterministic finite tree automaton which recognizes the relative complement of two expansive tree languages.[13]

Let $L_1$ and $L_2$ be two languages over $\Sigma_T$. The relative complement of $L_2$ with respect to $L_1$ is the set $L_1 \setminus L_2 = \{\alpha \in \Sigma_T^* : \alpha \in L_1 \text{ and } \alpha \notin L_2\}$.

Now, we can introduce the rule which allows one to construct a tree automaton which recognizes the relative complement of two expansive tree languages.

Let $A_1 = (Q_1, \Sigma_T, r, \delta_1, Q_{F,1})$ and $A_2 = (Q_2, \Sigma_T, r, \delta_2, Q_{F,2})$, $Q_1 \cap Q_2 = \emptyset$, be two frontier-to-root nondeterministic finite tree automata which recognize expansive tree languages $L_1$ and $L_2$, respectively. A tree automaton $A_3 = (Q_3, \Sigma_T, r, \delta_3, Q_{F,3})$ such that $L(A_3) = L(A_1) \setminus L(A_2) = L_1 \setminus L_2$ is constructed according to the following

---

[13] Expansive tree languages have been introduced in Sec. 7.1.

rule [Barrero (1991a)].

**Rule 8.2 (Tree Automaton for Difference of Tree Languages):**
1) Construct $\bar{A}_1 = (\bar{Q}_1, \Sigma_T, r, \bar{\delta}_1, \bar{Q}_{F,1}'$ in the following way:

- $\bar{Q}_1 = Q_1 \cup Q_2$,
- $\bar{\delta}_1 = \delta_1 \cup \delta_2$,
- $\bar{Q}_{F,1} = Q_{F,1}$.

2) Construct $\bar{A}_2 = (\bar{Q}_2, \Sigma_T, r, \bar{\delta}_2, \bar{Q}_{F,2}$ in the following way:

- $\bar{Q}_2 = Q_1 \cup Q_2$,
- $\bar{\delta}_2 = \delta_1 \cup \delta_2$,
- $\bar{Q}_{F,2} = Q_{F,2}$.

3) Construct a deterministic automaton $\bar{\bar{A}}_1 = (\bar{\bar{Q}}_1, \Sigma_T, r, \bar{\bar{\delta}}_1, \bar{\bar{Q}}_{F,1})$ such that
   $L(\bar{A}_1) = L(\bar{\bar{A}}_1)$.
4) Construct a deterministic automaton $\bar{\bar{A}}_2 = (\bar{\bar{Q}}_2, \Sigma_T, r, \bar{\bar{\delta}}_2, \bar{\bar{Q}}_{F,2})$ such that
   $L(\bar{A}_2) = L(\bar{\bar{A}}_2)$.
5) Construct $A_3 = (Q_3, \Sigma_T, r, \delta_3, Q_{F,3})$ in the following way:

- $Q_3 = \bar{\bar{Q}}_1$,
- $\delta_3 = \bar{\bar{\delta}}_1$,
- $Q_{F,3} = \bar{\bar{Q}}_{F,1} \setminus \bar{\bar{Q}}_{F,2}$.

Let us introduce the following definition [Barrero (1991a)].

Let $S_+$ be a sample, $Sub(S_+)$ be the set of subtrees[14] for $S_+$.

**Definition 8.6 (Canonical Expansive Tree Grammar for $S_+$):** The
canonical expansive tree grammar for $S_+$ is an expansive tree grammar

$$G = (\Sigma_N, \Sigma_T, r, P, S), \text{ where}$$

$\Sigma_N = Sub(S_+)$ is the set of nonterminal symbols,
$(\Sigma_T, r)$ is the ranked alphabet of terminal symbols which appear in $S_+$,
$P$ is the set of productions such that:

- $X \rightarrow a(X_1 X_2 \ldots X_n) \in P$, $n > 0$ iff $X \in \Sigma_N$ corresponds to the subtree $t \in Sub(S_+)$ such that $a \in \Sigma_{T,n}$ is the root of $t$ and $X_1, X_2, \ldots, X_n$ correspond to the descendants of this root or
- $X \rightarrow a \in P$ iff $X \in \Sigma_N$ corresponds to the subtree $t \in Sub(S_+)$ which consists of $a \in \Sigma_{T,0}$ (i.e., the subtree $t$ is a leaf),

$S = S_+$ is the start symbol.

---

[14]A set of subtrees has been defined in Sec. 8.2.

Let us notice the analogy between the canonical expansive tree grammar for $S_+$ and the subtree automaton for $S_+$ introduced in Sec. 8.2 (see Definition 8.2).

At the end of this section we shall introduce the generic rule of the informed learning of tree languages.

Let $(S_+, S_-)$ be a sample. An expansive tree grammar $G$ such that $S_+ \subseteq L(G)$ and $S_- \cap L(G) = \emptyset$ is constructed according to the following rule [Barrero (1991a)].

**Rule 8.3 (Informed Learning of Tree Languages):**
1) Construct a canonical grammar $G_C^+$ for $S_+$ according to Definition 8.6.
2) Construct a derived grammar $G_D^+$ for $S_+$ from the canonical grammar $G_C^+$.[15]
3) Construct a canonical grammar $G_C^-$ for $S_-$ according to Definition 8.6.
4) Construct tree automata $A_1$ and $A_2$ corresponding to $G_D^+$ and $G_C^-$, respectively.
5) Use Rule 8.2 to construct the automaton $A$ such that $L(A) = L(A_1) \setminus L(A_2)$.
6) Construct the grammar $G$ which corresponds to the automaton $A$.

One can easily notice that $L(G) = L(G_D^+) \setminus L(G_C^-)$.

## 8.5 Remarks on the Inference of Tree Languages

The first methods in the inference of tree languages, which were based on the $k$-tails technique, were defined independently in [Bhargava and Fu (1974b); Brayer and Fu (1977)] and [Gonzales and Thomason (1974); Gonzales *et al.* (1976)]. A tree-derivative-based inference algorithm was proposed in [Levine (1981, 1982)]. The equivalence of nonterminals in expansive tree grammars was studied in [Barrero *et al.* (1981)]. An inference algorithm which was based on the concept of $k$-followers of trees was presented in [Fukuda and Kamata (1984)]. The enhancement of Levine's algorithm by the use of semantic information was proposed in [Crimi *et al.* (1990)]. The generic method of the informed learning of expansive tree languages was introduced in [Barrero (1991a)]. An algebraic approach to the inference of tree languages was presented in [Knuutila and Steinby (1994)]. A stochastic tree language inference method was defined in [Carrasco *et al.* (2001)]. The model of an error-correcting tree language inference was proposed in [López and España (2002)]. The learning of decision trees and tree automata was studied in [Sempere and López (2003)]. The method of the inference of $k$-reversible tree languages was presented in [López *et al.* (2004)]. The learning of stochastic $k$-testable tree languages was presented in [Rico-Juan *et al.* (2005)]. An algorithm for the learning of tree languages from positive examples and membership queries was defined in [Besombes and Marion (2007)]. The concept of function distinguishability for tree languages was used to construct learning algorithms in [Fernau (2007)]. Query learning algorithms for tree languages were studied in [Drewes (2009)]. An algo-

---

[15]The generic rule of the constructing of a derived grammar from the corresponding canonical grammar has been presented in Sec. 5.5. In fact, any method presented in the previous sections of this chapter can be used for this purpose.

rithm for the incremental addition or removal of unranked ordered trees to minimal frontier-to-root deterministic finite tree automata was proposed in [Carrasco *et al.* (2009)].

A survey on the inference of tree languages was conducted in [Björklund and Fernau (2016)].

# Chapter 9

# Applications of Tree Methods

As we have mentioned in Chap. 2, tree languages allow us to represent much more complex structural objects/systems than do string ones. Therefore they have been applied in constructing syntactic pattern recognition methods in various application areas since the 1970s. We shall present them in the subsequent sections according to the following application areas: image analysis and processing, optical character recognition (OCR), structure analysis in bioinformatics, texture analysis, analysis of visual events and activities, pattern recognition in seismology, speech recognition and natural language processing (NLP). Similarly as in the case of string methods, the summary of these application in a tabular form is to be found in the last section.

## 9.1 Image Analysis and Processing

The applications of tree grammars and automata for image analysis and processing were studied by K. S. Fu and his collaborators in the 1970s and 1980s. The first research concerned interpreting data obtained from the LANDSAT earth resource technology satellite. Regular tree grammars, frontier-to-root finite automata, and an inference procedure for LANDSAT data interpretation were presented in [Fu (1976a); Li and Fu (1976)] and structure-preserved error-correcting tree automata (SPECTA) in [Fu (1980a)]. Parallel parsing with error-correcting tree automata for interpreting LANDSAT data was proposed in [Chang and Fu (1979)].

Fingerprint classification was performed with regular tree grammars and frontier-to-root finite automata in [Moayer and Fu (1976b)]. Stochastic tree grammars were used for image segmentation in [Don and Fu (1986)]. Weighted structure-preserved error-correcting tree automata (SPECTA) were applied for image segmentation in [Basu and Fu (1987)].

Fuzzy tree automata were proposed for image interpretation in [Lee (1982)]. Automatic scaling of ionograms was performed with the parsing of tree languages in [Guiducci *et al.* (1983)].

*Quadtrees* [Finkel and Bentley (1974)] are used as geometrical description models in computer vision [Dyer *et al.* (1979)]. Regular tree grammars were used for generating quadtrees and for the parallel recognition of multidimensional images in [Saoudi (1992)]. Tree Adjoining Grammars were extended to quadtree adjoining grammars for representing images in [Aizawa and Nakamura (1999b)]. Parsing algorithms for quadtree adjoining grammars were investigated in [Aizawa and Nakamura (1999a)]. A quadtree-like representation of document images and an error-correcting parsing of tree languages were proposed in [Perea and López (2004)].

Expansive tree grammars were used for the analysis of palm structures in X-ray images in [Ogiela *et al.* (2006)].

## 9.2   Optical Character Recognition

Tree grammars and automata were applied for optical character recognition (OCR) by K. S. Fu and his collaborators in the 1970s and 1980s. Tree grammars, transformations on trees and tree automata were used for the recognition of English characters in [Fu and Bhargava (1973)]. Error-correcting tree automata were defined for character recognition in [Lu and Fu (1978)]. Recognition of hand-printed characters was performed with minimum-distance error-correcting tree automata and maximum-likelihood error-correcting tree automata in [Shi and Fu (1982)]. Generalized error-correcting tree automata (GECTA) were used for hand-printed character recognition in [Fu (1982)].

Korean characters (Hangul) were represented and recognized with tree grammars in [Agui *et al.* (1979)]. Tree grammars were used for the high-accuracy recognition of handwritten numerals in [Shridhar and Badreldin (1985)]. A method of recognizing handwritten numerals with tree automata was presented in [Kamata *et al.* (1988)]. Error-correcting tree automata and tree language inference algorithms were applied for a handwritten digit recognition in [López and Piñaga (2000)]. Context-free tree grammars were used for the verification of mathematical formulae in an OCR system in [Fujiyoshi *et al.* (2000)].

## 9.3   Structure Analysis in Bioinformatics

A prediction of protein secondary structures with stochastic tree grammars was presented in [Mamitsuka and Abe (1994); Abe and Mamitsuka (1997)]. Tree Adjoining Grammars were used for RNA structure prediction in [Uemura *et al.* (1999)].

Extended simple linear Tree Adjoining Grammars (ESL-TAG) were defined for generating RNA secondary structure including pseudoknots in [Kato *et al.* (2004)]. Pseudoknot RNA structures were predicted with pair stochastic Tree Adjoining Grammars (PSTAG) in [Matsui *et al.* (2005)]. Tree Adjoining Grammars and related formalisms were considered as grammatical representations of macromolecular structures in [Chiang *et al.* (2006)]. An algorithm for tertiary interactions over pseudoknots, based on extended simple Tree Adjoining Grammars, for RNA secondary structure prediction was presented in [Hsu *et al.* (2013)]. Regular tree grammars were used for the mining of human-viral infection patterns in [Smoly *et al.* (2016)].

## 9.4 Texture Analysis

The first tree language-based model for texture analysis was proposed in [Carlucci (1972)]. Then, research in this area was led by K. S. Fu and his collaborators in the 1970s. Maximum-likelihood SPECTA were used for the discrimination of textures in [Lu and Fu (1978, 1979)]. Parallel parsing with ECTA for texture analysis was proposed in [Chang and Fu (1979)]. The summary of this research was presented in [Fu (1980b)]. The use of stochastic ECTA for recognizing tissues in cytopathology and histopathology was considered in [Prewitt (1979)]. Texture paths in images were recognized with tree grammars in [Vafaie and Bourbakis (1988)].

## 9.5 Analysis of Visual Events and Activities

Programmed context-free languages and tree grammars translation were proposed for time-varying image analysis in [Fan and Fu (1979)]. Minimum-distance SPECTA were used for an analysis of human motion in [Lin and Fu (1982)]. Generalized syntax-directed translation schemes for modelling vehicle motion patterns were applied in a traffic monitoring system in [Fu and Fan (1982)]. An analysis of time-varying image sequences was conducted using stochastic tree grammars and stochastic translation schemes in [Don (1992)].

## 9.6 Pattern Recognition in Seismology

Tree classifiers were used for the detection of bright spots in seismic signals in [Huang and Fu (1984)]. A tree automaton system for recognizing seismic patterns was described in [Huang and Sheen (1986)]. Structure-preserved and generalized error-correcting tree automata for seismic oil exploration were presented in [Huang (2002)]. A novel top-down error-correcting tree automaton for the recognition of nonstructural preserved seismic patterns was proposed in [Huang and Chao (2004)].

## 9.7 Speech Recognition and NLP

The method of error-correcting tree language inference for speech recognition was presented in [López and España (2002)]. Stochastic k-testable tree languages were used for natural language processing in [Verdú-Mas *et al.* (2005)]. Weighted finite tree automata were applied for machine translation, sentence compression and question answering in [May and Knight (2006)]. An overview of stochastic tree transducers for NLP can be found in [Knight and Graehl (2005)].

## 9.8 Summary

A summary of the applications of tree syntactic pattern recognition methods presented in the previous sections is contained in Table 9.1.

Table 9.1    The applications of tree-based methods.

| Applications | Models | References |
|---|---|---|
| Image analysis and processing | (Stochastic) regular tree grammars, Tree Adjoining Grammars, tree automata, error-correcting tree automata, fuzzy tree automata | [Fu (1976a)], [Li and Fu (1976)], [Fu (1980a)], [Moayer and Fu (1976b)], [Chang and Fu (1979)], [Lee (1982)], [Guiducci *et al.* (1983)], [Don and Fu (1986)], [Basu and Fu (1987)], [Saoudi (1992)], [Aizawa and Nakamura (1999b)], [Aizawa and Nakamura (1999a)], [Perea and López (2004)], [Ogiela *et al.* (2006)] |
| Optical character recognition | Regular tree grammars, tree automata, GECTA | [Fu and Bhargava (1973)], [Lu and Fu (1978)], [Agui *et al.* (1979)], [Shi and Fu (1982)], [Fu (1982)], [Shridhar and Badreldin (1985)], [Kamata *et al.* (1988)], [López and Piñaga (2000)], [Fujiyoshi *et al.* (2000)] |
| Structure analysis in bioinformatics | (Stochastic) regular tree grammars, Tree Adjoining Grammars | [Mamitsuka and Abe (1994)], [Abe and Mamitsuka (1997)], [Uemura *et al.* (1999)], [Kato *et al.* (2004)], [Matsui *et al.* (2005)], [Chiang *et al.* (2006)], [Hsu *et al.* (2013)], [Smoly *et al.* (2016)] |
| Texture analysis | (Stochastic) regular tree grammars, Maximum-Likelihood SPECTA | [Carlucci (1972)], [Lu and Fu (1978)], [Lu and Fu (1979)], [Chang and Fu (1979)], [Prewitt (1979)], [Fu (1980b)], [Vafaie and Bourbakis (1988)] |
| Analysis of visual events and activities | Stochastic tree grammars, tree transducers, Minimum-Distance SPECTA | [Fan and Fu (1979)], [Lin and Fu (1982)], [Fu and Fan (1982)], [Don (1992)] |
| Pattern recognition in seismology | Minimum-Distance SPECTA, Maximum-Likelihood SPECTA, GECTA | [Huang and Fu (1984)], [Huang and Sheen (1986)], [Huang (2002)], [Huang and Chao (2004)] |
| Speech recognition and NLP | Stochastic tree automata/transducres, error-correcting tree automata, weighted tree automata | [López and España (2002)], [Knight and Graehl (2005)], [Verdú-Mas *et al.* (2005)], [May and Knight (2006)] |

# PART 4
# GRAPH-BASED MODELS

# Chapter 10

# Pattern Analysis with Graph Grammars

Graph grammars are the strongest descriptive/generative formalism in the theory of formal languages [Pfaltz and Rosenfeld (1969); Montanari (1970); Pavlidis (1972a, 1980); Pfaltz (1972); Abe *et al.* (1973)], since one can define every kind of relation among the structure components. Therefore graph grammars have been used for the *synthesis/generation* of formal representations in various areas of computer science such as computer graphics and vision, programming languages and compiler design, software engineering, database design, distributed and concurrent computing etc., [Ehrig *et al.* (1999)] for more than half a century. On the other hand, only a few graph language parsers used as tools for the *analysis/recognition* of graph patterns in syntactic pattern recognition have been presented over the course of this time. It results from the intractability of the problem of parsing for graph grammars.[1] Graph-based syntactic pattern recognition models are presented in this chapter.

In the late 1970s and the early 1980s, graph-based models were developed at Purdue University, where K. S. Fu and his collaborators conducted research into the applications of graph grammars for syntactic pattern recognition. The model of Attributed Programmed Graph Grammars, *APGG*, [Bunke (1978, 1982a,b)], presented in the next section, was not based on graph language parsing, but used the programming mechanism for the interpretation of scenes represented by graphs. It was used for scene analysis, the interpretation of electronic circuit (EC) diagrams and flowcharts, and product family modelling in ERP systems.

Then, two graph parsers for syntactic pattern recognition were developed at Purdue University. The method of parsing, $\mathcal{O}(n)$ ($n$ is the number of graph nodes), and translation for expansive graph grammars was proposed in [Shi and Fu (1983)]. This was used for scene analysis and the recognition of Chinese characters. A parsing algorithm, $\mathcal{O}(n^3)$, for Attributed Tree-Graph Grammars was presented in [Sanfeliu and Fu (1983b)]. It was applied for the recognition of circuit diagrams and 3D complex objects. These methods are introduced in sections 10.2 and 10.3.

*ETPL(k)* and *ETPR(k)* graph languages [Flasiński (1988, 1989, 1990, 1993, 2018)], presented in Sec. 10.4, are the subclasses of the *edNLC* class of graph grammars [Janssens and Rozenberg (1980a)], which is a standard class in the the-

---

[1]This problem is discussed in Sec. 10.7.

231

ory of graph grammars. $ETPL(k)$ languages and their parsers were defined by
the analogy to $LL(k)$ (string) languages, whereas $ETPR(k)$ languages and their
parser were defined by the analogy to $LR(k)$ (string) languages.[2] These parsing
algorithms are highly efficient, $\mathcal{O}(n^2)$. The model was applied for scene analysis in robotics [Flasiński (1988, 1993)], the recognition of objects in vague images
[Flasiński (1990)], the analysis of features of machined parts in CAD/CAM integration systems [Flasiński (1995b)], the recognition of (Polish) sign language [Flasiński
and Myśliński (2010)], the analysis of configurations of hardware/software components in distributed systems [Flasiński and Kotulski (1992)] and the analysis
of semantic networks/frames in real-time expert systems [Behrens *et al.* (1994);
Flasiński (1994)].

The class of *plex grammars* [Feder (1971)] is also a standard class in the theory
of graph grammars. In section 10.5 two syntactic pattern recognition parsing models for plex grammars are introduced. Both parsing algorithms are efficient, i.e.,
they are of the polynomial complexity, and they are based on the Earley parser.[3]
The parser introduced in [Bunke and Haller (1990)] was applied for the analysis of
flowcharts. The parser introduced in [Peng *et al.* (1990)] was used for the interpretation of electronic circuits.

The *And-Or graph model* [Mumford (2002); Zhu (2003); Zhu and Mumford
(2006)] is a novel approach to graph-based syntactic pattern recognition. Generative rules are attributed and stochastic. A grammar is defined with the help of
an And-Or graph-like representation which specifies both the rules and their context
(an analog for embedding mechanisms in standard graph grammars). The model
has been very popular in computer vision since its publication. A lot of systems
have been developed on its basis including applications for: scene analysis [Han and
Zhu (2009); Lin *et al.* (2009b); Zhao and Zhu (2011); Zarchi *et al.* (2016); Yu *et al.*
(2017); Liu *et al.* (2018)], the analysis of visual events and human activities [Lin
*et al.* (2009a); Pei *et al.* (2011, 2013); Qi *et al.* (2017)] and the estimation of human
attributes,parts and poses [Rothrock *et al.* (2013); Park and Zhu (2015); Park *et al.*
(2018)]. The model is presented in Sec. 10.6.

The last section includes remarks on graph grammars, the problem of parsing
for graph grammars and the comparisons of standard graph grammars and their
parsers used for syntactic pattern recognition.


## 10.1   Bunke Attributed Programmed Graph Grammars

Attributed Programmed Graph Grammars, *APGGs*, were introduced in [Bunke
(1978, 1982a,b)] as a tool for the interpretation of structural patterns. The model
allowed one to analyze not only structural relations among pattern components,
but also their semantic characteristics. Instead of using a parsing technique, the
method made use of the programming mechanism to control derivations. A novelty

---

[2]The $LL(k)$ and $LR(k)$ languages have been introduced in sections 3.2.1 and 3.2.2, respectively.
[3]The Earley parser has been introduced in Sec. 3.2.4.

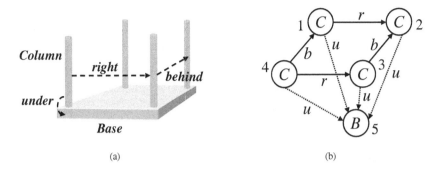

Fig. 10.1 (a) The exemplary scene and (b) its attributed graph representation.

of the approach consisted of constructing the programming mechanism with the help of production applicability predicates defined with semantic attributes.

In defining various types of graphs in the sections of this chapter, we assume denotation conventions as in Appendix A.3 for consistency sake.[4]

Let $A$ be a set of node attributes and $B$ be a set of edge attributes.

**Definition 10.1 (Attributed Graph):** A directed node- and edge-labelled attributed graph, *a-EDG* graph, over $\Sigma$ and $\Gamma$ is a septuple

$$H = (V, E, \Sigma, \Gamma, \phi, \alpha, \beta), \text{ where}$$

$V$ is a finite, non-empty set of nodes,
$\Sigma$ is a finite, non-empty set of node labels,
$\Gamma$ is a finite, non-empty set of edge labels,
$E$ is a set of edges of the form $(v, \gamma, v')$, in which $v, v' \in V, \gamma \in \Gamma$, and $E_w, w \in \Gamma$ denotes a subset of $w$-labelled edges of $E$,
$\phi : V \rightarrow \Sigma$ is a node-labelling function,
$\alpha : V \rightarrow 2^A$ is a function which associates a set of node attributes with each node,
$\beta = (\beta_w)_{w \in \Gamma}$ is a tuple of functions $\beta_w : E_w \rightarrow 2^B$ associating a set of edge attributes with each $w$-labelled edge, for each $w \in \Gamma$.

The family of the *a-EDG* graphs over $\Sigma$ and $\Gamma$ is denoted by *a-EDG*$_{\Sigma,\Gamma}$.

Let us consider the representing of the exemplary scene shown in Fig. 10.1a with a graph depicted in Fig. 10.1b. According to Definition 10.1, $\Sigma$ consists of the node labels $C$ (Column) and $B$ (Base). $\Gamma$ consists of the edge labels $r$ (right), $b$ (behind), and $u$ (under). For example, if every column has a radius $0.25m$ and a height $7.0m$, then $\alpha(k) = \{radius, height\}$, $k = 1, 2, 3, 4$ and $radius(k) = 0.25, height(k) = 7, 0$. If the distances between the pairs of neighboring columns are equal to $9.5m$, then $\beta(e) = \{dist\}$ for each edge $e$ labelled with $r$ or $b$ and, e.g., $dist(\ (4, r, 3)\ ) = 9.5$.

Now, we introduce the definition of a production. Let $D_a$, $a \in A$ denote the

---

[4]Thus, the form of graph definitions can differ a little from the original ones.

domain of a node attribute $a$ and $D_b$, $b \in B$ denote the domain of an edge attribute $b$. Let $g$ and $g'$ be graphs[5] such that $g' \subseteq g$. The edges between the subgraph $g'$ and the graph $g \setminus g'$ are called the embedding of $g'$ in $g$, denoted $EMB(g', g)$.

**Definition 10.2 (Production of *APGG*):** A production of *APGG* is a quintuple

$$p = (g_l, g_r, T, \pi, F), \text{ where}$$

$g_l = (V_l, E_l, \Sigma, \Gamma, \phi_l)$ , $g_r = (V_r, E_r, \Sigma, \Gamma, \phi_r) \in EDG_{\Sigma,\Gamma}$ are the left-hand side and right-hand side graphs, respectively,
$T = \{L_w, R_w : w \in \Gamma\}$, $L_w$ , $R_w \subseteq V_l \times V_r$ is the embedding transformation,
$\pi : a\text{-}EDG_{\Sigma,\Gamma} \to \{$ *TRUE, FALSE* $\}$ is the applicability predicate,
$F$ is a finite set of partial functions $f_a : V_r \to D_a$ and $f_b : E_r \cup EMB(g_r, g) \to D_b$,
$a \in A$, $b \in B$, $g \in a\text{-}EDG_{\Sigma,\Gamma}$, in which $f_a$ is the node attribute transfer function and $f_b$ is the edge attribute transfer function.

Let a transformed graph[6] after removing the left-hand side graph $g_l$ of a production be called the *rest graph*. The embedding transformation $T$ is interpreted in the following way:

(1) If $(v, v') \in L_w$, then a $w$-labelled edge between node $v$ of the left-hand side graph $g_l$ and node $v''$ of the rest graph, which *comes in* $v$ should be replaced by a $w$-labelled edge between node $v'$ of the right-hand side graph $g_r$ and node $v''$ of the rest graph.[7]

(2) If $(v, v') \in R_w$, then a $w$-labelled edge between node $v$ of the left-hand side graph $g_l$ and node $v''$ of the rest graph, which *goes out* from $v$ should be replaced by a $w$-labelled edge between node $v'$ of the right-hand side graph $g_r$ and node $v''$ of the rest graph.[8]

For example, let us consider the production shown in Fig. 10.2a. Let $T = \{R_u\}$[9] and $R_u = \{(1', 5'), (2', 6'), (3', 7'), (4', 8')\}$. Defining $T$ in such a way we ensure that the $u$-labelled edges coming out from nodes $1', 2', 3', 4'$ of the left-hand side graph $g_l$ (cf. Fig. 10.1b) will be "inherited" by nodes $5', 6', 7', 8'$, respectively, of the right-hand side graph $g_r$. If we apply this production to the graph depicted in Fig. 10.1b, we obtain a graph depicted in Fig. 10.2c which represents the scene shown in Fig. 10.2b.

Let us notice that the production defined can be interpreted as laying a slab on four columns. In reality, obviously, certain "semantic" conditions have to be fulfilled for this operation to be performed successfully. For example, all the columns should be the same height. We can define such a precondition for this production with the

---

[5]Basic notions and denotations concerning graphs are presented in Appendix A.3.
[6]A transformed graph means a graph being changed by the application of a production.
[7]The new edge should come in $v'$.
[8]The new edge should go out from $v'$.
[9]Let us remind ourselves that the edge label $u$ means *under*.

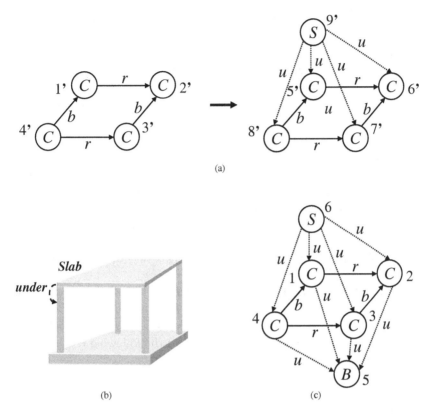

(a)

Slab

under

(b)

(c)

Fig. 10.2   (a) The exemplary production and (b) the scene after the application of the production with (c) its attributed graph representation.

applicability predicate $\pi$ : $height(1') = height(2') = height(3') = height(4')$.

Let us also note that the left-hand side and right-hand side graphs are not attributed graphs. Thus, after performing the syntactical part of the production we have to assign attributes to the right-hand side graph $g_r$ and to the edges of its embedding $EMB(g_r, g)$ in the transformed graph $g$. We do this with the help of node and edge attribute transfer functions. For example, $f_{height}(5') := height(1')$ etc.

Now, we can formalize our consideration with the following definition.

**Definition 10.3 (Derivation Step in *APGG*):** The direct derivation of a graph $g'$ from a graph $g$ by means of a production $p = (g_l, g_r, T, \pi, F)$, denoted $g \overset{p}{\Longrightarrow} g'$, is defined by the following procedure.
(1) Check whether $g_l \subseteq g$ and $\pi$ is *TRUE*. If so then go to step (2).
(2) Replace $g_l$ by $g_r$.
(3) Apply the embedding transformation $T$.
(4) Assign attributes according to the attribute transfer functions of $F$.

The graph grammar presented in this section is programmed with the control mechanism which is analogous to that introduced in [Rosenkrantz (1969)] and presented in Sec. 4.2.1. Instead of the success and failure fields ascribed to a production, the so-called control diagram is used for $APGGs$. This is an $EDG$ graph with nodes labelled with the indices of productions. If we are at a node labelled with a production index and this production is applied then we leave this node *via* an edge labelled with $Y$ (*Yes*), as in the case of the success field for Rosenkrantz grammars. If a production is not applied then we leave this node *via* an edge labelled with $N$ (*No*), as in the case of the failure field. Let us note, however, the fundamental difference between Rosenkrantz grammars and Bunke grammars. Whereas the applicability of a production depends on syntax solely for Rosenkrantz grammars, the production applicability depends on both syntax and semantics (the applicability predicate operating on attributes) in the case of Bunke grammars. Thus, the control of a derivation is more powerful for the latter.

Let us introduce the following definition [Bunke (1982a)].

**Definition 10.4 (Control Diagram of $APGG$):** Let $P$ be a finite set of productions. A control diagram over $P$ is an $EDG$ graph $C$ over $\Sigma$ and $\Gamma$ such that $\Sigma$ contains the indices of the productions of P as node labels and two additional node labels $I$ and $F$, $\Gamma = \{Y, N\}$ and the following conditions hold.
1) Exactly one initial node $v_l$ is labelled with $I$.
2) Exactly one final node $v_F$ is labelled with $F$.
3) No edge terminates at $v_l$.
4) No edge originates at $v_F$.

Now, we can define Attributed Programmed Graph Grammars [Bunke (1982a)].

**Definition 10.5 (Attributed Programmed Graph Grammar):** An attributed programmed graph grammar, $APGG$, is a septuple

$$G = (\Sigma, \Gamma, A, B, P, S, C), \text{ where}$$

$\Sigma$ is a finite, non-empty set of node labels,
$\Gamma$ is a finite, non-empty set of edge labels,
$A$ is a finite set of node attributes,
$B$ is a finite set of edge attributes,
$P$ is a finite set of productions,
$S$ is a finite, non-empty set of initial graphs,
$C$ is a control diagram over $P$.

As we will see below, completing a derivation in $APGGs$ is defined with the help of the final node of the control diagram. Therefore, a distinction between terminal and nonterminal labels is no needed in Definition 10.5.

The language of $APGG$ is defined in the following way [Bunke (1982a)]:

**Definition 10.6 (*APGG* Language):** Let $G$ be an attributed programmed graph grammar. The language of $G$ consists of all *a-EDG* graphs which can be derived in the following way:
(1) Start with an initial graph.
(2) Apply productions in an order defined by the control diagram.
(3) Stop the derivation sequence when the final node in the control diagram has been reached.

*APGG* languages can be used for the interpretation of vague/distorted patterns. Structural distortions can be handled with error transformation-based productions and semantic variations can be taken into account in applicability predicates.

## 10.2 Shi-Fu Parser for Expansive Graph Languages

Expansive graph grammars generate the graph family $\Omega$ which is suitable for syntactic pattern recognition. Analogously as in [Shi and Fu (1983)], we, firstly, introduce $\Omega$ graphs in an intuitive way.

Let $g$ be a directed node- and edge-labelled graph, *EDG* graph, over $\Sigma$ and $\Gamma^{10}$, i.e. $g = (V, E, \Sigma, \Gamma, \phi) \in EDG_{\Sigma,\Gamma}$.

An edge $e = (v, \gamma, w) \in E$ is called a *basic edge* iff on the *EDG* graph obtained by removing $e$ from $E$, $w$ is not a successor of $v$.

A partial graph $g_b = (V, E_b, \Sigma, \Gamma, \phi) \in EDG_{\Sigma,\Gamma}$ of $g$ is called a *basis graph* of $g$ iff
(1) for every $v \in V$, each successor of $v$ on $g$ is a successor of $v$ on $g_b$, and
(2) the set of edges $E_b$ is minimum in the sense that if any edge is removed from $E_b$, condition (1) is no longer satisfied.

Let us assume that $g$ has $n$ nodes. The Boolean adjacency matrix of $g$ is $M = [m_{ij}]_{n \times n}$, in which $m_{ij} = 1$ if there exists $(v_i, \gamma_{ij}, v_j) \in E$, and $m_{ij} = 0$ otherwise.

The graph family $\Omega$ is introduced as the family of acyclic *EDG* graphs such that for every $g \in \Omega$, the basis graph of $g$ should be a tree. Formally, the family $\Omega$ is specified by the following theorem in [Shi and Fu (1983)]:

**Theorem 10.1 (Characteristics of $\Omega$ Graph Family)**

*Given an n-node EDG graph $g$. A necessary and sufficient condition for $g$ belonging to $\Omega$ is that its nodes can be indexed to ensure its Boolean adjacency matrix $M = [m_{ij}]_{n \times n}$ satisfying:*
*(a) $m_{ij} = 0$ for all $i \geq j$,*
*(b) for each $j = 2, \ldots, n$, there exists $1 \leq k(j) < j$ such that $m_{k(j)j} = 1$ and $m_{ij} = 0$ for all $k(j) < i \leq n$, and*
*(c) for each $m_{ij}$ such that $m_{ij} = 1$ and $i \neq k(j)$, there exist $i < j_1 < j_2 < \ldots < j_r < j$ such that $i = k(j_1)$, $j_1 = k(j_2), \ldots$, and $j_r = k(j)$.*

---

[10]Basic notions and denotations concerning graphs are presented in Appendix A.3.

Let us consider the example of representing the Chinese character *river* by the $\Omega$ graph $g = (V, E, \Sigma, \Gamma, \phi)$. (This example is a modification of that introduced in [Shi and Fu (1983)].) The character is shown in Fig. 10.3a. The set of primitives $A, B, C, D$ which defines the set of node labels $\Sigma$ is shown in Fig. 10.3b. The set of edge labels $\Gamma$ is defined for relations: *right* ($r$), *under* ($u$) and *connected* ($c$). The $\Omega$ graph for the character is shown in Fig. 10.3c. (Obviously, we should use an attributed graph to obtain an adequate graph representation.)

The indexing of an $\Omega$ graph $g$ is performed according to the following scheme: Firstly, the basis graph of $g$, which is the tree $t_b$, is indexed according to the Polish prefix (pre-order) traversal scheme. Then, $g$ inherits node indexing from $t_b$. Let us notice that the $\Omega$ graph shown in Fig. 10.3c is indexed according to this scheme.

For indexed $\Omega$ graphs, the string representation was introduced in [Shi and Fu (1983)]. This string representation was adopted for the syntactic pattern recognition model based on $ETPL(k)/ETPR(k)$ graph languages [Flasiński (1988, 1993, 2018)].[11] Therefore, we will formulate it in a general way, i.e., with respect to indexed $EDG$ graphs.

**Definition 10.7 (Characteristic Description of Node):** Let $v_k \in V$ be the node of an indexed $EDG$ graph $g = (V, E, \Sigma, \Gamma, \phi)$. A characteristic description of $v_k$ is the quadruple

$$( a, \; r, \; (e_1 \ldots e_r), \; (i_1 \ldots i_r) ), \text{ where}$$

$a$ is the label of the node $v_k$, i.e., $\phi(v_k) = a$,
$r$ is the out-degree of $v_k$ (the out-degree of the node designates the number of edges going out from this node),
$(i_1 \ldots i_r)$ is the string of node indices to which edges going out from $v_k$ come (in increasing order),
$(e_1 \ldots e_r)$ is the string of edge labels ordered in such a way that the edge having the label $e_x$ comes into the node having the index $i_x$.

Now, we shall define the characteristic description of a graph.

**Definition 10.8 (Characteristic Description of Graph):** Let $g = (V, E, \Sigma, \Gamma, \phi)$ be an indexed $EDG$ graph, where $V = \{v_1, \ldots, v_n\}$ is the set of nodes indexed such that $v_i$ is indexed with $i$ and $I(i), i = 1, \ldots, n$ is the characteristic description of the node $v_i$.
The string $I(1) \ldots I(n)$ is called the characteristic description of the graph $g$.

In the case of $\Omega$ graphs nonbasic edges are marked with $*$. For example, the characteristic description of the $\Omega$ graph shown in 10.3c is defined in the following way:

---

[11]The $ETPL(k)/ETPR(k)$ model is presented in the next section.

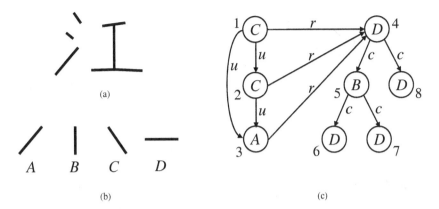

Fig. 10.3    (a) The Chinese character *river*, (b) the set of primitives and (c) its Ω graph representation.

$$C \qquad C \quad A \quad D \quad B \quad D\,D\,D$$

$$3 \qquad 2 \quad 1 \quad 2 \quad 2 \quad 0\ 0\ 0$$

$$(u\ u^*\ r^*)\ (u\ r^*)\ (r)\ (c\ c)\ (c\ c) - - -$$

$$(2\ 3\ 4)\quad (3\ 4)\ (4)\ (5\ 8)\ (6\ 7) - - -$$

Now, we can define expansive graph grammars [Shi and Fu (1983)].

**Definition 10.9 (Expansive Graph Grammar):** An expansive graph grammar is a quintuple

$$G = (\Sigma_N, \Sigma_T, \Gamma, P, S), \text{ where}$$

$\Sigma_N$ is a finite set of nonterminal node labels,
$\Sigma_T$ is a finite set of terminal node labels,
$\Gamma$ is a finite set of edge labels,
$P$ is a finite set of productions of the expansive form

$$A \rightarrow a x_1 B_1 x_2 B_2^{e_2} \dots x_r B_r^{e_r} \text{ (see Fig. 10.4a)}$$

or the reduced form $A \rightarrow a$, in which $a \in \Sigma_T$, $A, B_k \in \Sigma_N$, $k = 1, 2, \dots, r$, $x_k \in \Gamma, k = 1, 2, \dots, r$, and $e_k \in \{*, \lambda\}, k = 2, \dots, r$ are embedding operators, the ordering of $B_k$'s is defined as follows: each $B_k$ without $*$ has a distinct order starting from 1 and increasing from left to right and each $B_k$ with $*$ has an order the same as that of the nonterminal laying on its left side and nearest to it, $S \in \Sigma_N$ is the start symbol.

A derivation according to an expansive grammar $G = (\Sigma_N, \Sigma_T, \Gamma, P, S)$ is defined recursively in the following way:

(1) The first graph $g$ in a derivation sequence consists of one node of order 0 and

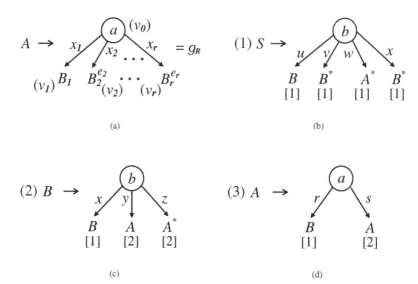

Fig. 10.4    (a) The form of an expansive production and (b)-(d) the exemplary expansive productions.

labelled by $S$.

(2) A derivation step according to a rule $A \to a$ (the reduced form) applied to a node $v$ of $g$ labelled by $A$ consists of the replacement of $A$ by $a$ for $v$.

(3) A derivation step according to a rule of the expansive form shown in Fig. 10.4a applied to a node $v$ of $g$ labelled by $A$ consists of two stages.

    (a) The node $v$ is replaced by the right-hand side of the production $g_R$ (i.e., the node $v_0$ labelled by $a$ of $g_R$ is attached to the node $v$). The order of $v$ is assigned to $v_0$. The successors $v_1, v_2, \ldots, v_k$ of $v_0$ labelled by $B_1, B_2, \ldots, B_k$ obtain new orders in $g$ according to the following rule: the successor $v_k$ labelled by $B_k$ obtains the order $p \cdot l_k$, where $p$ is the (new) order of $v_0$ in $g$, $l_k$ is the order of $v_k$ in $g_R$.

    (b) (*The embedding mechanism.*) If any node $v'$ of $g$ is labelled by the same nonterminal as $v_k$ which is marked with $*$, the order of $v_k$ is a multiple of the order of $v'$, and no edge so far has been incident to the predecessor of $v'$ and incident to $v_k$, then:

        • $v'$ should be removed, if there is only one $v'$ which fulfills this precondition; if there is more than one node fulfilling this precondition, then one of them should be removed, and

        • all the edges which were originally incident to $v'$ should be transformed to be incident to $v_k$.

The language generated by an expansive graph grammar is defined in a standard way.[12]

---

[12]See Definition A.15, point (3) in Appendix A.3.

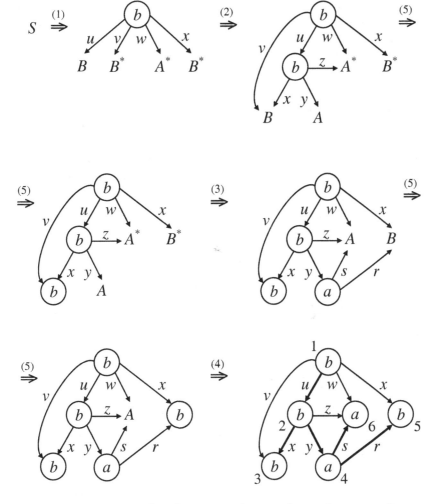

Fig. 10.5   The exemplary derivation in the expansive graph grammar $G$.

Let us define the exemplary expansive graph grammar $G = (\Sigma_N, \Sigma_T, \Gamma, P, S)$, where:

$\Sigma_N = \{S, A, B\}$, $\Sigma_T = \{a, b\}$, $\Gamma = \{r, s, u, v, w, x, y, z\}$, and $P$ consists of the following productions.

(1) $S \rightarrow buBvB^*wA^*xB^*$    (3) $A \rightarrow arBsA$    (5) $B \rightarrow b$

(2) $B \rightarrow bxByAzA^*$    (4) $A \rightarrow a$

The first three productions are shown in Fig. 10.4b-d. (The node orders are included in square brackets.) The example of a derivation in $G$ is shown in Fig. 10.5. The node indices are shown in the final graph and the basic edges are thickened.

At the end of this section we will present the parsing algorithm for expansive graph grammars. The parser constructs the set of parsing lists $I$ for a graph $g$ in an analogous way as the minimum-distance SPECTA (cf. Scheme 7.2 in Sec. 7.2). The set $I$ is constructed according to frontier-to-root parsing of the basis graph/tree $t_b$ of $g$. The parsing list $I(k)$ is defined for the node $v_k$ indexed with $k$. The item of the parsing list is of the form $[A, \alpha, l]$, where $A$ is the left hand side of a production which generates $v_k$ as the root of the right hand side, $l$ is the index of this production, and $\alpha$ is a string of productions applied to the successors of $v_k$ during the derivation.

The input to the parsing algorithm is the grammar $G = (\Sigma_N, \Sigma_T, \Gamma, P, S)$ and a graph $g \in \Omega$ represented by the following characteristic description.

$$
\begin{array}{llll}
a(1) & a(2) & \dots & a(n) \\[2mm]
r(1) & r(2) & \dots & r(n) \\[2mm]
y(1) & y(2) & \dots & y(N) \\[2mm]
i(1) & i(2) & \dots & i(N), \quad \text{where } N = \sum_{t=1}^{n} r(t)
\end{array}
$$

Before we present the Shi-Fu parsing algorithm [Shi and Fu (1983)], we shall introduce its functions.

- $add([A, \alpha, l], I(k))$ - the function adds item $[A, \alpha, l]$ to the parsing list $I(k)$,[13]
- $reduction\_possible(l, j, I)$ - for a production of the form

$$
(l) \quad A \to a(k) x_1 B_1 x_2 B_2^{e_2} \dots x_{r(k)} B_{r(k)}^{e_{r(k)}}
$$

  the function checks whether there exist $[C_1, \beta_1, l_1] \in I(i(j+1))$, $[C_2, \beta_2, l_2] \in I(i(j+2)), \dots, [C_{r(k)}, \beta_{r(k)}, l_{r(k)}] \in I(i(j+r(k)))$ such that for $t = 1, 2, \dots, r(k)$:

  - $(x_t, B_t) = (y_{j+t}, C_t)$, whenever $e_t = \lambda$, and
  - the set $\{(x_{t+1}^*, B_{t+1}), \dots, (x_{t+w}^*, B_{t+w})\}$ is the same as the set $\{(y_{j+t+1}^*, C_{t+1}), \dots, (y_{j+t+w}^*, C_{t+w})\}$, whenever $e_{t+1} = \dots = e_{t+w} = *$ and $e_t = e_{t+w+1} = \lambda$,

- $string\_of\_productions(l, j, I)$ - for a production of the form

$$
(l) \quad A \to a(k) x_1 B_1 x_2 B_2^{e_2} \dots x_{r(k)} B_{r(k)}^{e_{r(k)}}
$$

  which fulfills the conditions defined in the item above (the definition of the function $reduction\_possible(l, j, I)$), the function gives the string $\alpha$ which consists of successively those $l_t$'s such that the corresponding $e_t = \lambda$, $t = 1, 2, \dots, r(k)$,
- $is\_empty(W)$ - the Boolean function which checks whether set $W$ is empty,
- $first\_list\_from\_S(I)$ - the Boolean function which checks whether there is the first list, $I(1)$, with $S$ as the first element in the set of parsing lists $I$.

---

[13]$\alpha$ can be the empty string $\lambda$.

---

**Parsing Scheme 10.1: Shi-Fu Parser**

$error := 0;$
$accept := 0;$
$k := n;$
$j := N;$
**repeat**
  **if** $r(k) = 0$ **then**
    **for each** $(l)$ $A_{(l)} \rightarrow a(k)$ **in** $P$ **do** $add([A_{(l)}, \lambda, l], I(k));$
  **else** /* $r(k) > 0$ */
    **begin**
      $j := j - r(k);$
      **for each** $(l)$ $A_{(l)} \rightarrow a(k)x_{(l,1)}B_{(l,1)}x_{(l,2)}B_{(l,2)}^{e_2} \ldots x_{(l,r(k))}B_{(l,r(k))}^{e_{r(k)}}$ **in** $P$ **do**
        **if** $reduction\_possible(l, j, I)$ **then**
          **begin**
            $\alpha := string\_of\_productions(l, j, I);$
            $add([A_{(l)}, \alpha, l], I(k));$
          **end;**
    **end;**
  **if** $is\_empty(I(k))$ **then** $error := 1;$
  **if** $k = 1$ **then if** $first\_list\_from\_S(I)$ **then** $accept := 1$ **else** $error := 1;$
  $k := k - 1;$
**until** $accept = 1$ **or** $error = 1;$

---

Let us present the following theorem.

**Theorem 10.2 ([Shi and Fu (1983)] Parser Complexity)**

*The running time of the Shi-Fu parsing algorithm for expansive graph grammars is $\mathcal{O}(n)$, where $n$ is the number of graph nodes.*

One can easily notice that the parser accepts a graph $g$ derived in Fig. 10.5 and generates the following parsing lists for $g$:

$$I(1) = [S, \ 2, \ 1] \quad I(3) = [B, \ \lambda, \ 5] \quad I(5) = [B, \ \lambda, \ 5]$$
$$I(2) = [B, \ 53, \ 2] \quad I(4) = [A, \ 54, \ 3] \quad I(6) = [A, \ \lambda, \ 4]$$

The variety of extensions were defined for expansive graph languages, including attributed grammars (and the corresponding parser), programmed grammars, and their syntax-directed translation [Shi and Fu (1983)].

## 10.3   Sanfeliu-Fu Parser for Attributed Tree-Graph Grammars

The idea of defining graph grammars by the extension of tree grammars, used in the Shi-Fu model, was also applied for constructing the class of Tree-Graph Grammars (*TGGs*) [Sanfeliu and Fu (1983b)]. Tree-Graph Grammars have greater generative power than expansive graph grammars because of the use of graphs in the right-hand sides of productions and a stronger embedding mechanism than in the case of expansive graph grammars. Let us introduce the following definition.

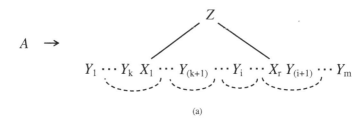

(a)

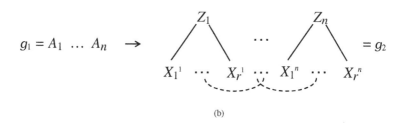

(b)

Fig. 10.6   (a) The type 1 of a TGG production and (b) the type 4 of a TGG production.

**Definition 10.10 (Tree-Graph Grammar):** A Tree-Graph Grammar, *TGG*, is a quintuple

$$G = (\Sigma_N, \Sigma_T, \Gamma, P, S), \text{ where}$$

$\Sigma_N$ is a finite nonempty set of nonterminal node labels,
$\Sigma_T$ is a finite nonempty set of terminal node labels, $\Sigma = \Sigma_N \cup \Sigma_T$,
$\Gamma$ is a finite nonempty set of edge labels,
$P$ is a finite set of productions; the following types of productions are defined:
• type 1, which is depicted in Fig. 10.6a, in which $A \in \Sigma_N$, $Z$, $X_s$, $Y_j \in \Sigma$, $s = 1,\ldots,r$, $j = 1,\ldots,m$; $Z$ is a predecessor of each $X_s$ and $Z$ is not a predecessor of any $Y_j$; $X_s$ can be connected to any other $X_t$ or any other $Y_j$,
• type 2, $A \longrightarrow Z$, in which $A, Z \in \Sigma_N$,
• type 3, $A \longrightarrow a$, in which $A \in \Sigma_N$, $a \in \Sigma_T$,
• type 4, which is depicted in Fig. 10.6b, in which $A_s \in \Sigma_N$, $Z_s, X_{j_s} \in \Sigma$, $s = 1,\ldots,n$,
$S \in \Sigma_N$ is the start symbol or the start graph.

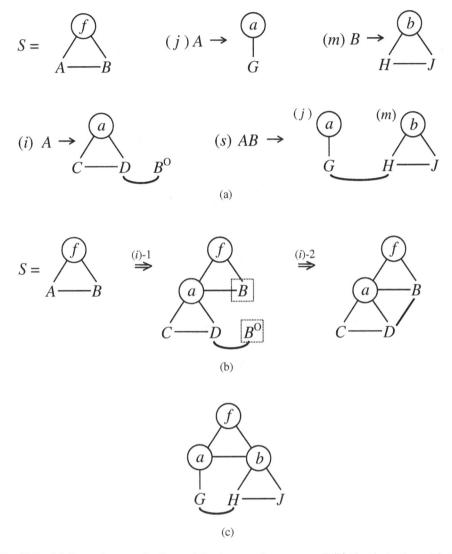

(a)

(b)

(c)

Fig. 10.7 (a) Exemplary productions of the tree-graph grammar $G$ (b) the derivation with the production of type 1 of $G$ and (c) the result of the applying of the production of type 4 of $G$.

Now, we characterize a derivation in a Tree-Graph Grammar. We shall use the exemplary grammar $G = (\Sigma_N, \Sigma_T, \Gamma, P, S)$, for which some productions are shown in Fig. 10.7a. Let us define the following rules [Sanfeliu and Fu (1983b)].

**Type 1.** The nodes $X_s$ and $Y_j$ are grouped into two classes:

NEW: the nodes which are added as new nodes to the derived graph,

OLD: the nodes which are *superimposed* on the existing nodes of the derived graph. The nodes $Y_j$ are always of type OLD (marked with the upper index "O"), whereas the nodes $X_s$ can be NEW or OLD. For example, the application of the production

($i$) of the grammar $G$ with the superimposition of the OLD-type node $B^O$ on the node $B$ is shown in Fig. 10.7b.

**Type 4.**[14] If graph nodes are indexed,[15] then the nonterminals $A_1, A_2, \ldots, A_n$ of $g_1$ are arranged in an increasing order. No superimposition on the nodes $A_1, A_2, \ldots, A_n$ can be made in the following steps of the derivation. For each $A_s$ there is only one right-hand side of the production of the type 1 in $g_2$. Each right-hand side of the production of the type 1 - $rhs_s$ in $g_2$ must have at least one *external horizontal contextual edge*, denoted $HC$, which connects $rhs_s$ with the other right-hand side of the production of the type 1 - $rhs_u$. The nodes $X_{j_s}$ of $g_2$ are NEW.

Summing up, a production of the type 4 is used to connect the nodes of some right-hand sides with $HC$ edges. For example, the graph shown in Fig. 10.7c can be derived from the start graph $S$ with the help of the production ($s$) of the type 4.

Analogously as in the case of the Bunke and Shi-Fu models, Tree-Graph Grammars are extended to their attributed version, namely Attributed Tree-Graph Grammars ($ATGGs$). For $ATGGs$ a parsing algorithm is defined. The Sanfeliu-Fu parser is based on the Earley parsing scheme. Therefore, a string representation of an indexed graph is proposed.[16] For the reason of efficiency, some "technical" constraints are also imposed on $ATGGs$.[17]

In the Sanfeliu-Fu parsing scheme the Earley parser is modified slightly in order to check the vertical and horizontal edges. Additionally, some items (productions) in state sets have to be deleted because either they relate to superimposed nodes or relate to $HC$ edges.

Before we present the Sanfeliu-Fu parsing algorithm, we shall introduce the following functions and assumptions concerning its data structures.

As in the case of the (standard) Earley parser, a table $I$ contains a sequence of state sets $I(0), I(1), \ldots, I(n)$. It is assumed that $n$ is the sum of the number of graph nodes and the number of superimposed nodes.

- *modified_Earley_parser*($I$) - the function is a modified Earley parser which serves superimposition and verifies edges additionally; if the parser cannot add a new nonempty state set then it returns 1 (which means *error*),
- *delete_productions_due_to_superimposition*($I$) - the function deletes redundant items/productions due to superimposition,
- *delete_productions_due_to_HC_edges*($I$) - the function deletes redundant items/productions due to $HC$ edges; if the valid $HC$ edge is not found then it returns 1 (which means *error*),
- *final_state_from_S*($I$) - the function which checks whether there is the final state with $S$ in the left-hand side in the state set $I$.

---

[14]The interpretation is given for types 1 and 4. For types 2 and 3, the interpretation is trivial.

[15]The indexing of graph nodes in this model is from top to bottom and from left to right.

[16]This string representation is analogous to that defined in the Shi-Fu model.

[17]We do not present here the "technical" details of the parsing scheme. Hence, we do not discuss these constraints. The reader is referred to [Sanfeliu and Fu (1983b)].

---

**Parsing Scheme 10.2: Sanfeliu-Fu Parser**

/* $n$ is the number of graph nodes + the number of superimposed nodes */
$error := 0;$
$accept := 0;$
$error := modified\_Earley\_parser(I);$
**if not** $error$ **then**
   **begin**
      $delete\_productions\_due\_to\_superimposition(I);$
      $error := delete\_productions\_due\_to\_HC\_edges(I);$
   **end;**
**if not** $error$ **then if** $final\_state\_from\_S(I(n))$ **then** $accept := 1$ **else** $error := 1;$

---

Let us present the following theorem.[18]

---

**Theorem 10.3 ([Sanfeliu and Fu (1983b)] Parser Complexity)**

*The running time of the Sanfeliu-Fu parsing algorithm for Attributed Tree-Graph Grammars (ATGGs) is $\mathcal{O}(n^3)$, where $n$ is the number of graph nodes.*

---

Attributed Tree-Graph Grammars were used for the analysis of circuit diagrams [Sanfeliu and Fu (1983b)] and the recognition of hidden and deformed 3D complex objects [Sanfeliu (1984)].

## 10.4 Recognition of ETPL(k) and ETPR(k) Graph Languages

The lack of the ordering of a graph structure and the complexity of a graph grammar derivation are two main reasons of difficulties with constructing efficient graph grammar parsers.[19]

The first problem is solved in the $ETPL(k)/ETPR(k)$ model [Flasiński (1988, 1989, 1993, 2018)] by imposing the linear (total) order on the set of graph nodes $V$ of an $EDG$ graph[20] $h = (V, E, \Sigma, \Gamma, \phi)$. For this purpose, a rule for the unambiguous indexing of the nodes, performed on the basis of the properties of a structure represented by $h$, should be defined. In computer vision applications, such a rule can be based, e.g., on the placement of objects in 2D/3D space [Flasiński (1988, 1989, 1993)]. For example, we can index the objects of the scene shown in Fig. 10.8a moving from left to right, i.e., according to the (less) $x$-coordinate.[21] Then,

---

[18]We assume that the starting node is fixed in the parsed graph.
[19]Both problems are discussed in Sec. 10.7 in a more detailed way.
[20]Basic notions and denotations concerning graphs are presented in Appendix A.3.
[21]If two objects have the same $x$-coordinate, the $y$-coordinate can be used to establish the precedence relation.

the object indices are ascribed to the corresponding graph nodes as is shown in Fig. 10.8.[22]

Having the graph nodes uniquely indexed, the graph edges are defined on the basis of the objects' inter-relations[23] in an unambiguous way. The following property of the set of edge labels $\Gamma$ is assumed: there exists the edge label $\gamma^{-1} \in \Gamma$ for each label $\gamma \in \Gamma$ such that the edges connecting nodes $v, w \in V$: $(v, \gamma, w) \in E$ and $(w, \gamma^{-1}, v) \in E$ describe the same relation between the objects of the structure represented by these nodes. The edges $(v, \gamma, w)$ and $(w, \gamma^{-1}, v)$ are called *semantically equivalent*, denoted $(v, \gamma, w) \stackrel{sem}{=} (w, \gamma^{-1}, v)$. Two graphs which differ one from another in semantically equivalent edges only are also called semantically equivalent. For example, for the graphs $g_1$ and $g_2$ shown in Figs. 10.8 c and d, respectively, the following holds: $g_1 \stackrel{sem}{=} g_2$. This assumption is not restrictive in practical applications. For example, for the set of spatial relations: *left* (*l*), *right* (*r*), *behind* (*b*), *in-front-of* (*f*), *behind-left* (*bl*), *in-front-of-right* (*fr*), *behind-right* (*br*), *in-front-of-left* (*fl*) depicted in Fig. 10.8b, the set $\Gamma = \{ l, r, b, f, bl, fr, br, fl \}$ obviously fulfills this assumption.[24] Now, we can define the *edge-unambiguous* graph in such a way that every edge is directed from the node with a smaller index to the node with a greater index. For example, the graph $g_2$ shown in Fig. 10.8d is edge-unambiguous, whereas the graph $g_1$ shown in Fig. 10.8c is not.

Now, we shall formalize our considerations. Since we have referred to the *semantic aspect* of a graph representation, we shall make this formalization on the basis of Tarski's (semantic) model theory approach. Firstly, we shall introduce the definition of a relational structure, which corresponds to a structure to be represented by an *EDG* graph.

**Definition 10.11 (Relational Structure):** Let $\mathcal{U}$ be a finite set of individual objects called a universe, $\mathcal{N}_\mathcal{U}$ be a set of their names, $\mathcal{A}_\mathcal{U}$ be a set of their attributes.

Let each object $o^k, k = 1, \ldots K$ of $\mathcal{U}$ be represented by its name $n_u^k \in \mathcal{N}_\mathcal{U}$ and the set of its attributes $a_u^k \in 2^{\mathcal{A}_\mathcal{U}}$.

Let $\mathcal{R} \subset 2^{\mathcal{U} \times \mathcal{U}}$ be a set of binary relations such that for a pair of objects at most one relation is established, $\mathcal{N}_\mathcal{R}$ be a set of their names, $\mathcal{A}_\mathcal{R}$ be a set of their attributes, $\mathcal{R} = \{(n_r, a_r) : n_r \in \mathcal{N}_\mathcal{R}, a_r \in 2^{\mathcal{A}_\mathcal{R}}\}$.

A relational structure is a sextuple $\mathfrak{S} = (\mathcal{U}, \mathcal{R}, \mathcal{N}_\mathcal{U}, \mathcal{N}_\mathcal{R}, \mathcal{A}_\mathcal{U}, \mathcal{A}_\mathcal{R})$.

---

[22]The definition of an indexing rule depends mainly on the specificity of an application field. The formulating of this rule is not difficult in practice. The $ETPL(k)/ETPR(k)$ model has been used for a *variety of applications* like scene analysis in robotics, the recognition of objects in vague images, the analysis of features of machined parts in CAD/CAM integration systems, the recognition of (Polish) sign language, the analysis of configurations of hardware/software components in distributed systems and the analysis of semantic networks/frames in real-time expert systems.

[23]These inter-relations are marked with dashed white lines in Fig. 10.8a.

[24]Besides, if for some relation *rel* no semantic "opposite counterpart" exists, a formal trick is applied in the model, which consists in defining the opposite edge label $rel^{-1}$, i.e. the label *rel* marked by $^{-1}$.

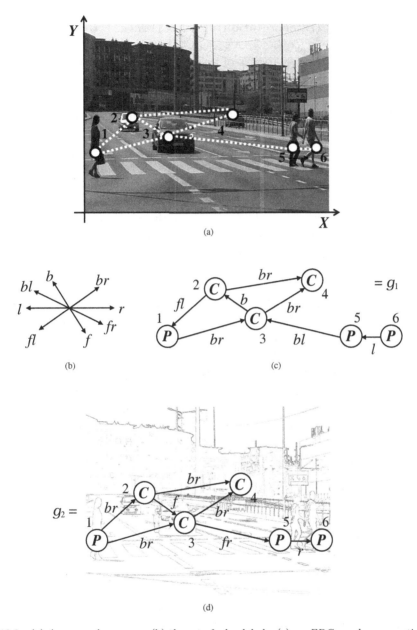

Fig. 10.8 (a) An exemplary scene, (b) the set of edge labels, (c) an *EDG* graph representing the scene, and (d) the edge-unambiguous graph representing the scene.

Now, we can define the interpretation of an *EDG* graph over a relational structure.

**Definition 10.12 (Interpretation):** Let $h = (V, E, \Sigma, \Gamma, \phi)$ be an *EDG* graph over $\Sigma$ and $\Gamma$, $\mathfrak{S} = (\mathcal{U}, \mathcal{R}, \mathcal{N_U}, \mathcal{N_R}, \mathcal{A_U}, \mathcal{A_R})$ be a relational structure, $\Sigma \subset \mathcal{N_U}, \Gamma \subset \mathcal{N_R}$. An interpretation $\mathcal{I}$ of the graph $h$ over the structure $\mathfrak{S}$ is a pair

$$\mathcal{I} = (\mathfrak{S}, \mathcal{F}), \text{ where:}$$

$\mathcal{F} = (\mathcal{F}_1, \mathcal{F}_2)$ is the *denotation function* defined in the following way:
- $\mathcal{F}_1$ assigns an object $u \in \mathcal{U}$ having a name $a \in \mathcal{N_U}$ to each graph node $v \in V, \phi(v) = a, a \in \Sigma$,
- $\mathcal{F}_2$ assigns a pair of objects $(u', u'') \in r, r \in \mathcal{R}$ to each graph edge $(v, \gamma, w) \in E$, $v, w \in V, \gamma \in \Gamma$ such that $\mathcal{F}_1(v) = u'$, $\mathcal{F}_1(w) = u''$ and $r$ has the name $\gamma$.

Finally, we introduce the definition of an interpreted *EDG* graph.

**Definition 10.13 (Interpreted *EDG* Graph):** Let $h$ be an *EDG* graph over $\Sigma$ and $\Gamma$, $\mathfrak{S}$ be a relational structure, $\mathcal{I}$ be the interpretation of $h$ over $\mathfrak{S}$ defined as in Definition 10.12. An interpreted *EDG* graph is a triple $h^\mathcal{I} = (\mathfrak{S}, h, \mathcal{I})$.

Obviously, we can define an *attributed* interpreted *EDG* graph by analogy to the Bunke's model presented in Sec. 10.1. Then attributes of the elements of a relational structure (i.e., the objects and the relations) are ascribed to the corresponding components of a graph (i.e., the nodes and the edges).

The model presented in this section is based on top-down parsable *ETPL(k)* graph languages [Flasiński (1988, 1989, 1993)] and bottom-up parsable *ETPR(k)* graph languages [Flasiński (2018)]. For graphs belonging to these language families various indexing schemes are applied. Therefore, we introduce two classes of graphs: *IE* graphs belonging to the *ETPL(k)* family and *rIE* graphs belonging to the *ETPR(k)* family.

**Definition 10.14 (*IE* Graph):** Let $h^\mathcal{I} = (\mathfrak{S}, h, \mathcal{I})$ be an interpreted *EDG* graph over $\Sigma$ and $\Gamma$. An indexed edge-unambiguous graph, *IE*, graph over $\Sigma$ and $\Gamma$ defined on the basis of the graph $h^\mathcal{I}$ is an *EDG* graph $g = (V, E, \Sigma, \Gamma, \phi)$ which is isomorphic to $h$ up to the direction of the edges, such that the following conditions are fulfilled:
1. $g$ contains a directed spanning tree $t$ such that the nodes of $t$ have been indexed due to the Level Order Tree Traversal (LOTT).
2. The nodes of $g$ are indexed in the same way as the nodes of $t$.
3. Every edge in $g$ is directed from the node having a smaller index to the node having a greater index.

(Let us recall that LOTT means that for each node firstly the node is visited, then its child nodes are put into the FIFO queue. This type of a tree traversal is also known as the Breadth First Search (BFS) scheme.)
The family of all the IE graphs over $\Sigma$ and $\Gamma$ is denoted by $IE_{\Sigma, \Gamma}$.
An exemplary *IE* graph $h_1$ is shown in Fig. 10.9a. The edges of the spanning tree

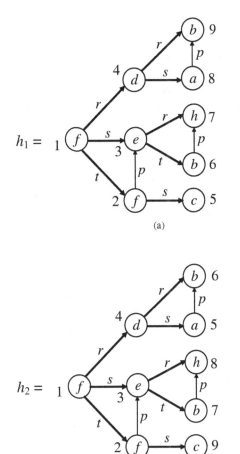

Fig. 10.9 (a) An exemplary *IE* graph and (b) *rIE* graph.

$t$ are thickened.

Now, we shall define *rIE* graphs belonging to the *ETPR(k)* family.

**Definition 10.15 (*rIE* Graph):** Let $h^{\mathcal{I}} = (\mathfrak{S}, h, \mathcal{I})$ be an interpreted *EDG* graph over $\Sigma$ and $\Gamma$. A reversely indexed edge-unambiguous graph, *rIE*, graph over $\Sigma$ and $\Gamma$ defined on the basis of the graph $h^{\mathcal{I}}$ is an *EDG* graph $g = (V, E, \Sigma, \Gamma, \phi)$ which is isomorphic to $H$ up to the direction of the edges, such that the following conditions are fulfilled:
1. $g$ contains a directed spanning tree $t$ such that the nodes of $t$ have been indexed due to the Reverse Level Order Tree Traversal (RLOTT).
2. The nodes of $g$ are indexed in the same way as the nodes of $t$.
3. Every edge in $g$ is directed from the node having a smaller index to the node having a greater index.

(The RLOTT scheme is analogous to the LOTT (BFS) scheme, however it uses a LIFO queue (i.e., a stack) instead of a FIFO queue.)

The family of all the *rIE* graphs over $\Sigma$ and $\Gamma$ is denoted by $rIE_{\Sigma,\Gamma}$.

An exemplary *rIE* graph $h_2$ is shown in Fig. 10.9b.

Now, we shall present a solution to the second problem, i.e., the complexity of a graph grammar derivation. Both classes used in the model presented here, i.e., the class of *ETPL(k)* graph grammars and the class of *ETPR(k)* graph grammars, are subclasses of the standard family of *edNLC* graph grammars [Janssens and Rozenberg (1980a,b)].[25] Therefore, firstly, we shall introduce *edNLC* graph grammars. Since their formal definition is rather complex, we shall do this in an intuitive way. (The corresponding formal definitions are included in Appendix A.3.)

Let us consider the following *edNLC* graph grammar $G = (\Sigma, \Sigma_T, \Gamma, P, Z)$, where $\Sigma = \{b, d, f, A, B\}$ is the set of node labels, $\Sigma_T = \{b, d, f\}$ is the set of terminal node labels, $\Gamma = \{p, s, t, u\}$ is the set of edge labels, $Z \in EDG_{\Sigma,\Gamma}$ is the start graph shown in Fig. 10.10a. Productions of the set $P$ are of the form $(l, D, C)$, in which $l \in \Sigma \setminus \Sigma_T$ is the nonterminal node label of the left-hand side of the production, $D \in EDG_{\Sigma,\Gamma}$ is the graph of the right-hand side of the production, and $C$ is the embedding transformation. The left- and right-hand sides of an exemplary production of the grammar $G$ are shown in Fig. 10.10b. The embedding transformation of this production is defined as follows:

(i) $C(p, out) = \{(d, A, u, in)\}$,
(ii) $C(t, in) = \{(b, f, t, in)\}$.

The graph $g$ which is the result of applying this production to the start graph $Z$ is shown in Fig. 10.10c.

The derivational step is performed in two parts. During the first stage, the node labelled with $B$ of the graph $Z$ is removed, and the graph of the right-hand side replaces the removed node. The transformed graph obtained by removing the node and its adjacent edges is called the rest graph. During the second stage, the embedding transformation is used in order to connect certain nodes of the right-hand side graph with the rest graph. The item $(i)$ is interpreted in the following way.

(1) Each edge labelled with $p$ and going *out* from the node corresponding to the left-hand side of a production, i.e. $B$, should be replaced by
(2) the edge:

    (a) connecting the node of the graph of the right-hand side of the production and labelled with $d$ with the node of the rest graph and labelled with $A$,

    (b) labelled with $u$,

    (c) and coming *in* the node $d$.

---

[25] A brief overview of graph grammars theory is included in Sec. 10.7.

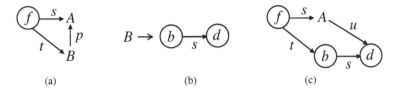

Fig. 10.10 (a) The start graph $Z$ of the edNLC grammar $G$, (b) a production of $G$ and (c) the derived graph $g$.

Thus the item $(i)$ of the embedding transformation generates the edge of the graph $g$, shown in Fig. 10.10c, which is labelled with $u$ and connects the nodes labelled with $d$ and $A$ on the basis of the edge of the graph $Z$ which is labelled with $p$ and connects the nodes labelled with $B$ and $A$. The item $(ii)$ preserves the edge labelled with $t$.

Now, we shall impose subsequent constraints on the class of edNLC graph grammars in order to obtain the efficiently parsable subclasses $ETPL(k)$ and $ETPR(k)$. Since the corresponding constraints for both subclasses differ only slightly, they will be formalized by single definitions with modifications. (The modifications for $ETPR(k)$ grammars will be written in brackets in the definitions.) The examples will be defined for $ETPL(k)$ grammars. (The examples for $ETPR(k)$ grammars can be defined in an analogous way.)

For the purpose of the standardization of the right-hand side graphs we formulate the following definition. Firstly, however, we shall introduce the notion of node level. We say that a node $v$ of the *IE* (*rIE*) graph is on level $n$, if $v$ is on level $n$ of the spanning tree $t$ constructed as in Definition 10.14 (Definition 10.15).

**Definition 10.16 (*TLP* Grammar):** Let $G = (\Sigma, \Sigma_T, \Gamma, P, Z)$ be an *edNLC* graph grammar. The grammar $G$ is called a *TLP* graph grammar, abbrev. from *Two-Level Production*, if the right-hand side of every production from $P$ (and the axiom $Z$) is an $(r)IE$ graph having nodes of level at most 2 and the node on level 1 is labelled with a terminal symbol.

Now, we shall introduce two constraints which allow one to perform a derivation according to the linear ordering imposed on *IE* (*rIE*) graphs.

**Definition 10.17 (Closed *TLP* (*rTLP*) Grammar):** A *TLP* graph grammar $G$ is called a closed *TLP* (*rTLP*) graph grammar $G$ if for each derivation of this grammar

$$Z = g_0 \underset{G}{\Longrightarrow} g_1 \underset{G}{\Longrightarrow} \dots \underset{G}{\Longrightarrow} g_n$$

each graph $g_i$, $i = 0, \dots, n$ is an *IE* (*rIE*) graph.

**Definition 10.18 (Closed *TLPO* (*rTLPO*) Grammar):** Let there be given a derivation of a closed *TLP* (*rTLP*) graph grammar $G$:

$$Z = g_0 \underset{G}{\Longrightarrow} g_1 \underset{G}{\Longrightarrow} \ldots \underset{G}{\Longrightarrow} g_n.$$

This derivation is called a regular left-hand (right-hand) side derivation, denoted $\underset{rl(G)}{\Longrightarrow}$ ( $\underset{rr(G)}{\Longrightarrow}$ ) if:

(1) for each $i = 0, \ldots, n-1$ a production for a nonterminal node having the least (greatest) index in a graph $g_i$ is applied,

(2) node indices do not change during a derivation.

A closed *TLP* (*rTLP*) graph grammar which rewrites graphs according to the regular left-hand (right-hand) side derivation is called a closed *TLPO* (*rTLPO*) graph grammar, abbrev. from (reverse) Two-Level Production-Ordered.

In order to illustrate the definitions introduced above, let us consider the following simple closed *TLPO* graph grammar[26] $G = (\Sigma, \Sigma_T, \Gamma, P, Z)$, where $\Sigma = \{a, b, d, e, f, A, B\}$, $\Sigma_T = \{a, b, d, e, f\}$, $\Gamma = \{p, r, s, t\}$, the left- and right-hand sides of three productions of $P$ and the axiom $Z$ are shown in Fig. 10.11a, the embedding transformations $C_1$, $C_2$ and $C_3$ of the productions (1), (2) and (3), respectively, are defined as follows:

- $C_1(s, in) = \{(a, f, s, in)\}$, $C_1(p, in) = \{(a, b, p, in)\}$,
  $C_1(t, out) = \{(a, e, t, out), (a, f, t, out)\}$, $C_1(p, out) = \{(a, B, p, out)\}$,
- $C_2(t, in) = \{(b, f, t, in)\}$, $C_2(r, in) = \{(b, f, r, in)\}$,
  $C_2(p, out) = \{(b, A, p, out), (e, A, t, in)\}$, $C_2(p, in) = \{(b, a, p, in)\}$,
- $C_3(t, in) = \{(b, f, t, in)\}$, $C_3(r, in) = \{(b, f, r, in)\}$,
  $C_3(p, out) = \{(b, A, p, out), (f, A, t, in)\}$, $C_3(p, in) = \{(b, a, p, in)\}$.

Let us notice that $G$ is a *TLP* grammar since the right-hand side of every production and the axiom $Z$ is an $(r)IE$ graph having nodes of level at most 2 and the node on level 1 is labelled with a terminal symbol. $G$ is also a closed *TLP* grammar because each graph belonging to any derivation in $G$ is an $IE$ graph (e.g., see Figs. 10.11b-e). Finally, $G$ is a closed *TLPO* grammar since at any derivational step a production is applied to a node having the least index, and node indices do not change during a derivation.

*ETPL(k)* and *ETPR(k)* graph grammars are analogous to (string) *LL(k)* and *LR(k)* grammars, respectively, introduced in Sections 3.2.1 and 3.2.2. For *LL(k)* and *LR(k)* grammars, the fundamental *properties of an unambiguous choice of a production during a parsing* have been defined in order to make their parsers deterministic. These properties have been defined with the help of the notion of *the k-length prefix*, denoted $FIRST_k$. The notions of *k-TL* and *CTL* graphs, which are analogous to $FIRST_k$, must be defined in the case of graph grammars. These notions will be used for extracting handles in parsed graphs which are matched against

[26]Examples of more complex graph grammars of this type are considered in Sec. 11.2.

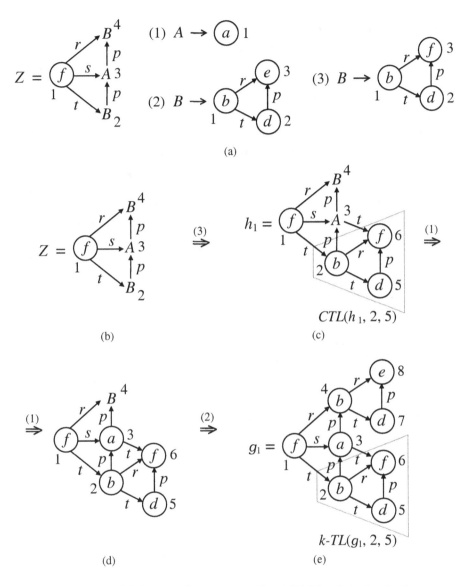

Fig. 10.11   (a) An exemplary grammar $G$ and (b)-(e) a derivation in $G$.

right-hand sides of productions. We assume that *IE* (*rIE*) graphs are represented with characteristic descriptions introduced in the Fu-Shi model in Sec. 10.2 (cf. Definitions 10.7 and 10.8).[27]

---

[27] The reader is encouraged to recall these definitions and the corresponding example.

**Definition 10.19 ($k$-$TL$ Graph):** Let $g$ be an $IE$ ($rIE$) graph, $t$ the index of the node $v$ of $g$ defined by a characteristic description $(b, r, (e_1 \ldots e_r), (i_1 \ldots i_r))$, $\phi(v) = b$. A subgraph $h$ of the graph $g$ consisting of the node indexed with $t$, nodes having indices $i_{a+1}, i_{a+2}, \ldots, i_{a+k}$, $a \geq 0$, $a + k \leq r$, and edges connecting the nodes indexed with: $t, i_{a+1}, i_{a+2}, \ldots, i_{a+k}$ is called a $k$-successors two-level graph originated in the node $v$ and beginning with the $(i_{a+1})$th successor, denoted $h = k\text{-}TL(g, l, i_{a+1})$. By $0\text{-}TL(g, l, -)$ we denote the subgraph of $g$ consisting only of the node $v$.

**Definition 10.20 ($CTL$ Graph):** Let $g$ be an $IE$ ($rIE$) graph, $t$ the index of the node $v$ of $g$ defined by a characteristic description $(b, r, (e_1 \ldots e_r), (i_1 \ldots i_r))$, $\phi(v) = b$. A subgraph $h$ of the graph $g$ consisting of the node indexed with $t$, nodes having indices $i_{a+1}, i_{a+2}, \ldots, i_r$, $a \geq 0$, and edges connecting the nodes indexed with: $t, i_{a+1}, i_{a+2}, \ldots, i_r$ is called a complete two-level graph originated in the node $v$ and beginning with the $(i_{a+1})$th successor, denoted $h = CTL(g, l, i_{a+1})$.

For example, a $k$-$TL$ graph for $k = 2$, i.e., $2\text{-}TL(g_1, 2, 5)$ is marked in Fig. 10.11e.

Now, we can impose the constraint which is analogous to that used in the definition of string $LL(k)$ grammars [Lewis II and Stearns (1968); Rosenkrantz and Stearns (1970)] (cf. Definition 3.1). This allows us to construct a deterministic top-down parsing scheme for edNLC grammars.

**Definition 10.21 ($PL(k)$ Grammar):** Let $G = (\Sigma, \Sigma_T, \Gamma, P, Z)$ be a closed $TLPO$ graph grammar. The grammar $G$ is called a $PL(k)$, abbrev. Production-ordered $k$-Left nodes unambiguous, graph grammar if the following condition is fulfilled: Let

$$Z \xrightarrow[rl(G)]{*} X_1 A X_2 \xrightarrow[rl(G)]{} h_1 \xrightarrow[rl(G)]{*} g_1$$

and

$$Z \xrightarrow[rl(G)]{*} X_1 A X_2 \xrightarrow[rl(G)]{} h_2 \xrightarrow[rl(G)]{*} g_2 \,,$$

where $\xrightarrow[rl(G)]{*}$ is the transitive and reflexive closure of $\xrightarrow[rl(G)]{}$, be two regular left-hand side derivations, such that $A$ is a characteristic description of a node indexed with $t$, and $X_1$ and $X_2$ are substrings of characteristic descriptions. Let $max$ be the number of nodes of the graph $X_1 A X_2$. If

$$k\text{-}TL(g_1, t, max + 1) \cong k\text{-}TL(g_2, t, max + 1)$$

then

$$CTL(h_1, t, max + 1) \cong CTL(h_2, t, max + 1).$$

Let us notice that our exemplary grammar $G$ is a $PL(2)$ grammar since at the derivation step shown in Fig. 10.11b one has to analyze the 2-*TL* graph of the input graph shown in Fig. 10.11e in order to identify which production should be used during the derivation (i.e., production (2) or production (3)). The grammar $G$ is not a $PL(1)$ grammar because 1-*TL* graphs for productions (2) and (3) are the same.

For the purpose of constructing a deterministic bottom-up parsing scheme, we impose the constraint which is analogous to that used in the definition of string $LR(k)$ grammars [Knuth (1965)] (cf. Definition 3.2).

**Definition 10.22 ($PR(k)$ Grammar):** Let $G = (\Sigma, \Sigma_T, \Gamma, P, Z)$ be a closed *rTLPO* graph grammar. The grammar $G$ is called a $PR(k)$, abbrev. Production-ordered $k$-Right nodes unambiguous, graph grammar if the following condition is fulfilled. Let

$$ Z \xrightarrow[rr(G)]{*} X_1 A X_2 \xrightarrow[rr(G)]{} X_1 g X_2 \, , $$

$$ Z \xrightarrow[rr(G)]{*} X_3 B X_4 \xrightarrow[rr(G)]{} X_1 g X_5 \, , $$

and

$$ k\text{-}TL(X_2, 1, 2) \cong k\text{-}TL(X_5, 1, 2) \, , $$

where $\xrightarrow[rr(G)]{*}$ is the transitive and reflexive closure of $\xrightarrow[rr(G)]{}$ , $A$, $B$ are characteristic descriptions of certain nodes, $X_1$, $X_2$, $X_3$, $X_4$, $X_5$ are substrings of characteristic descriptions, $g$ is the right-hand side of a production: $A \longrightarrow g$. Then:

$$ X_1 = X_3 \, , \quad A = B \, , \quad X_4 = X_5 \, . $$

Let us note that if an edge goes out from some node $v$ and comes into a node $w$ which is labelled by a nonterminal symbol,[28] then the embedding transformation of a production applied to the node $w$ can delete this edge. It means that after accepting the characteristic description of the node $v$ this description can be changed during the next steps of parsing. In order to disable such an unwanted effect we impose the following constraint:

**Definition 10.23 (Potential Previous Context):** Let $G = (\Sigma, \Sigma_T, \Gamma, P, Z)$ be a $PL(k)$ ($PR(k)$) graph grammar. A pair $(b, x), b \in \Sigma_T, x \in \Gamma$, is called a potential previous context for a node label $a \in \Sigma \setminus \Sigma_T$, if there exists the *IE* (*rIE*) graph $g = (V, E, \Sigma, \Gamma, \phi)$ belonging to a certain regular left-hand (right-hand) side derivation in $G$ such that : $(v, x, w) \in E, \phi(v) = b$, and $\phi(w) = a$.

---

[28] Let us also note that the index of $v$ is less than the index of $w$.

**Definition 10.24 (*ETPL(k)* (*ETPR(k)*)) Grammar):** A *PL(k)* (*PR(k)*) graph grammar $G$ is called an *ETPL(k)* (*ETPR(k)*), abbrev. from Embedding Transformation-preserving Production-ordered $k$-Left ($k$-Right) nodes unambiguous, graph grammar if for each production $(l, D, C) \in P$ the following condition is fulfilled.
Let $l = A$, $X_1, X_2, \ldots, X_m$, where $X_i \neq X_j, i, j = 1, \ldots, m$, be the labels of nodes indexed with $1, 2, \ldots, m$ of the right-hand side graph $D$. For each potential previous context $(b, y)$ for $A$, there exists $(X_i, b, z, in) \in C(y, in), i \in \{1, \ldots, m\}$. If $i = 1$, then $z = y$, i.e. $(X_1, b, y, in) \in C(y, in)$.

The language generated by an *ETPL(k)* (*ETPR(k)*) graph grammar is defined in a standard way.[29]
Before we present the parsing algorithm for *ETPL(k)* graph grammars [Flasiński (1993)], we shall mention the following issue which is taken into account during a parsing.[30] Let us assume that the *ETPL(k)* parser analyzes an $n$-node *IE* graph $G$ which is represented by its characteristic description. Since the parser is generative (i.e. top-down), it derives the working graph $H$ during a parsing. Its scheme consists merely in reading the characteristic description of the succeeding node of $G$ indexed with $i = 1, \ldots, n$ and comparing it with the characteristic description of the node of $H$ having the index $i$. If the node of $H$ is nonterminal, the proper production is found and applied to $H$. If it is terminal, the characteristic descriptions of both nodes should be *compatible*. The compatibility means that they are the same or they are *potentially context-identical* [Flasiński (1993)]. The nodes indexed with $i$ of the graphs $G$ and $H$ are potentially context-identical, if their characteristic descriptions are the same up to the edges which go out of the node of $G$ and come into the nodes which have not yet been generated in $H$. The descriptions of these edges are stored by the parser and verified once these edges are generated in $H$. Let us introduce the following functions of the parser.

- *is_terminal*($A$) - the Boolean function which checks whether $A$ is terminal,
- *nodes_compatible*($G, H, i$) - the function checks whether the nodes indexed with $i$ of the graphs $G$ and $H$ are the same or they are potentially context-identical; if not, the function returns 1 (which means *error*); if they are potentially context-identical the function stores the descriptions of the missing edges,
- *choose_production*($G, i$) - the function returns the index of a production which should be applied to the node indexed with $i$ of the graph $H$ according to Definition 10.21; if such a production does not exist, the function returns 0,
- *production*($H, i, k$) - the function applies the production indexed with $k$ to the node indexed with $i$ of the graph $H$; the function verifies also the descriptions

---

[29]See Definition A.15, point (3) in Appendix A.3.
[30]We do not present here the "technical" details of the parsing scheme. Hence, we do not discuss the issue of a *potential context identity* of nodes in detail. The reader is referred to [Flasiński (1993)].

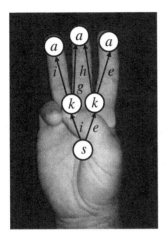

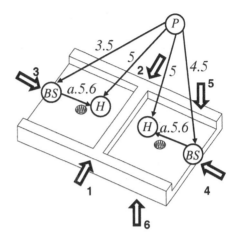

(a)                                                                                      (b)

Fig. 10.12   The applications of the $ETPL(k)/ETPR(k)$ model: (a) the recognition of Polish Sign Language ([Flasiński and Myśliński (2010)]) and (b) the recognition of machined parts for the CAD/CAM integration ([Flasiński (1995b)]).

of the newly generated edges according to the descriptions of the edges of the potential context-identical nodes and in the case of their incompatibility the function returns 1 (which means *error*).

---

**Parsing Scheme 10.3: $ETPL(k)$ Parser**

$H := Z$;
$i := 1$;
$err := 0$;
**while** $err = 0$ **and** $i \leq n$ **do**
   **begin**
      **if** *is_terminal*$(\phi_H(i))$ **then** $err := nodes\_compatible(G, H, i)$
      **else**
         **begin**
            $k := choose\_production(G, i)$;
            **if** $k = 0$ **then** $err := 1$ **else** $err := production(H, i, k)$;
         **end**;
      $i := i + 1$;
   **end**;

---

The parsing scheme for $ETPR(k)$ graph grammars [Flasiński (2018)] is a slight modification of Scheme 10.3. Firstly, *reductions* are performed instead of *produc-*

*tions.* (At the beginning the graph $H$ is set to $G$, not $Z$.) Secondly, instead of the choosing of the succeeding nodes indexed with $i = 1, \ldots, n$ (according to LOTT, cf. Definition 10.14), the nodes are to be analyzed according to RLOTT (cf. Definition 10.15) and in a bottom-up (reductive) mode. Thus, a stack has to be used by the parser.

Let us present the following theorem [Flasiński (1993, 2018)].

**Theorem 10.4 ($ETPL(k)$ and $ETPR(k)$ Parsers Complexity)**

*The running time of the parsing algorithms for $ETPL(k)$ and $ETPR(k)$ graph grammars is $\mathcal{O}(n^2)$, where $n$ is the number of graph nodes.*

The $ETPL(k)/ETPR(k)$ model was applied, among others, for scene analysis in [Flasiński (1988, 1989, 1993)], CAD/CAM integration in [Flasiński (1995b)] (see, e.g., Fig. 10.12b), the recognition of Polish Sign Language in [Flasiński and Myśliński (2010)] (see, e.g., Fig. 10.12a). The error-correcting $ETPL(k)$ parser [Flasiński (1990, 1991)] and its attributed version based on polynomial discriminant functions [Flasiński and Lewicki (1991)] were used for the recognition of objects in vague images. Stochastic $ETPL(k)$ grammars were applied for manufacturing quality control in [Flasiński and Skomorowski (1998)] and scene analysis in [Skomorowski (1999, 2007)]. Attributed programmed $ETPL(k)$ grammars were used for process monitoring and control in [Flasiński and Kotulski (1992); Flasiński (1994)].

## 10.5 Recognition of Plex Languages

As we have mentioned in Chap. 2, graph representations generalize string representations in syntactic pattern recognition. *Plex structures*, introduced in [Feder (1971)] on the basis of an idea presented in [Narasimhan (1966)], extend strings as well. They are constructed out of components called $N$ *attaching point entities*, NAPEs (see Fig. 10.13b). While a symbol in a string can be treated as a 2 attaching-point entity, i.e., having two attaching points - one on its left side and one on its right side - NAPE has an arbitrary number of attaching points for connecting to other components. Let us introduce the following definition [Feder (1971)]

**Definition 10.25 (Plex Structure):** A plex structure is a triple

$$\Pi = (X, \Gamma_X, \Delta_X), \text{ where}$$

$X = (\chi_1, \ldots, \chi_k)$ is a list of NAPEs,
$\Gamma_X = (\gamma_1, \ldots, \gamma_m)$ is a list of internal connections for $X$,
$\Delta_X = (d_1, \ldots, d_n)$ is a list of external connections for $X$ such that each attaching point of each NAPE belongs to exactly one internal or external connection.

For example, for generating the structure of the polyvinyl chloride shown in

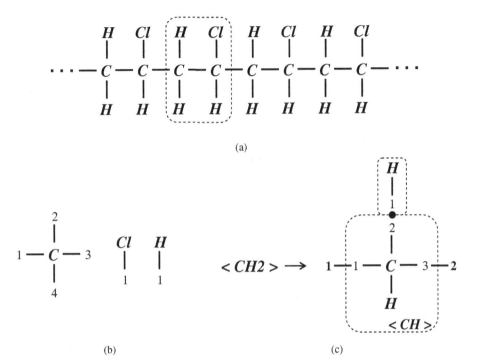

(a)

(b)                                                     (c)

Fig. 10.13    (a) The structure of polyvinyl chloride (b) the NAPEs for carbon, chlorine and hydrogen, (c) the exemplary production of the plex grammar $G$.

Fig. 10.13a, the NAPEs which represent carbon, chlorine and hydrogen are shown in Fig. 10.13b. The sets of plex structures are treated as plex languages which, in turn, are generated by plex grammars.[31] Plex grammars create a hierarchy which is analogous to the Chomsky hierarchy for string grammars. In syntactic pattern recognition context-free plex grammars are usually used.

**Definition 10.26 (CF Plex Grammar):** A context-free plex grammar is a sextuple

$$G = (\Sigma_T, \Sigma_N, P, S, I, i_0), \text{ where}$$

$\Sigma_T$ is a finite nonempty set of terminal NAPEs,
$\Sigma_N$ is a finite nonempty set of nonterminal NAPEs,
$P$ is a set of productions of the form:  $A\Delta_A \rightarrow X\Gamma_X\Delta_X$, in which $A \in \Sigma_N$,
$\Delta_A$ is a list of external connections for $A$, $(X, \Gamma_X, \Delta_X)$ is a plex structure,
$S \in \Sigma_N$ is the start NAPE,
$I$ is a finite set of symbols called identifiers,
$i_0 \in I$ is a special identifier, called the null identifier.

---

[31] In the theory of graph grammars plex structures, generated by plex grammars, are sometimes considered as hypergraphs. Then, NAPEs may be viewed as hyperedges.

We assume that $\Sigma_N \cap \Sigma_T = \emptyset$, $\Sigma = \Sigma_T \cup \Sigma_N$ and each terminal NAPE has the nonempty set of attaching points.

Let us consider the context-free plex grammar $G = (\Sigma_T, \Sigma_N, P, S, I, i_0)$ which generates the structures of polyvinyl chloride shown in Fig. 10.13a.

The terminal NAPEs of $\Sigma_T$: $<C>$, $<Cl>$ and $<H>$ are shown in Fig. 10.13b.

$P$ consists of the following productions.

(1) $<CHAIN>$ (**1, 2**) $\rightarrow$ $<UNIT>$ $<CHAIN>$ (2 1) (10, 02),
(2) $<CHAIN>$ (**1, 2**) $\rightarrow$ $<UNIT>$ ( ) (1, 2),
(3) $<UNIT>$ (**1, 2**) $\rightarrow$ $<CH2>$ $<CHCl>$ (2 1) (10, 02),
(4) $<CHCl>$ (**1, 2**) $\rightarrow$ $<CH>$ $<Cl>$ (2 1) (10, 30),
(5) $<CH2>$ (**1, 2**) $\rightarrow$ $<CH>$ $<H>$ (2 1) (10, 30),
(6) $<CH>$ (**1, 2, 3**) $\rightarrow$ $<C>$ $<H>$ (4 1) (10, 20, 30).

$\Sigma_N = \{ <CHAIN>, <UNIT>, <CHCl>, <CH2>, <CH> \}$.

The start NAPE $S = <CHAIN>$.

The set $I = \{0, 1, 2, 3, 4\}$ is used to identify attaching points of the NAPEs, and the null identifier $i_0 = 0$.

Let us explain the application of a production with the help of production (5) shown in Fig. 10.13c. The nonterminal $<CH2>$ denotes the new NAPE which is constructed out of two NAPEs: $<CH>$ and $<H>$. The list of internal connections (2 1) defines how these NAPEs should be connected, i.e., the attaching point 2 of $<CH>$ should be connected to the attaching point 1 of $<H>$ (see Fig. 10.13c).

The newly created NAPE $<CH2>$ has two attaching points indexed with **1** and **2**: $<CH2>$ (**1, 2**). The list of external connections (10 30) defines them in the following way. The attaching point **1** (in bold in Fig. 10.13c) of $<CH2>$ corresponds to the attaching point 1 of $<CH>$. (The first element of the list, i.e., the two-element string 10, says that the attaching point 1 of the first nonterminal of the right-hand side of the production ($<CH>$) should be used.)[32] The attaching point **2** (in bold in Fig. 10.13c) of $<CH2>$ corresponds to the attaching point 3 of $<CH>$. (The second element of the list, i.e., the two-element string 30, says that the attaching point 3 of the first nonterminal of the right-hand side of the production ($<CH>$) should be used.)[33]

A plex language is defined in a standard way as the set of the plex structures which consist of terminal NAPEs only and are derivable from the start NAPE $S$.

## 10.5.1   *Bunke-Haller Parser*

The Bunke-Haller parser [Bunke and Haller (1990)] is an extension of the Earley parser [Earley (1970)]. Although its general scheme is analogous to the Earley

---

[32] The null identifier 0 at the second position of the string 10, says that the second nonterminal of the right-hand side of the production ($<H>$) is not used for determining the attaching point **1** of the left-hand side of the production.

[33] The null identifier 0 at the second position of the string 30, says that the second nonterminal of the right-hand side of the production ($<H>$) is not used for determining the attaching point **2** of the left-hand side of the production.

parser scheme presented in Sec. 3.2.4 (Parsing Scheme 3.4), its data structures and functions are extended remarkably in order to process more complex structures than strings.

Let $G = (\Sigma_T, \Sigma_N, P, S, I, i_0)$ be a context-free plex grammar. For a plex structure $\Pi = (Y, \Gamma_Y, \Delta_Y)$, $Y = y_1 \ldots y_n$, to be parsed, the parser generates the sequence of states $I(1), \ldots, I(n)$. The items of the state set are defined in the following way [Bunke and Haller (1990)]. Let the production $p : A\Delta_A \to X\Gamma_X\Delta_X$ belong to the set $I(k)$ defined after reading the input terminals $y_1, \ldots, y_k$.
A state set $I(k)$ contains the following *additional data*.

(1) *A mapping* showing which of $y_1, \ldots, y_k$ can be identified as instances of the terminals of $X$. It contains the information whether $p$ has been recognized completely, as well.
(2) *A mapping* for external and internal connections which is analogous to that described in point (1).
(3) *All the productions* which contain $A$ in their right-hand sides (taking $y_1, \ldots, y_k$ into account).
(4) For each nonterminal $B \in X$: *all the productions* of the form $B\Delta_B \to Z\Gamma_Z\Delta_Z$ (taking $y_1, \ldots, y_k$ into account).
(5) For each item $i \in I(k)$, if $i$ has been generated from the item $i' \in I(k-1)$ - *the pointer to the item $i'$*.

The item $i$ of $I(k)$ is of the form $i = [p : A\Delta_A \to X\Gamma_X\Delta_X, < \text{additional data} >]$, where $< \text{additional data} >$ have been characterized above.

Three basic operations of the parser are modified with respect to the string version presented in Sec. 3.2.4 in the following way:

- *predict* - for each $i_1 = [p_1 : A\Delta_A \to X_1 B X_2 \Gamma_X \Delta_X, \ldots] \in I(k)$, $X_1, X_2 \in \Sigma^*, B \in \Sigma_N$, for each $p_2 : B\Delta_B \to Z\Gamma_Z\Delta_Z \in P$ do:
  - nothing, if $i_2 = [p_2 : B\Delta_B \to Z\Gamma_Z\Delta_Z, \ldots] \in I(k)$,
  - if $i_2 = [p_2 : B\Delta_B \to Z\Gamma_Z\Delta_Z, \ldots] \in I(k-1)$ and $i_2 \notin I(k)$, then update $i_2$ by information about $y_k$ and add the updated item to $I(k)$,
  - if $i_2 = [p_2 : B\Delta_B \to Z\Gamma_Z\Delta_Z, \ldots] \notin I(k-1)$ and $i_2 \notin I(k)$, then if $B$ shares a common attaching point with $y_k$ then add $i_2$ to $I(k)$.[34]

- *scan* - for each $i = [p : A\Delta_A \to X_1 x X_2 \Gamma_X \Delta_X, \ldots] \in I(k)$, $X_1, X_2 \in \Sigma^*, x \in \Sigma_T$ such that $x = y_{(k+1)}$ and it is compatible with $y_1, \ldots, y_k$, update the additional information of the item $i$ in order to take into account that $y_{(k+1)}$ has been read, and add the updated item to $I(k+1)$.

- *complete* - for each $i_1 = [p_1 : A\Delta_A \to \ldots , \ldots] \in I(k)$
  for each $i_2 = [p_2 : A\Delta_A \to \ldots , \ldots] \in I(k-1)$
  such that the item $i_1$ has been generated from the item $i_2$:
  if $i_3 = [p_3 : B\Delta_B \to X_1 A X_2 \Gamma_X \Delta_X, \ldots] \in I(k-1)$,

---

[34]Otherwise, the function do nothing.

then update the item $i_3$ by information about $y_k$, and add the updated item to $I(k)$.

One can easily notice that the functions *predict*, *scan* and *complete* defined above for plex structures are analogous to those presented for the string Earley parser (cf. Sec. 3.2.4). As we have mentioned above, the scheme of the Bunke-Haller parser is also analogous to that of the Earley parser. The only difference consists in processing the input according to the multidimensional structure of plexes, not to the linear structure of strings.

The same concerns the function *final_state_from_S*$(I(n))$ used for the completion of parsing (cf. Parsing Scheme 3.4). The plex structure $\Pi$ is accepted by the parser, i.e., $\Pi \in L(G)$, if this function confirms that:

- the item of the form $[p : S\Delta_S \rightarrow W\Gamma_W\Delta_W, \ldots] \in I(n)$, S is the start NAPE,
- all the terminals and all the connections of $\Pi$ either occur in $W\Gamma_W\Delta_W$ or they can be derived in $G$ from the nonterminals of $W$, and
- $W\Gamma_W\Delta_W$ has been recognized.

Similarly as in the case of the Earley parser, derivation sequences can be reconstructed on the basis of state sets.

The Bunke-Haller parser is efficient.[35] Let us present the following theorem.

**Theorem 10.5 ([Bunke and Haller (1990)] Parser Complexity)**

*The running time of the Bunke-Haller parsing algorithm for plex grammars is* $\mathcal{O}(n^5)$, *where n is the number of graph nodes.*

The Bunke-Haller parser was used for the analysis of flowcharts [Bunke and Haller (1990)].

### 10.5.2  *Peng-Yamamoto-Aoki Parser*

An interesting approach to the parsing of multidimensional structures was proposed in [Peng *et al.* (1990)]. Connections among symbols constituting a plex structure are treated as syntactic constraints imposed on these symbols. In consequence, the parsing scheme is divided into two phases. During the first phase the input symbols are analyzed without considering the syntactic constraints. If the set of input symbols cannot constitute any structure generated by a given plex grammar, then the input plex structure is rejected. Otherwise, the parser generates all the possible plex structures which can be constructed out of these input symbols. During the second phase the connections are examined in order to find such a structure from among the generated structures which matches the input plex structure.

Let $G = (\Sigma_T, \Sigma_N, P, S, I, i_0)$ be a context-free plex grammar and $\Pi = (\bar{X}, \Gamma_{\bar{X}}, \Delta_{\bar{X}})$ be a plex structure to be parsed, $X = \{x_i : x_i$ is the element of

---

[35]The best complexity is assumed [Bunke and Haller (1990)].

$\bar{X}$, $i = 1, \ldots, n\}$. The items of a state set are defined in the following way.[36] Let the production $p : A^p \Delta_A \rightarrow X_1^p \ldots X_t^p \Gamma_X \Delta_X$, $A^p \in \Sigma_N$, $X_1^p, \ldots, X_t^p \in \Sigma_T$ be given. The item $s$ of a state set related to the production $p$ is a quintuple

$$s = [p, \ d, \ j, \ \mathbf{Y}, \ \mathbf{Z}], \text{ where}$$

- $p$ is the production (as in the Earley parser),
- $d$ is a pointer which is analogous to the position of the *dot* in the Earley parser; let us note that a *final state* of the form $[A \rightarrow \omega_\bullet, \ i]$ in the Earley parser corresponds to a state for which $d = t$ in the Peng-Yamamoto-Aoki parser,
- $j$ denotes the number of symbols in $X$ which have been recognized before the application of the production $p$,[37]
- $\mathbf{Y} = (Y_1, \ldots, Y_m)$ is a list of the strings of the recognized symbols of $X$,
- $\mathbf{Z} = (Z_1, \ldots, Z_m)$ is a list of the unrecognized subsets of $X$.

Now, we can present the modified operations of the Peng-Yamamoto-Aoki (PYA) parser with respect to the Earley parser operations [Peng *et al.* (1990)]. They are defined in the following way. Let $s = [p, \ d, \ j, \ \mathbf{Y}, \ \mathbf{Z}] \in I(k)$ be defined as above. Let $\odot$ denote the concatenation operation.

- *predict* - for each non-final item $s$ such that $X_{(d+1)}^p \in \Sigma_N$,
  for each $q : B^q \Delta_B \rightarrow W^q \Gamma_W \Delta_W \in P$ such that $X_{(d+1)}^p = B^q$,
  add the item $s = [q, \ 0, \ k, \ \mathbf{Y}, \ \mathbf{Z}]$ to $I(k)$, if it is not already in $I(k)$.
- *scan* - for each non-final item $s$ such that $X_{(d+1)}^p \in \Sigma_T$, search each $Z_a \in \mathbf{Z}$, $1 \leq a \leq m$, for this terminal. If $X_{(d+1)}^p \in Z_a$, then add $[p, \ (d+1), \ j, \ \mathbf{Y'}, \ \mathbf{Z'}]$ to $I(k+1)$, where $\mathbf{Y'} = (Y_1, \ldots, Y_b)$ is such that $Y_i = Y_a \odot X_{(d+1)}^p$, $Y_i \in \mathbf{Y'}$, $Y_a \in \mathbf{Y}$ and $\mathbf{Z'} = (Z_1, \ldots, Z_b)$ is such that $Z_i = Z_a \setminus X_{(d+1)}^p$, $Z_i \in \mathbf{Z'}$, $Z_a \in \mathbf{Z}$.
- *complete* - for each final item $s$, for each $[q, \ e, \ h, \ \mathbf{Y'}, \ \mathbf{Z'}] \in I(j)$, where $q : B^q \Delta_B \rightarrow W_1^q \ldots W_u^q \Gamma_W \Delta_W \in P$, such that $W_{(e+1)}^q = A^p$ do:
  if $[q, \ (e+1), \ h, \ \mathbf{Y}, \ \mathbf{Z}]$ is not in $I(k)$ then add it to $I(k)$, otherwise update $\mathbf{Y}$ and $\mathbf{Z}$ only.

It can be easily noticed that the operations of the PYA parser are analogous to those of the Earley parser (cf. Sec. 3.2.4). The scheme of the first phase of the PYA parser is analogous to that of the Earley parser as well.

For the initialization/completion purpose, the 0th production of the form $0 : A^0 \rightarrow S$ is added to the set P. The function *final_state_from_S*$(I(n))$ finishes the analysis positively (cf. Parsing Scheme 3.4) at the first phase, if $[0, \ 1, \ 0, \ \mathbf{Y}, \ ()] \in I(n)$. After the generating of the state sets, the set $\{\Pi_1, \ldots, \Pi_N\}$ of the plex structures derivable with these state sets is constructed.

---

[36] We do not present here the "technical" details of the parsing scheme (e.g., matrix descriptions of lists of internal and external connections etc.). The reader is referred to [Peng *et al.* (1990)] for such details.

[37] It is a pointer which is analogous to the pointer $j$ used in the description of a state item of the Earley parser in Sec. 3.2.4.

As we have mentioned, during the second phase the plex structures $\Pi_1, \ldots, \Pi_N$ are matched to the input structure $\Pi$, i.e., the connections are examined. The matching is performed with the help of matrices which represent the connections.

The PYA parser is efficient.[38] Let us present the following theorem:

**Theorem 10.6 (PYA Parser Complexity)**

*The running time of the Peng-Yamamoto-Aoki parsing algorithm for plex grammars is $\mathcal{O}(n^4)$, where $n$ is the number of graph nodes.*

The PYA parser was used for the analysis of circuit diagrams [Peng *et al.* (1990)].

## 10.6   And-Or Graph Model

The methodological foundations of the And-Or graph model were presented in [Mumford (1996, 2002); Zhu (2003); Zhu and Mumford (2006)]. The model has been used for implementing many applications in computer vision. Consequently, many versions of this model have been developed to date. In this section we present its basic methodological concepts.

Let us begin with the following definition (cf. [Zhu and Mumford (2006); Park *et al.* (2018)]).

**Definition 10.27 (And-Or Graph):** An (attributed) And-Or graph is a quintuple

$$G = (S, V, E, X, \mathcal{P}), \text{ where}$$

$V$ is a set of nodes which consists of the following three subsets, $V = V_{and} \cup V_{or} \cup V_T$:
- $V_{and}$ is a set of nonterminal nodes which represent the decomposition of a structure into substructures,
- $V_{or}$ is a set of nonterminal nodes which represent the branching to alternative decompositions,
- $V_T$ is a set of terminal nodes which represent the pattern features (attributed primitives),
$S \in V \setminus V_T$ is the root node of a pattern representation,
$E$ is a set of edges,
$X$ is a set of attributes,
$\mathcal{P}$ is the probability model on the graphical representation.

And-Or graphs introduced in [Slagle (1963)] are used in artificial intelligence for the decomposing of problems to be solved by state space search strategies [Slagle (1971); Pearl (1984)]. In [Zhu and Mumford (2006)] they are interpreted in a different way from that assumed in artificial intelligence. An And-Or graph is used here

---

[38]The best complexity is assumed [Peng *et al.* (1990)].

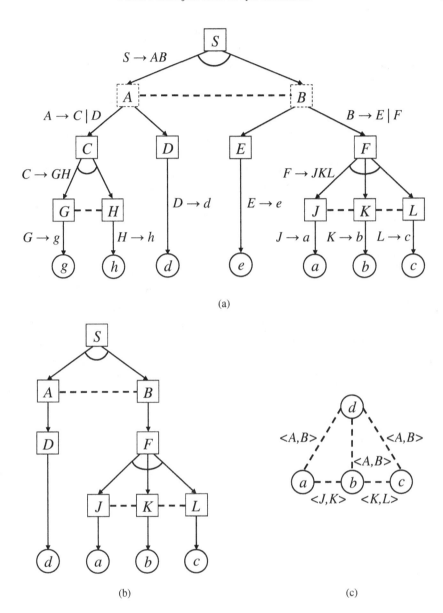

Fig. 10.14 The components of the And-Or graph model: (a) an And-Or graph, (b) a parse graph and (c) the lowest level configuration for the parse graph.

as a formalism for the representation of an attributed stochastic graph grammar. Let us consider the following example. The exemplary And-Or graph $G$ for a grammar $\mathcal{G}$ is shown in Fig. 10.14a. (The productions of the grammar $\mathcal{G}$ are also shown in Fig. 10.14a.) Nonterminal And-nodes (belonging to $V_{and}$ in Definition 10.27) are marked with solid squares, whereas nonterminal Or-nodes (belonging to $V_{or}$) are marked with dashed squares. For example, the And-node $S$ decomposes the whole structure into the substructures $A$ and $B$, which corresponds to the production $S \to AB$. The Or-node $A$ represents the branching to alternative decompositions: $C$ or $D$, which corresponds to the production $A \to C \mid D$.[39] The terminal nodes (belonging to $V_T$) are marked with circles.

The set of edges $E = E_{gram} \cup E_{rel}$ consists of the following two subsets. The vertical edges of the subset $E_{gram}$ (marked with solid arrows in Fig. 10.14a) correspond to the productions of the grammar represented.[40] The horizontal (relational) edges of the subset $E_{rel}$ (marked with dashed lines) are used to define relations between substructures. The set $X$ in Definition 10.27 is used to ascribe attributes to the nodes of $V$. The probability model $\mathcal{P}$ plays an analogous role as in stochastic grammars presented in Sec. 3.3.1. $S$ corresponds to the start symbol in a generative grammar. Summing up, the And-Or graph $G$ represents the grammar $\mathcal{G}$ in a holistic and compact way.

We can define a derivation tree for any graph derived in $\mathcal{G}$ in an analogous way as we have done this for string grammars in Sec. 3.2. In the And-Or graph model a derivation tree is called a parse tree. Let us note that a parse tree contains terminal nodes and nonterminal And-nodes only, since it describes a generation of one instance of $L(\mathcal{G})$ only. For defining a parse tree the subset $E_{gram}$ of $E$ is used only. Thus, it can be defined formally as $PT = (S, V_{and}, V_T, E_{gram}, X)$. However, a parse (derivation) tree defined in such a way does not represent the relations between substructures. Therefore, it has to be augmented with these relations. Let us introduce the following definition (cf. [Zhu and Mumford (2006); Park *et al.* (2018)]).

**Definition 10.28 (Parse Graph):** Let $G = (S, V, E, X, \mathcal{P})$, $V = V_{and} \cup V_{or} \cup V_T$, $E = E_{gram} \cup E_{rel}$, be an attributed And-Or graph representing a grammar $\mathcal{G}$, $h$ be a graph derived in $\mathcal{G}$ and $PT = (S, V_{and}, V_T, E_{gram}, X)$ be a parse tree for $h$. A parse graph $PG$ for $h$ is a triple

$$PG = (PT, E'_{rel}, X'), \text{ where}$$

$X' \subseteq X$ is a set of attributes used for $PG$,
$E'_{rel} \subseteq E_{rel}$ is a set of the relational edges such that if two nodes $v_1$ and $v_2$ of $G$ are connected with the edge $e \in E_{rel}$ then the corresponding nodes $v'_1$ and $v'_2$ of $PG$ are connected with the corresponding edge $e' \in E'_{rel}$.

The exemplary parse graph for our And-Or graph is shown in Fig. 10.14b.

Before we define the language defined by an And-Or graph, we introduce the concept of a configuration [Zhu and Mumford (2006)]. A *configuration* $\mathcal{C}$ is a structural (often: spatial) layout of the components (i.e., substructures, primitives) of a pattern (e.g., image, scene) which is defined at a certain level of abstraction in the

---

[39]In this section we use the following notational convention. If $A \to \alpha_1, A \to \alpha_2, \ldots, A \to \alpha_n$ are the productions which start with the same nonterminal $A$, then we denote this by $A \to \alpha_1 \mid \alpha_2 \mid \ldots \mid \alpha_n$.

[40]They are analogous to the edges of a derivation tree introduced in Sec. 3.2 (cf. Fig. 3.8a).

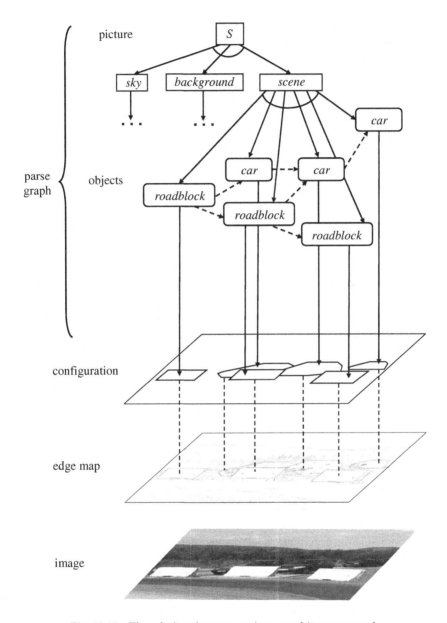

Fig. 10.15   The relations between an image and its parse graph.

form of an attributed graph. The graph consists of these components, represented by elements of $V$, and the links among them, represented by edges of $E_{rel}$. The links between the components of $\mathcal{C}$ defined at a given level of abstraction are inherited from the relations between ancestor nodes in the parse graph. For example, the configuration $\mathcal{C}$ at the lowest level of abstraction, for the parse graph $PG$ shown in Fig. 10.14b, is shown in Fig. 10.14c.

As stated by Definition 10.27, an And-Or graph is augmented with the probability model $\mathcal{P}$. In the And-Or graph model, configurations are treated as Markov networks [Zhu and Mumford (2006)] and a probability is computed for each configuration.

Now, we can introduce the following definition [Zhu and Mumford (2006)]:

**Definition 10.29 (And-Or Graph Language):** The language generated by the And-Or graph $G = (S, V, E, X, \mathcal{P})$ is the set

$$L(G) = \{ \mathcal{C} : \mathcal{S} \xRightarrow[G]{*} \mathcal{C}, \mathcal{C} \text{ is a configuration } \}.$$

The And-Or graph model is very popular in computer vision and a lot of successful applications have been developed on its basis [Han and Zhu (2009); Lin *et al.* (2009b); Pei *et al.* (2011); Zhao and Zhu (2011); Pei *et al.* (2013); Rothrock *et al.* (2013); Park and Zhu (2015); Zarchi *et al.* (2016); Qi *et al.* (2017); Yu *et al.* (2017); Liu *et al.* (2018); Park *et al.* (2018)]. This results mainly from the holistic approach of the model. Due to the holistic approach the high-level formal syntactic formalisms are integrated with the low-level image characteristics in one compact model (see Fig. 10.15). Its great descriptive/discriminating power, resulting from the use of the stochastic and attributed linguistic formalisms, is the second advantage of the And-Or graph model.

## 10.7 Remarks on Graph Languages and Their Parsing

In the theory of graph grammars [Rozenberg (1997); Ehrig *et al.* (1999)], a graph grammar production is defined as a triple[41] $(L, R, E)$, where $L$ is the left-hand side graph,[42] $R$ is the right-hand side graph and $E$ is some embedding mechanism.[43] The embedding mechanism is the "heart" of a graph grammar [Janssens *et al.* (1982)] and it is so important that the taxonomy of graph grammars is defined merely according to various types of embedding mechanisms.

Graph grammars are grouped into two large families according to the embedding mechanism: *grammars with connecting embedding* (the set theoretic approach, the algorithmic approach) and *grammars with gluing embedding* (the algebraic approach). The *VR* (vertex replacement) grammars, including the families of *NLC* (Node Label Controlled) grammars [Janssens and Rozenberg (1980a)] and *NCE* (Neighbourhood Controlled Embedding) grammars [Janssens and Rozenberg (1982)], are standard grammars of the connecting embedding approach. *Plex grammars* [Feder (1971)] and *hyperedge replacement grammars* [Bauderon and Courcelle (1987); Habel and Kreowski (1987)] are classic examples of grammars of the gluing

---

[41]This distinguishes graph grammars from string and tree grammars, in which a production is a pair.

[42]Usually, $L$ consists of one node only in practical applications.

[43]A production means here a *core* of (a syntactic part of) a production. Of course, there can be more components of a graph grammar production, e.g., the set of attributing functions for an attributed graph grammar, the predicate of applicability for a programmed graph grammar etc.

embedding approach.

The issue of parsing for graph languages is much more difficult than for string or tree languages. The studies of the issue conducted in the 1980s [Janssens and Rozenberg (1980b); Slisenko (1982); Turan (1982); Brandenburg (1983)] revealed a hard membership problem, PSPACE-complete or NP-complete [Garey and Johnson (1979)], for graph grammars. We can identify the following fundamental reasons for the intractability of this problem [Flasiński (1998)] which are useful for formulating methodological recommendations for developing efficient syntactic pattern recognition models.

First of all, let us note that a graph structure is unordered in general, whereas linear ordering is defined by a string structure, and we have at least partial ordering for a tree structure. The main concept of any syntax analysis scheme consists of analyzing the sentence/structure in order to identify consecutive subphrases/substructures, called *handles* in the theory of compilers design, and matching them against predefined phrases/structures[44] stored in a parsing table.[45] Having any kind of ordering whatsoever, one can try to answer the question: *what is a succeeding handle?* In case of the lack of any ordering in a graph structure, this means to look for a subgraph (a handle) that is isomorphic to a given graph, i.e. resolving the subgraph isomorphism problem, which is known to be NP-complete.

The second reason for the problem intractability, results from the form of a graph grammar production. In the case of string and tree grammars we know how (or rather *where*) to embed the right hand-side of a production applied because ithis is determined by a uniform rigid structure of strings and trees. In the case of graph grammars we have to specify how to embed the right-hand side graph in a graph transformed with the embedding mechanism. The embedding mechanism operates at the border between the left- and right-hand sides of a production and their context. Thus, we do not have the important *context freeness* property stating that a reordering of the derivation steps does not influence the result of the derivation. The lack of the order-independence property, related to the *finite Church-Rosser, fCR,* property (non-overlapping steps can be done in any order), results in the intractability of the parsing. Therefore, the power of the embedding mechanism must be restricted in order to obtain the *fCR* property and to guarantee the efficiency of parsing. (Two additional properties of graph languages, namely the *connectivity* of graphs generated and the *bounded degree* of a language,[46] are identified in the theory of graph grammars as necessary for the tractability of the problem [Brandenburg (1988)]. These requirements, however, usually can be fulfilled easily in syntactic pattern recognition.)

---

[44]These phrases/structures are predefined on the basis of right-hand sides of grammar productions.

[45]In top-down (generative) parsing handles are used to find the appropriate production to be applied. In bottom-up (reductive) parsing handles are consumed (reduced) to the left-hand sides of the appropriate productions.

[46]The degree of a graph node is the number of edges incident to the node. A graph language $L$ is degree-bounded if there exists $k \geq 1$ such that for every node $v$ in every graph of $L$, the degree of $v$ is less than or equal to $k$.

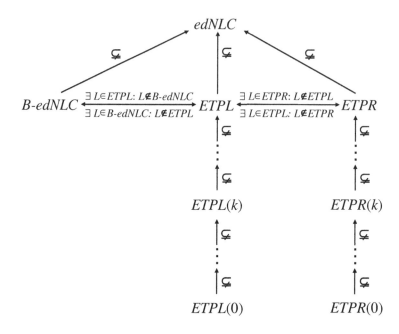

Fig. 10.16  The relations among the parsable subclasses of *edNLC* languages.

Despite the intractability of the membership problem for graph grammars a variety of parsing algorithms for graph languages have been developed for half a century. The web automata were defined in [Rosenfeld and Milgram (1972)] and the web parser in [Brayer (1977)] for web grammars [Pfaltz and Rosenfeld (1969)]. The precedence relations-based syntax analyzer,[47] $\mathcal{O}(n^2)$, was presented in [Franck (1978)] for *NLC*-like grammars [Janssens and Rozenberg (1980a)] with restricted embedding transformations. The parser, $\mathcal{O}(n^2)$, for grammars based on the Pratt model [Pratt (1971)] was proposed in [Della Vigna and Ghezzi (1978)]. The precedence relations-based parser, $\mathcal{O}(n^2)$, was constructed in [Kaul (1983)] for *NLC*-like grammars [Janssens and Rozenberg (1980a)]. The parser, $\mathcal{O}(n^3)$, for tree-graph grammars was proposed in [Sanfeliu and Fu (1983b)]. The parsing algorithm, $\mathcal{O}(n^2)$, for expansive graph grammars was defined in [Shi and Fu (1983)].[48] The polynomial parsing algorithm for boundary *NLC* languages was presented in [Rozenberg and Welzl (1986)]. Three top-down parsing algorithms, $\mathcal{O}(n^2)$, based on the analogy to *LL(k)* parsers were proposed; for the regular *ETL(1)* subclass of *edNLC* languages [Flasiński (1988, 1989)], the error-correcting parser [Flasiński (1990)] and for the context-free *ETPL(k)* subclass of *edNLC* languages [Flasiński (1993)].[49]

The polynomial parser for hyperedge replacement grammars [Bauderon and Courcelle (1987); Habel and Kreowski (1987)] was constructed in [Lautemann

---

[47]The time complexities of parsers are stated with respect to the number of graph nodes $n$.
[48]This parsing algorithm has been presented in Sec. 10.2.
[49]This parsing model has been presented in Sec. 10.4.

Table 10.1 The comparison of graph parsers used for syntactic pattern recognition.

| Embedding | Class | Parser | Running time |
|---|---|---|---|
| (specific) | Tree-graph | [Sanfeliu and Fu (1983b)] | $\mathcal{O}(n^3)$ |
| (specific) | Expansive | [Shi and Fu (1983)] | $\mathcal{O}(n)$ |
| connecting | *NLC* | *ETPL(k)*: [Flasiński (1988, 1993)] | $\mathcal{O}(n^2)$ |
| | | *ETPR(k)*: [Flasiński (2018)] | $\mathcal{O}(n^2)$ |
| gluing | Plex | [Bunke and Haller (1990)] | $\mathcal{O}(n^5)$ |
| | | [Peng, Yamamoto and Aoki (1990)] | $\mathcal{O}(n^4)$ |

(1988)]. The succeeding parsers for this class of graph grammars were proposed in [Vogler (1991)], $\mathcal{O}(n^3)$, (the Cocke-Younger-Kasami-based parser), in [Seifert and Fischer (2004)], $\mathcal{O}(n^3)$, (the Earley-based parser), in [Mazanek and Minas (2008)] (a method based on polynomial graph parser combinators), in [Drewes *et al.* (2015)], $\mathcal{O}(n^2)$, (for the predictively top-down parsable subclass of hyperedge replacement grammars) and in [Drewes *et al.* (2017)] (for the predictively shift-reduce parsable subclass of hyperedge replacement grammars). Two polynomial syntax analyzers for plex grammars [Feder (1971)] were defined independently in [Bunke and Haller (1990)] and in [Peng *et al.* (1990)].[50] The exponential Earley-based parsing for attributed flow graph grammars was presented in [Wills (1996)]. The exponential parser for layered graph grammars was constructed in [Rekers and Schürr (1997)] and its improved version was defined in [Fürst *et al.* (2011)]. The polynomial syntax analyzer for reserved graph grammars was proposed in [Zhang *et al.* (2001)]. The automata for *NCE* graph languages [Janssens and Rozenberg (1982)] were defined in [Brandenburg and Skodinis (2005)]. The bottom-up parsable, $\mathcal{O}(n^2)$, *ETPR(k)* subclass of *edNLC* languages [Janssens and Rozenberg (1980a)], based on the analogy to *LR(k)* string languages, was defined in [Flasiński (2018)].[51]

The great *descriptive* power of *ETPL(k)* and *ETPR(k)* graph grammars has been verified in the practical applications presented in Sec. 10.4. At the same time, theoretical studies of their *generative* power[52] properties have resulted in their formal characteristics [Flasiński (1998, 2018)], which are summarized in Fig. 10.16. Firstly, let us note a nice analogy between the triad of *CF - LL(k) - LR(k)* string languages (cf. Fig. 3.14 in Sec. 3.2.6) and the triad of *NLC - ETPL(k) - ETPR(k)* graph languages. Secondly, let us note that whereas the class of *LL* languages is strictly contained in the class of *LR* languages, the families *ETPL* and *ETPR* are not comparable. The insufficient descriptive power of *ETPL* languages for solving certain syntactic pattern recognition problems was the original motivation for conducting research into the bottom-up parsable subclass of *edNLC* grammars.

---

[50] These parsing algorithms are presented in Sec. 10.5.

[51] This parsing model is presented in Sec. 10.4.

[52] A difference between a *descriptive power* and a *generative power* of a class of grammars/languages is introduced at the beginning of Chap. 4.

Ultimately it has turned out that both parsable subclasses are required from the practical point of view and that they complement each other. Thirdly, *ETPL(k)* grammars have been compared to the important *boundary NLC* subclass of *NLC* grammars,[53] which is a kind of a formal benchmark for any class of *NLC* grammars with a polynomial membership problem [Rozenberg and Welzl (1986)]. As one can see in Fig. 10.16, these classes are not comparable as well.

The comparison of graph grammar parsing algorithms which have been used for syntactic pattern recognition is presented in Table 10.1.[54]

---

[53]In the case of edge-labelled and directed graphs considered in this chapter, this class is denoted by *B-edNLC*.

[54]The best complexity is assumed for parsers for tree-graph and plex grammars.

## Chapter 11

# Inference (Induction) of Graph Languages

As we have mentioned in Chap. 2, a syntactic pattern recognition model is complete if a corresponding language inference algorithm is defined. Unfortunately, the problem of grammatical inference for graph languages is even more difficult than that for tree grammars. The main issue in the case of graph grammar induction consists in handling the embedding transformation.

Syntactic pattern recognition models based on parsing for graph grammars were presented in the previous chapter. For two of them the inference algorithms have been constructed. Inferring expansive graph grammar productions from an $\Omega$ graph was proposed in [Shi and Fu (1983)]. For the parsable $ETPL(k)$ graph languages [Flasiński (1988, 1993)] the polynomial inference algorithm was defined in [Flasiński (2007)]. These inference methods are presented in the following sections. Section 11.3 contains the remarks on the inference of graph languages.

## 11.1 Inference of Expansive Graph Languages

A method for the inference of an expansive graph grammar from an $\Omega$ graph was defined in [Shi and Fu (1983)]. First of all, let us remind ourselves that every $\Omega$ graph can be indexed in such a way that its Boolean adjacency matrix fulfills the conditions of Theorem 10.1 introduced in Sec. 10.2. (The indexing algorithm of $\Omega$ graphs was presented in [Shi and Fu (1983)].)

Let $g = (V, E, \Sigma_T, \Gamma, \phi)$ be an n-node $\Omega$ graph, $M = [m_{ij}]_{n \times n}$ be its Boolean adjacency matrix. For any node index $j = 2, \ldots, n$, let $k(j)$ be defined as in Theorem 10.1. That is, for the node indexed with $j$, $k(j)$ defines the maximum index among from the indices of its predecessors. Thus, the set $\{m_{k(j)j} : j = 2, \ldots, n\}$ corresponds to the set of basic edges of $g$.

The inference algorithm is defined with the help of the labelled adjacency matrix $M_L = [m_{ij}]_{n \times n}$ of $g$, in which $m_{ij} = \gamma_{ij}$ if there exists $(v_i, \gamma_{ij}, v_j) \in E$, and $m_{ij} = 0$ otherwise. For the exemplary graph $g$ depicted in Fig. 11.1a, the labelled adjacency matrix $M_L$ is shown in Fig. 11.1b. The basic edges in Fig. 11.1a are thickened and the nonbasic edges are marked with $*$ in Fig. 11.1b.

Let us define the following functions of the inference algorithm.

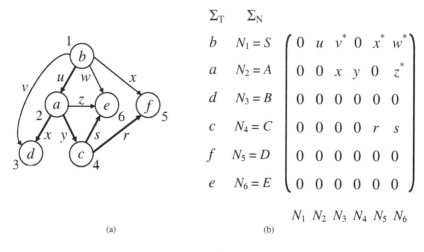

$$\begin{array}{cc} \Sigma_{\mathrm{T}} & \Sigma_{\mathrm{N}} \\ b & N_1 = S \\ a & N_2 = A \\ d & N_3 = B \\ c & N_4 = C \\ f & N_5 = D \\ e & N_6 = E \end{array} \left(\begin{array}{cccccc} 0 & u & v^* & 0 & x^* & w^* \\ 0 & 0 & x & y & 0 & z^* \\ 0 & 0 & 0 & 0 & 0 & 0 \\ 0 & 0 & 0 & 0 & r & s \\ 0 & 0 & 0 & 0 & 0 & 0 \\ 0 & 0 & 0 & 0 & 0 & 0 \end{array}\right)$$

$$N_1 \ N_2 \ N_3 \ N_4 \ N_5 \ N_6$$

(a)                                    (b)

Fig. 11.1 (a) The exemplary $\Omega$ graph $g$ and (b) its labelled adjacency matrix $M_L$.

- $rank(i)$ - the function gives the out-degree of the node indexed with $i$,
- $max\_pred(j)$ - the function gives the maximum index from among the indices of the predecessors of the node indexed with $j$. (This is denoted $k(j)$ according to Theorem 10.1.)

An expansive graph grammar $G = (\Sigma_N, \Sigma'_T, \Gamma', P, S)$ which generates a graph $g = (V, E, \Sigma_T, \Gamma, \phi)$ is inferred with the following scheme.

---

**Induction Scheme 11.1: Expansive Graph Grammar Inference**

$\Sigma'_T := \Sigma_T;$
$\Gamma' := \Gamma;$
$\Sigma_N := \{N_1, N_2, \ldots, N_n\};$
$S := N_1;$
$P := \emptyset;$
**for** $i := 1$ **to** $n$ **do**
  **if** $rank(i) = 0$ **then** $P := P \cup \{ (i) \ N_i \rightarrow \phi(v_i) \};$
  **else** /* $rank(i) > 0$ */
  $P := P \cup \{ (i) \ N_i \rightarrow \phi(v_i) m_{ij_1} N_{j_1} m_{ij_2} N_{j_2}^{e_{j_2}} ... m_{ij_{rank(i)}} N_{j_{rank(i)}}^{e_{j_{rank(i)}}},$
  $m_{ij_t} \neq 0 , \ e_{j_t} = *$ for $i \neq max\_pred(j_t) , \ e_{j_t} = \lambda$ for $i = max\_pred(j_t),$
  $t = 1, 2, \ldots, rank(i) \};$

---

For our exemplary graph, Induction Scheme 11.1 generates the following expansive graph grammar. $G = (\Sigma_N, \Sigma_T, \Gamma, P, S)$, where: $\Sigma_N = \{N_1 = S, N_2 = A, N_3 = B, N_4 = C, N_5 = D, N_6 = E, \}$, (cf. Fig. 11.1b) $\Sigma_T = \{a, b, c, d, e, f\}$, $\Gamma = \{r, s, u, v, w, x, y, z\}$, and $P$ consists of the following productions.

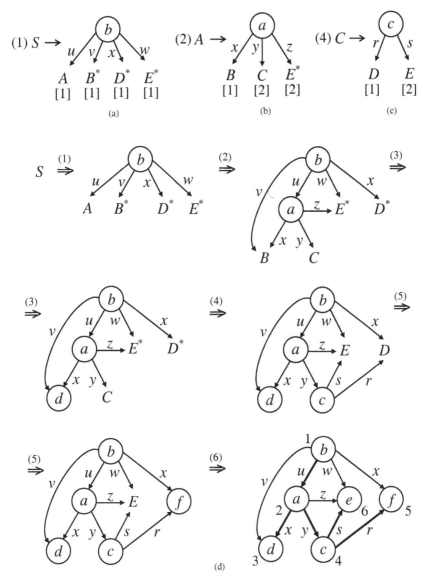

Fig. 11.2 (a)-(c) The exemplary productions inferred from the graph $g$ and (d) the derivation of the graph $g$ in the inferred grammar $G$.

(1) $S \rightarrow buAvB^*xD^*wE^*$     (3) $B \rightarrow d$     (5) $D \rightarrow f$

(2) $A \rightarrow axByCzE^*$     (4) $C \rightarrow crDsE$     (6) $E \rightarrow e$

Productions (1), (2) and (4) are shown in Fig. 11.2a-c. (The node orders are included in square brackets.) The derivation of $g$ in $G$ is shown in Fig. 11.2d.

## 11.2    Inference of ETPL(k) Graph Languages

An inference algorithm [Flasiński (2007)] for $ETPL(k)$ graph languages [Flasiński (1988, 1993)] introduced in Sec. 10.4 is presented in this section. Firstly, a method for inferring an $ETPL(k)$ graph grammar from an $IE$ graph is defined in Sec. 11.2.1. Secondly, we construct the algorithm of the inference of an $ETPL(k)$ graph grammar from a sample of $IE$ graphs in Sec. 11.2.2.

### 11.2.1    *Inference from IE Graph*

Firstly we introduce the auxiliary notions concerning $IE$ graphs defined in Sec. 10.4. Let $g = (V, E, \Sigma, \Gamma, \phi)$ an $IE$ graph. The node $v_1 \in V$ of the $k$th level[1] is the *direct predecessor* of the node $w \in V$ of the $(k + 1)$th level, if for each edge $(v_i, \gamma_i, w) \in E, i = 2, \ldots, n$ the index of $v_1$ is less than the index of $v_i, i = 2, \ldots, n$. The node $w$ is called the *direct successor* of $v_1$. A node $v_0$ is a *predecessor* of a node $v_m$, if there exists a string of edges $(v_i, \gamma_i, v_{i+1}) \in E, i = 0, \ldots m - 1$ such that $v_i$ is a direct predecessor of $v_{i+1}$. Then the node $v_m$ is called a *successor* of the node $v_0$.

Now, we shall introduce the structural indices of $IE$ graph nodes on the basis of their (common) indices (see Sec. 10.4). The node $w \in V$ indexed with 1 has the structural index 0. Let $v \in V$ be the node of the $k$th level having the structural index $x$. Let $v_1, \ldots v_p$ be its direct successors of the $(k+1)$th level having (common) indices $x_1, \ldots x_p, x_1 < \ldots < x_p$. Then the node $v_i, i = 1, \ldots, p$ has the structural index $x_\bullet i$. Each structural index of the form $0_\bullet s$ is denoted $s$. For example, structural indexing is shown in Fig. 11.3. (Common indices are placed in brackets.)

According to the definition of *edNLC* graph grammar (cf. definitions: A.14 and A.15 in Appendix A.3 and the discussion in Sec. 10.4) some of edges can be defined explicitly with right-hand side graphs. However, some of them cannot be determined in this way and they have to be generated with the embedding transformation. For the purpose of grammatical inference we shall introduce the following types of edges.

The edge connecting the node with its direct successor is called the *indexing edge*. (Indexing edges are of the form $(x_1 \bullet x_2 \bullet \ldots \bullet x_n, \gamma, x_1 \bullet x_2 \bullet \ldots \bullet x_n \bullet x_{n+1})$.)
The edge connecting two nodes having the common direct predecessor is called the *directly generated edge*. (Directly generated edges are of the form $(x_1 \bullet x_2 \bullet \ldots \bullet x_n \bullet z, \gamma, x_1 \bullet x_2 \bullet \ldots \bullet x_n \bullet y)$.)
The edge which is neither an indexing edge nor a directly generated edge is called the *indirectly generated edge*. For example, in Fig. 11.3 indexing edges are thickened and indirectly generated edges are dashed.

Let us notice that both indexing edges and directly generated edges can be defined with right-hand side graphs of an $ETPL(k)$ grammar, since these graphs are two-level graphs (cf. Definition 10.16 in Sec. 10.4). However, indirectly generated edges are to be generated with the help of the embedding transformation.

---

[1]As we have defined in Sec. 10.4, the levels in an $IE$ graph correspond to the levels of its spanned tree.

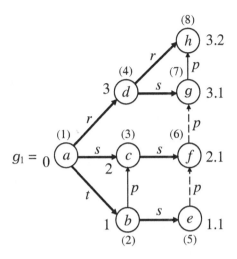

Fig. 11.3   The example of the *IE* graph and its structural indices.

Firstly, we introduce formalisms allowing us to infer productions from an *IE* graph which does not have indirectly generated edges. So, let us assume that the graph $g_1$ in Fig. 11.3 does not have edges $(1.1, p, 2.1)$ and $(2.1, p, 3.1)$ (marked with dashed arrows).

The inference is performed in two steps. At the first step *rests* are constructed.

**Definition 11.1 (Rest):** Let $g = (V, E, \Sigma, \Gamma, \phi)$ be an *IE* graph without indirectly generated edges. Let $v \in V$ be a node of the $k$th level having the structural index $i$. Let $v$ have $p$ successors $v_1, v_2, \ldots, v_p$.
The $i$th rest in the graph $g$ is a triple

$$R_i = (N_i, G_i, ET_i),$$

where $N_i$ is the unique nonterminal label assigned to the node $v$ by the nonterminal-generating function denoted by $\overline{\phi}_N$, i.e. $\overline{\phi}_N(v_i) = N_i$,
$G_i \in IE_{\Sigma,\Gamma}$ is the graph consisting of nodes $v, v_1, v_2, \ldots, v_p$ indexed structurally as in $g$, and all the edges among these nodes,
$ET_i$ is a set of all the edges of the form:
a) $(v', \gamma, v) \in E$ or
b) $(v, \beta, v'') \in E$, where $v''$ is a node of the $k$th level.

Nonterminals $N_i$ and graphs $G_i$ for the graph $g_1$ shown in Fig. 11.3 are presented in Fig. 11.4. $G_0 = g_1$. For example, according to Definition 11.1, $ET_1 = \{(0, t, 1), (1, p, 2)\}$.

At the second step *productions* are defined on the basis of rests. In defining embedding transformations we firstly use node structural indices and further on we assign node labels.

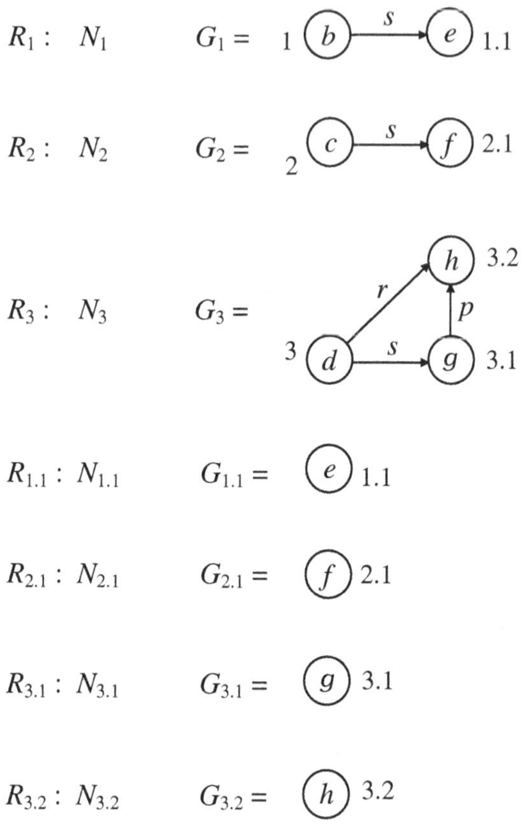

$$R_1: \quad N_1 \qquad G_1 = \quad 1 \;\;\text{(b)} \xrightarrow{\;s\;} \text{(e)} \;\; 1.1$$

$$R_2: \quad N_2 \qquad G_2 = \quad 2 \;\;\text{(c)} \xrightarrow{\;s\;} \text{(f)} \;\; 2.1$$

$$R_3: \quad N_3 \qquad G_3 =$$

$$R_{1.1}: \; N_{1.1} \qquad G_{1.1} = \quad \text{(e)} \;\; 1.1$$

$$R_{2.1}: \; N_{2.1} \qquad G_{2.1} = \quad \text{(f)} \;\; 2.1$$

$$R_{3.1}: \; N_{3.1} \qquad G_{3.1} = \quad \text{(g)} \;\; 3.1$$

$$R_{3.2}: \; N_{3.2} \qquad G_{3.2} = \quad \text{(h)} \;\; 3.2$$

Fig. 11.4   Rests for the *IE* graph $g_1$.

**Definition 11.2 (Rest-Based Production):** Let $g = (V, E, \Sigma, \Gamma, \phi)$ be an *IE* graph without indirectly generated edges, $R_i = (N_i, G_i, ET_i)$, $G_i = (V_i, E_i, \Sigma, \Gamma, \phi)$ be the $i$th rest in $g$, where $i$ is the structural index of the node $v_i \in V_i$. Let the node $v_i$ have $r$ direct successors $v_{i\bullet 1}, v_{i\bullet 2}, \ldots, v_{i\bullet r} \in V_i$. The $i$th production generating the graph $g$ is a triple

$$p_i = (l_i, D_i, C_i),$$

where $l_i = N_i$,
$D_i = (V_i^D, E_i^D, \Sigma_i^D, \Gamma, \phi_i^D)$, in which
$V_i^D = \{v_i, v_{i\bullet 1}, v_{i\bullet 2}, \ldots, v_{i\bullet r}\}$,
$E_i^D = \{(w, \gamma, u) : w \in V_i^D, u \in V_i^D, \gamma \in \Gamma\}$,
$\phi_i^D(v_i) = \phi(v_i)$,
$\phi_i^D(v_k) = \overline{\phi}_N(v_k) = N_k, \; k = i_\bullet 1, i_\bullet 2, \ldots, i_\bullet r$,
$\Sigma_i^D = \{\phi_i^D(v_i)\} \cup \{N_k : k = i_\bullet 1, i_\bullet 2, \ldots, i_\bullet r\}$,
if $(u, \gamma, v_i) \in ET_i$, then $(v_i, u, \gamma, in) \in C_i(\gamma, in)$,
if $(v_i, \gamma, u) \in ET_i$, then $(v_i, u, \gamma, out) \in C_i(\gamma, out)$.

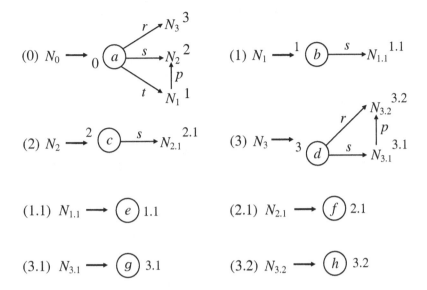

Fig. 11.5 Productions for the $IE$ graph $g_1$.

The right-hand side graph $D_i$ contains the node $v_i$, its direct successors, and edges among them. The node $v_i$ is labelled with a terminal and its direct successors with nonterminals. The productions generated on the basis of rests in the graph $g_1{}^2$ are shown in Fig. 11.5. The embedding transformation $C_i$ has to preserve edges connecting the $D_i$ with the remaining nodes of the graph during its derivation.[3] For example, since $ET_1 = \{(0, t, 1), (1, p, 2)\}$, then $C_1$ is (temporarily) defined as follows: $C_1(t, in) = \{(1, 0, t, in)\}$, $C(p, out) = \{(1, 2, p, out)\}$.

Now, we shall ascribe labels to nodes in items of the embedding transformation.

**Rule 11.1 (Labelling of Nodes in Embedding Transformation - I):**
1. In the *in-in* type embedding transformation $C(\gamma, in) = \{(w, u, \gamma, in)\}$ $w$ is labelled with a terminal symbol and $u$ is labelled with a terminal symbol.
2. In the *out-out* type embedding transformation $C(\gamma, out) = \{(w, u, \gamma, out)\}$ $w$ is labelled with a terminal symbol and $u$ is labelled with a nonterminal symbol.

Indeed $w$ as the node of the first level of the right-hand side graph has to be labelled with a terminal symbol. In point 1 the node $u$ has the less (common) index than the node $w$, so it is already the terminal node. In point 2 the node $u$ has the greater (common) index than the node $w$, so it is still the nonterminal node[4]. After labelling of all nodes with the help of Rule 11.1 we obtain the embedding transformation as seen in Table 11.1.

---

[2]The graph $g_1$ itself is the rest $R_0$.
[3]These edges are contained in the set $ET_i$.
[4]All nodes of the second level of right-hand side graphs are nonterminal ones.

Table 11.1   Elements $ET_i$ and $C_i$ for the graph $g_1$.

| Rest $(i)$ | $ET_i$ | $C_i$ |
|---|---|---|
| 0 | $\emptyset$ | $\emptyset$ |
| 1 | $\{(0,t,1),(1,p,2)\}$ | $C(t,in)=\{(b,a,t,in)\}$ |
| | | $C(p,out)=\{(b,N_2,p,out)\}$ |
| 2 | $\{(0,s,2),(1,p,2)\}$ | $C(s,in)=\{(c,a,s,in)\}$ |
| | | $C(p,in)=\{(c,b,p,in)\}$ |
| 3 | $\{(0,r,3)$ | $C(r,in)=\{(d,a,r,in)\}$ |
| $1_\bullet 1$ | $\{(1,s,1_\bullet 1)\}$ | $C(s,in)=\{(e,b,s,in)\}$ |
| $2_\bullet 1$ | $\{(2,s,2_\bullet 1)\}$ | $C(s,in)=\{(f,c,s,in)\}$ |
| $3_\bullet 1$ | $\{(3,s,3_\bullet 1),(3_\bullet 1,p,3_\bullet 2)\}$ | $C(s,in)=\{(g,d,s,in)\}$ |
| | | $C(p,out)=\{(g,N_{3_\bullet 2},p,out)\}$ |
| $3_\bullet 2$ | $\{(3,r,3_\bullet 2),(3_\bullet 1,p,3_\bullet 2)\}$ | $C(r,in)=\{(h,d,r,in)\}$ |
| | | $C(p,in)=\{(h,g,p,in)\}$ |

The derivation of the graph $g_1$ (with removed indirectly generated edges) with productions inferred is shown in Fig. 11.6.

Now, we consider the inference of the embedding transformation items used for generating indirectly generated edges. For a generation of an indirectly generated edge a certain directly generated edge is used, as it is shown, for example, in Fig. 11.7 in which the derivation of the (lower) part of the graph $g_1$, this time including its indirectly generated edges (cf. Fig. 11.3), is presented. Firstly, on the basis of the directly generated edge $(1,p,2)$ the auxiliary edge $(2,X,1_\bullet 1)$ is defined with the embedding transformation. Secondly, it is somehow being "moved"[5] along two paths which end with nodes of the indirectly generated edge $(1_\bullet 1,p,2_\bullet 1)$.

> **Definition 11.3 (First Bridge):** Let $g = (V,E,\Sigma,\Gamma,\phi)$ be an *IE* graph,
> $ige = (x_1{}_\bullet x_2{}_\bullet \ldots {}_\bullet x_n{}_\bullet z_1{}_\bullet z_2{}_\bullet \ldots {}_\bullet z_k, \pi, x_1{}_\bullet x_2{}_\bullet \ldots {}_\bullet x_n{}_\bullet y_1{}_\bullet y_2{}_\bullet \ldots {}_\bullet y_m) \in E$ be an
> indirectly generated edge.
> An edge $fb = (x_1{}_\bullet x_2{}_\bullet \ldots {}_\bullet x_n{}_\bullet z_1, \pi_0, x_1{}_\bullet x_2{}_\bullet \ldots {}_\bullet x_n{}_\bullet y_1) \in E$ is called the first
> bridge for $ige$.

Let us notice that the first bridge for any indirectly generated edge $ige = (v,\gamma,w)$ is the edge which connects direct successors $v_1$ and $w_1$ of the common predecessor[6] of nodes $v$ and $w$, and additionally $v_1$ is the predecessor of $v$ and $w_1$ is the predecessor of $w$. For example, for the indirectly generated edge $(1_\bullet 1,p,2_\bullet 1)$ in Fig. 11.7, the edge $(1,p,2)$ is its first bridge.

---

[5]The auxiliary edge is being "moved" with the embedding transformations.

[6]This common predecessor has the greatest (common) index from out of the common predecessors of nodes $v$ and $w$.

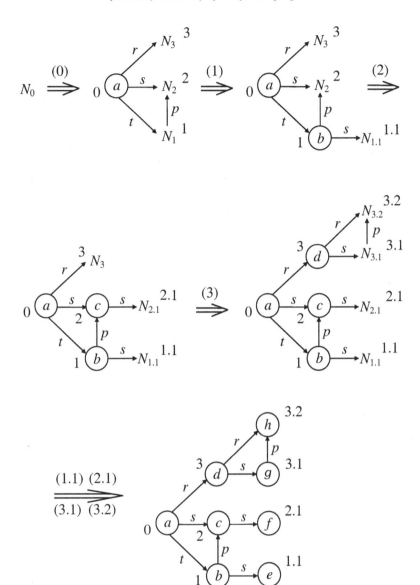

Fig. 11.6   The derivation of the *IE* graph $g_1$ without indirectly generated edges.

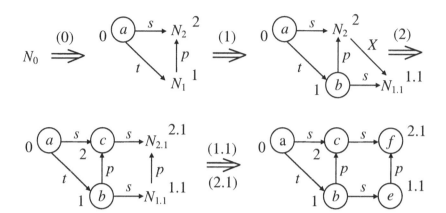

Fig. 11.7    The derivation of the part of the *IE* graph $g_1$ with the indirectly generated edge.

**Definition 11.4 (Sequence of Bridges):** Let $g = (V, E, \Sigma, \Gamma, \phi)$ be an *IE* graph, $ige = (x_1 \bullet x_2 \bullet \ldots \bullet x_n \bullet z_1 \bullet z_2 \bullet \ldots \bullet z_k, \ \pi, x_1 \bullet x_2 \bullet \ldots \bullet x_n \bullet y_1 \bullet y_2 \bullet \ldots \bullet y_m)$ be an indirectly generated edge, $fb = (x_1 \bullet x_2 \bullet \ldots \bullet x_n \bullet z_1, \ \pi_0, x_1 \bullet x_2 \bullet \ldots \bullet x_n \bullet y_1) \in E$ is the first bridge for $ige$. Let $z_1 < y_1$. A string of edges

$$((x_1 \bullet x_2 \bullet \ldots \bullet x_n \bullet z_1, \ \pi_0, x_1 \bullet x_2 \bullet \ldots \bullet x_n \bullet y_1),$$
$$(x_1 \bullet x_2 \bullet \ldots \bullet x_n \bullet y_1, \ \Pi, x_1 \bullet x_2 \bullet \ldots \bullet x_n \bullet z_1 \bullet z_2),$$
$$(x_1 \bullet x_2 \bullet \ldots \bullet x_n \bullet z_1 \bullet z_2, \ \Pi, x_1 \bullet x_2 \bullet \ldots \bullet x_n \bullet y_1 \bullet y_2),$$
$$(x_1 \bullet x_2 \bullet \ldots \bullet x_n \bullet y_1 \bullet y_2, \ \Pi, x_1 \bullet x_2 \bullet \ldots \bullet x_n \bullet z_1 \bullet z_2 \bullet z_3), \ldots,$$
$$(x_1 \bullet x_2 \bullet \ldots \bullet x_n \bullet z_1 \bullet z_2 \bullet \ldots \bullet z_k, \ \pi, x_1 \bullet x_2 \bullet \ldots \bullet x_n \bullet y_1 \bullet y_2 \bullet \ldots \bullet y_m))$$

is called a sequence of bridges generating the edge $ige$.

The last edge in the sequence of bridges is called the *target bridge*. Every edge in the sequence of bridges except the first bridge and the target bridge is called an *internal bridge*.

For example, for the indirectly generated edge $(1 \bullet 1, p, 2 \bullet 1)$ in Fig. 11.7, its sequence of bridges is defined as follows $((1, p, 2), (2, X, 1 \bullet 1), (1 \bullet 1, p, 2 \bullet 1))$.

Finally, let us define the rule of defining embedding transformation items used for generating an indirectly generated edge. (In Fig. 11.8 a dotted arrow represents a bridge used for generating the next bridge denoted with a dashed arrow.) As previously, defining embedding transformation items we firstly use node structural indices (Rule 11.2) and further on we assign node labels (Rules 11.1 and 11.3).

**Rule 11.2 (Embedding Transformation for Indirectly Generated Edge):**
Let $e = (v, \pi, w)$ be an indirectly generated edge, $p_i = (l_i, D_i, C_i)$ denote the $i$th production.
1. If $b = (m, \pi_0, n)$ is the first bridge for $e$, then
$C_m(\pi_0, out) = \{(m \bullet x, n, \Pi, in)\}$ is added to $C_m$, where $\Pi$ is the unique auxiliary edge label defined for $e$ (see Fig. 11.8(a)).

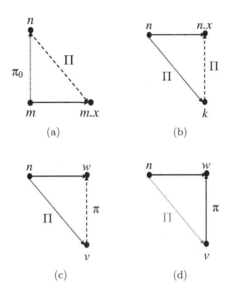

Fig. 11.8   The scheme of generation of indirectly generated edge.

2. If $b = (n, \Pi, k)$ is an internal bridge that is not the last internal bridge for $e$, then
$C_n(\Pi, out) = \{(n_\bullet x, k, \Pi, in)\}$ is added to $C_n$ (see Fig. 11.8(b)).
c) If $b = (n, \Pi, v)$ is the last internal bridge for $e$, then
$C_n(\Pi, out) = \{(w, v, \pi, in)\}$ is added to $C_n$, (see Fig. 11.8(c)).
d) If $b = (v, \pi, w)$ is the target bridge, then
$C_v(\pi, out) = \{(v, w, \pi, out)\}$ is added to $C_v$, and
$C_w(\pi, in) = \{(w, v, \pi, in)\}$ is added to $C_w$ (see Fig. 11.8(d)).

The labelling of embedding transformation items of the *in-in* type and the *out-out* type has been defined by Rule 11.1. Since in generating indirectly generated edges the *out-in* type is used, we introduce the following rule:

**Rule 11.3 (Labelling of Nodes in Embedding Transformation - II):**
In the *out-in* type embedding transformation $C(\beta, out) = \{(w, u, \gamma, in)\}$ $w$ is labelled with a nonterminal and $u$ is labelled with a nonterminal symbol.

Let us notice that a node $w$ in Rule 11.3 is the second-level node of a production applied. Therefore, it is labelled with a nonterminal. A node $u$ is a node of the same level as the node that a production is applied at. However, it has a greater (common) index, so a production has not been applied at it, and it is still nonterminal. Let us come back to our example shown in Fig. 11.7. According to Definition 11.4 and the rules of node labelling we define *additionally* the following items of the embedding transformation: $C_1(p, out) = \{(N_{1.1}, N_2, X, in)\}$, $C_2(X, out) = \{(N_{2.1}, N_{1.1}, p, in)\}$, $C_{1.1}(p, out) = \{(e, N_{2.1}, p, out)\}$, $C_{2.1}(p, in) = \{(f, e, p, in)\}$.

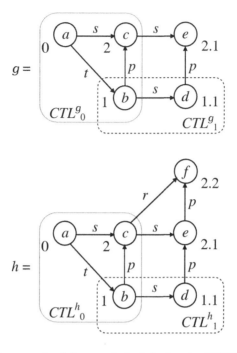

Fig. 11.9   The example of the sample for inferring the $ETPL(k)$ grammar.

At the end of this section, let us notice that for an indirectly generated edge the first bridge may not exist. In such a case we have to add the directly generated edge with the (unique) auxiliary label to a right-hand side graph of a proper production as the first bridge. We have to remember that this edge is temporal and it should not be preserved.

### 11.2.2   *Inference from a Sample of IE Graphs*

For a sample of *IE* graphs $S_+ = \{g^1, \ldots, g^s\}$ we can infer a set of $ETPL(k)$ grammars $SGG = \{GG^1, \ldots, GG^s\}$ such that $L(GG^i) = \{g^i\}, i = 1, \ldots, s$. Now, we show how to define one $ETPL(k)$ grammar $GG$ on the basis of $SGG$ such that $L(GG) = S_+$. At the first step we perform the *unification of the axioms,*[7] i.e., we replace $N_0^1, \ldots, N_0^s$ with one $N_0$. This operation, however, can violate the fundamental property of the $ETPL(k)$ grammar introduced by Definition 10.21. Let us analyze this problem with the following example:

In our considerations we assume that for the rest $R_i^g = (N_i^g, G_i^g, ET_i^g)$, its complete two-level graph originated in the starting node of the rest and beginning with its first successor, i.e. the graph $CTL(G_i^g, i, i_\bullet 1)$ is denoted $CTL_i^g$. Let the sample $S$ consist of two graphs $g$ and $h$ shown in Fig. 11.9. Productions of $ETPL(2)$ gram-

---

[7]In the case of the method presented in the previous section the axiom is the starting one-node graph.

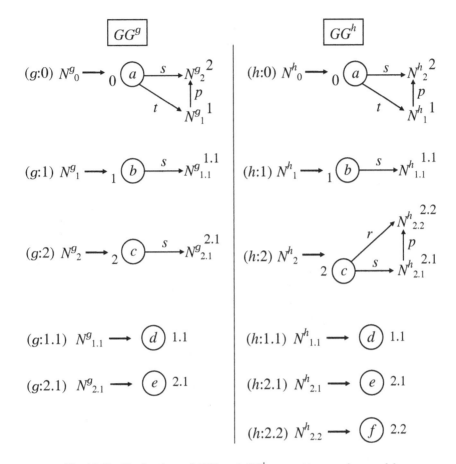

Fig. 11.10    Productions of $GG^g$ and $GG^h$ generating graphs $g$ and $h$.

mars $GG^g$ and $GG^h$ are shown in Fig. 11.10. After the unification of the axioms, since $2 - TL(g,0,1) \cong 2 - TL(G^h,0,1)$, i.e. $CTL_0^g = CTL_0^h$ (cf. Fig. 11.9). However, it means that, in order to fulfill Definition 10.21, we have to unify productions $(g:0)$ and $(h:0)$ (cf. Fig. 11.10) as well. This unification operation consists in:
- removing the second production, i.e., $(h:0)$, assuming that for the generation of both graphs $g$ and $h$, the first production, i.e., $(g:0)$ is used (see the unified production $(g - h:0)$ in Fig. 11.11),
- replacing, in the left-hand sides of all productions of the grammar $G^h$ nonterminals that have occurred in the right-hand side graph of a removed production (in our example: $N_1^h$ and $N_2^h$ in productions $(h:1)$ and $(h:2)$) with corresponding nonterminals of the unified production (i.e. $N_1^g$ and $N_2^g$).
One can easily notice that this unification causes another derivational ambiguity, this time for productions $(g:1)$ and $(h:1)$. So we have to continue the unification process. The final result of the process is shown in Fig. 11.11.

Now we can formalize our considerations.

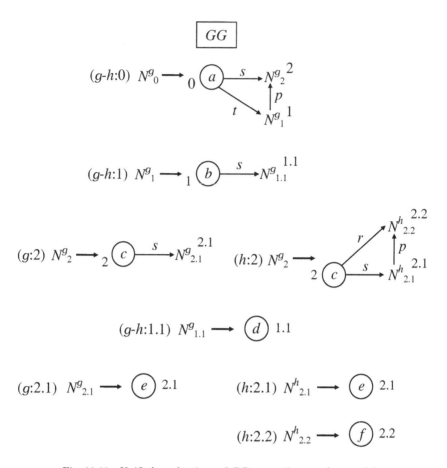

Fig. 11.11   Unified productions of $GG$ generating graphs $g$ and $h$.

**Definition 11.5 (Conflicting Productions):** Let productions $p_i^g = (l_i^g, D_i^g, C_i^g) \in GG^g, p_i^{h_1} = (l_i^{h_1}, D_i^{h_1}, C_i^{h_1}) \in GG^{h_1}, \ldots, p_i^{h_k} = (l_i^{h_k}, D_i^{h_k}, C_i^{h_k}) \in GG^{h_k}$ such that $g < h_1 < \ldots < h_k$ be generated for the rests $R_i^g = (N_i^g, G_i^g, ET_i^g), R_i^{h_1} = (N_i^{h_1}, G_i^{h_1}, ET_i^{h_1}), \ldots, R_i^{h_k} = (N_i^{h_k}, G_i^{h_k}, ET_i^{h_k})$ such that $CTL_i^g \cong CTL_i^{h_1} \cong \ldots \cong CTL_i^{h_k}$.
If $l_i^g = l_i^{h_1} = \ldots = l_i^{h_k}$, then $p_i^g, p_i^{h_1}, \ldots, p_i^{h_k}$ are called conflicting productions. The production $p_i^g$ is called the basic production for conflicting productions. The set $SCP_i = \{p_i^g, p_i^{h_1}, \ldots, p_i^{h_k}\}$ is called a set of conflicting productions (for the index i).

In our example pairs of isomorphic subgraphs: $CTL_0^g$ and $CTL_0^h$ $CTL_1^g$ and $CTL_1^h$, $CTL_{1.1}^g$ and $CTL_{1.1}^h$[8] cause ambiguity conflicts in the case of unifying the

---

[8]The last pair consists of one-node graphs labelled with $d$. Let us notice that the one-node subgraph which is last in the path can be treated formally as a (reduced) complete two-level graph according to Definition 10.20.

axioms (cf. Fig. 11.9). So sets of conflicting productions are defined as follows: $SCP_0 = \{p_0^g, p_0^h\}$, $SCP_1 = \{p_1^g, p_1^h\}$, $SCP_{1\bullet1} = \{p_{1\bullet1}^g, p_{1\bullet1}^h\}$.

**Definition 11.6 (Unification of Nonterminals):** Let $SCP_i = \{p_i^{h_1}, \ldots, p_i^{h_k}\}$ be a set of conflicting productions defined as in Definition 11.5. Let $V_i^g = \{v_i^g, N_{i\bullet1}^g, \ldots, N_{i\bullet m}^g\}, V_i^{h_1} = \{v_i^{h_1}, N_{i\bullet1}^{h_1}, \ldots, N_{i\bullet m}^{h_1}\}, \ldots, V_i^{h_k} = \{v_i^{h_k}, N_{i\bullet1}^{h_k}, \ldots, N_{i\bullet m}^{h_k}\}$ be sets of the nodes of graphs $D_i^g, D_i^{h_1}, \ldots D_i^{h_k}$. An operation consisting in replacing nonterminals $N_s^{h_1}, \ldots, N_s^{h_k}$ with the nonterminal $N_s^g$ for each $s = i_\bullet1, \ldots, i_\bullet m$ in grammars $GG^g, GG^{h_1}, \ldots, GG^{h_k}$ is called a unification of node nonterminals of the set $SCP_i$.

The unification of node nonterminals influences, obviously, the process of the generation of indirectly generated edges.[9] Let us notice that after unifying node nonterminals we should unify the auxiliary edge labels, as well. (Otherwise, we would generate multiple edges.) However, we can do so only if the indirectly generated edges involved in conflicting productions are the same, i.e., they have the same label and connect a pair of nodes having the same structural indices. Therefore, we shall introduce the following definitions:

**Definition 11.7 (Unifiability w.r.t. Indirectly Generated Edges):** Let $SCP_i = \{p_i^{h_1}, \ldots, p_i^{h_k}\}$ be a set of conflicting productions defined as in Definition 11.5. The set $SCP_i$ is unifiable with respect to indirectly generated edges, if the following condition holds.
If there exists an indirectly generated edge $(v, \gamma, w)$ in one of the rests $G_i^g, G_i^{h_1}, \ldots, G_i^{h_k}$, then for any other rest there exists an indirectly generated edge $(\overline{v}, \overline{\gamma}, \overline{w})$ such that $v = \overline{v}$, $w = \overline{w}$, $\phi(v) = \phi(\overline{v})$, $\phi(w) = \phi(\overline{w})$, $\gamma = \overline{\gamma}$.

A set of indirectly generated edges

$$\{(v^g, \gamma^g, w^g) \in E^g, (v^{h_1}, \gamma^{h_1}, w^{h_1}) \in E^{h_1}, \ldots, (v^{h_k}, \gamma^{h_k}, w^{h_k}) \in E^{h_k}\}$$

fulfilling the condition of Definition 11.7 is called *a set of equivalent indirectly generated edges*.
A set

$$\{Y^g, Y^{h_1}, \ldots, Y^{h_k}\}$$

of nonterminal edge labels of internal bridges used for the generation of edges $(v^g, \gamma^g, w^g) \in E^g, (v^{h_1}, \gamma^{h_1}, w^{h_1}) \in E^{h_1}, \ldots, (v^{h_k}, \gamma^{h_k}, w^{h_k}) \in E^{h_k}$ is called *a set of equivalent nonterminal bridge labels*, and the label $Y^g$ is called *the basic label* for this set.

---

[9]This issue is analyzed in detail in [Flasiński (2007)].

**Definition 11.8 (Unification of Embedding Transformations):** Let $SCP_i = \{p_i^{h_1}, \ldots, p_i^{h_k}\}$ be a set of conflicting productions defined as in Definition 11.5 which is unifiable with respect to indirectly generated edges, $\{(v^g, \gamma^g, w^g) \in E^g, (v^{h_1}, \gamma^{h_1}, w^{h_1}) \in E^{h_1}, \ldots, (v^{h_k}, \gamma^{h_k}, w^{h_k}) \in E^{h_k}\}$ be a set of equivalent indirectly generated edges with a set of equivalent nonterminal bridge labels $\{Y^g, Y^{h_1}, \ldots, Y^{h_k}\}$.

An operation of replacing labels $Y^{h_1}, \ldots, Y^{h_k}$ with the basic label $Y^g$ in the embedding transformations of the grammars $GG^g, GG^{h_1}, \ldots, GG^{h_k}$ is called a unification of embedding transformations for the set of equivalent indirectly generated edges.

The unification of axioms may also cause another undesired effect, called a combination of unified rests.[10] Let us consider the following example. Let the sample $S$ consist of two $IE$ graphs $g$ and $h$ as shown in Fig. 11.12. One can easily notice that the unification of the pair of rests: $R_1^g$ - $R_1^h$ and $R_2^g$ - $R_2^h$ results in defining the grammar, which additionally generates the graphs $h_1$ and $h_2$ shown in Fig. 11.12. In order to avoid such an effect, we have to test whether conflicting productions are unifiable with respect to rests combinations. Let us introduce the following definition:

**Definition 11.9 (Unifiability w.r.t. Combination of Rests):** Let $S_+ = \{g^1 \in IE_{\Sigma_T, \Gamma}, \ldots, g^s \in IE_{\Sigma_T, \Gamma}\}$ be a sample. Let a set of conflicting productions $SCP_0 = \{p_0^{s_1} = (l_0^{s_1}, D_0^{s_1}, C_0^{s_1}) \in GG^{s_1}, \ldots, p_0^{s_k} = (l_0^{s_k}, D_0^{s_k}, C_0^{s_k}) \in GG^{s_k}\}$, in which $p_0^{s_1}$ is the basic production, $l_0^{s_1}, \ldots, l_0^{s_k}$ are the axioms, be unified according to definitions: 11.6 and 11.8. Let

$$l_0^{s_1} \underset{rl(G)}{\Longrightarrow} D_0^{s_1} \underset{rl(G)}{\overset{*}{\Longrightarrow}} g^{t_1} \in IE_{\Sigma_T, \Gamma}, \; \ldots \; , l_0^{s_1} \underset{rl(G)}{\Longrightarrow} D_0^{s_1} \underset{rl(G)}{\overset{*}{\Longrightarrow}} g^{t_p} \in IE_{\Sigma_T, \Gamma}$$

be all the derivations in the unified grammar starting from the basic production $p_0^{s_1}$ after this unification.

The set $SCP_0$ is unifiable with respect to the combinations of rests, if

$$g^{t_1}, \ldots, g^{t_p} \in S_+.$$

Now, we can introduce the algorithm of the grammatical inference of $ETPL(k)$ graph grammar. Firstly, we shall define the following functions, and data structures.

- $g^s$ - the succeeding $IE$ graph that productions are inferred for,
- $rests^s$ - the set containing rests generated with the algorithm for $g^s$; the rests are of the form $rest_i^s = (N_i^s, G_i^s, ET_i^s)$,
- $productions^s$ - the set containing productions generated with the algorithm for $g^s$; the productions are of the form $production_i^s = (l_i^s, D_i^s, C_i^s)$,

---

[10]This issue is analyzed in detail in [Flasiński (2007)].

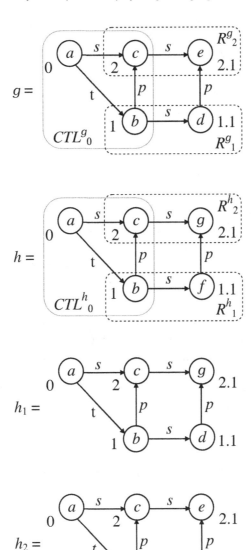

Fig. 11.12 The example of the problem of combination of unified rests.

- *productions* - the set containing productions of the unified grammar,
- *number_of_nodes*($g^s$) - the function gives the number of nodes of $g^s$,
- *structural_index*($g^s, j$) - the function gives the structural index of the node of $g^s$ having the common index $j$,
- *define_rest*($s, i, g^s, rests^s$) - the function generates the $i$th rest for $g^s$ (according to Definition 11.1) and stores it as the $rest_i^s$ in the set $rests^s$,

- *define_production(s, i, rests$^s$, productions$^s$)* - the function:
  - generates the *production$_i^s$* for the rest *rest$_i^s$* (according to Definition 11.2 and Rule 11.1),
  - stores it in the set *productions$^s$*,
- *define_embed_transf_for_ige(g$^s$, productions$^s$)* - the function:
  - places all temporary first bridges in *g$^s$*, if necessary,
  - defines items of embedding transformations for all indirectly generated edges of *g$^s$* (according to rules: 11.2 and 11.3), and places them to proper productions in the set *productions$^s$*,
- *unify_axioms(productions)* - the function replaces the axioms $N_0^1, \ldots, N_0^m$ defined for grammars $GG^1, \ldots, GG^m$ generating graphs $g^1, \ldots, g^m$ with one axiom $N_0$ for the unified grammar,
- *conflicting_productions(productions, index)* - the recursive function handling conflicting productions; it performs the following steps:
  - finds sets of conflicting productions (according to Definition 11.5),
  - unifies node nonterminals (according to Definition 11.6),
  - tests whether sets of conflicting productions are unifiable with respect to indirectly generated edges (according to Definition 11.7,
  - unifies embedding transformations (according to Definition 11.8),
  - tests whether sets of conflicting productions are unifiable with respect to combinations of rests (according to Definition 11.9),
  - if any test results in failure, then the function returns **false**.

---

**Induction Scheme 11.2: *ETPL(k)* Grammar Inference Algorithm**

**for** $s := 1$ **to** *sample_size* **do**
  **begin**
    **for** $j := 1$ **to** *number_of_nodes(g$^s$)* **do**
      **begin**
        $i := structural\_index(g^s, j)$;
        *define_rest(s, i, g$^s$, rests$^s$)*;
        *define_production(s, i, rests$^s$, productions$^s$)*;
      **end**;
    *define_embed_transf_for_ige(g$^s$, productions$^s$)*;
  **end**;
*unify_axioms(productions)*;
*inference_successful* := **true**;
*inference_successful* := *conflicting_productions(productions, 0)*;

---

At the end of this section we present the following theorem.

**Theorem 11.1 ($ETPL(k)$) Inference Complexity [Flasiński (2007)])**

*The running time of the algorithm of grammatical inference for ETPL(k) graph grammars is $\mathcal{O}(||S_+||^3 \cdot n^3)$, where $S_+$ is the sample, $n$ is the maximum number of nodes of a graph in the sample.*

## 11.3 Remarks on the Inference of Graph Languages

The model of syntactic pattern recognition based on the expansive graph grammars [Shi and Fu (1983)] contained the first inference method for graph grammars in the field. An inference algorithm for a special class of grammar grammars which generated chain- and star-like graphs was defined in [Bartsch-Spörl (1983)]. An inference method for hyperedge replacement graph grammars[11] was proposed in [Jeltsch and Kreowski (1991)]. An inference algorithm for web grammars was defined in [López and Sempere (1998)]. The connectionist learning approach for the inference of regular graph grammars was presented in [Fletcher (2001)]. This approach was extended with the use of concurrent processing in [Lam and Fletcher (2009)]. An inference method for stochastic context-free graph grammars was proposed in [Doshi *et al.* (2002); Oates *et al.* (2003)]. An algorithm for the inference of context-free graph grammars based on the MDL (minimum description length) principle was defined in [Jonyer *et al.* (2004)]. Two inference algorithms for node- and edge- replacement graph grammars were proposed in [Kukluk *et al.* (2007)] and [Kukluk *et al.* (2008)], respectively. An inference method for parsable $ETPL(k)$ graph grammars for syntactic pattern recognition was presented in [Flasiński (2007)].[12] An inference algorithm for $k$-testable graph languages was defined in [López *et al.* (2012); Gallego-Sánchez *et al.* (2018)].

---

[11] Hyperedge replacement graph grammars were introduced in Sec. 10.7.

[12] A preliminary version of the $ETPL(k)$ graph grammar inference algorithm was presented in: Flasiński M. (1993). Theoretical foundations of inference of edNLC-graph grammars, *Schedae Informaticae* (Series: *Universitas Iagellonica Acta Scientiarum Litterarumque*) **5**, pp. 114-164.

Chapter 12

# Applications of Graph Methods

The development of syntactic pattern recognition models based on graph grammars was to start nearly twenty years after the invention of the first string and tree methods. Graph-based methods are usually used if string and tree structural descriptions are simply too weak to represent patterns. In the subsequent sections we shall present the following application areas of graph methods: scene analysis, picture and diagram analysis, feature recognition for computer aided design and manufacturing, analysis of visual events and activities, structure analysis in chemistry, optical character recognition, structure analysis for process monitoring and control, and structure analysis in bioinformatics and medicine. The last section includes a summary of these applications in a tabular form.

## 12.1 Scene Analysis

The fundamental generic models for scene analysis were introduced in the seminal papers [Guzman (1968); Clowes (1971); Huffman (1971); Gips (1974); Waltz (1975); Haralick and Shapiro (1979a,b); Haralick (1980); Kanade (1980, 1981); Herman and Kanade (1986); Kirousis and Papadimitriou (1988)].

The use of Attributed Programmed Graph Grammars for the interpretation of scenes represented by graphs was proposed in [Bunke (1978, 1982a)]. The method of parsing and translation for expansive graph grammars for scene analysis was proposed in [Shi and Fu (1983)]. Plex grammars were used for the analysis of 3-D complex objects in [Lin and Fu (1984a,b, 1986)]. The recognition of hidden and deformed 3-D complex objects with the help of Attributed Tree-Graph Grammars was presented in [Sanfeliu (1984)]. $ETPL(k)$ and $ETPR(k)$ graph grammars and their parsing algorithm were defined for scene analysis in [Flasiński (1988, 1989, 1993, 2018)]. The error-correcting extension of the $ETPL(k)/ETPR(k)$ model for scene analysis was presented in [Flasiński (1990, 1991)], whereas its stochastic version was proposed in [Skomorowski (1999, 2007)].

The And-Or graph model [Mumford (2002); Zhu (2003); Zhu and Mumford (2006)] was developed for scene analysis applications by S. C. Zhu and his collaborators in [Han and Zhu (2009); Zhao and Zhu (2011); Yu et al. (2017); Liu et al.

(2018)]. An And-Or graph representation was also used for scene analysis in [Lin et al. (2009b); Zarchi et al. (2016)].

## 12.2 Picture and Diagram Analysis

Attributed Tree-Graph Grammars [Bunke (1978, 1982b)] were applied for the analysis of circuit diagrams and flowcharts in [Bunke (1982a)]. The recognition of circuit diagrams with the help of Attributed Tree-Graph Grammars was presented in [Sanfeliu and Fu (1983b)]. The analysis of distorted structural pictures was performed with error-correcting $ETPL(k)$ parsing [Flasiński (1990, 1991)] in the attributed version based on polynomial discriminant functions [Flasiński and Lewicki (1991)]. The parsing of plex grammars was used for the recognition of flowcharts in [Bunke and Haller (1990)] and circuit diagrams in [Peng et al. (1990)]. Dimensions in engineering drawings were recognized using web grammars in [Min et al. (1993)]. Path-controlled graph grammars and their parsing based on the $ETPL(k)$ model were defined in [Aizawa and Nakamura (1994)]. The analysis of technical drawing dimensions with the help of plex languages was presented in [Collin and Colnet (1994)]. Structural textures were analyzed with the help of the error-correcting graph grammar-based model in [Sánchez et al. (2002)]. The inference of $k$-testable graph languages was used for the analysis of drawings in [Gallego-Sánchez et al. (2018)].

## 12.3 Feature Recognition for CAD/CAM

Bond graph grammars were used for recognizing features in mechanical design in [Finger and Rinderle (1989)]. Compound feature recognition was performed with web grammar parsing in [Chuang and Henderson (1991)]. Augmented topology graph grammars were applied for feature recognition in [Finger et al. (1992)]. A syntactic pattern recognition scheme based on the $ETPL(k)$ graph grammar parsing model for the recognition of 3D solids modelled in CAD systems was presented in [Jakubowski and Flasiński (1992)]. Boundary solid grammars were used for reasoning about 3D solids in [Heisserman and Woodbury (1993)]. Feature-based modelling and reasoning based on graph grammar parsing was presented in [Fu and Pennington de (1994)]. The parsing of attributed node-labelled feature graph grammars was applied for computer integrated manufacturing in [Klauck and Mauss (1994)]. The $ETPL(k)$ graph grammar parsing model was proposed for the integration of CAD/CAM in [Flasiński (1995b)]. Stochastic $ETPL(k)$ graph grammars were applied for manufacturing quality control in [Flasiński and Skomorowski (1998)]. Graph grammar parsing was used for the converting of design geometrical features into manufacturing geometrical features in [Ben-Arieh (1999)]. Attributed Programmed Graph Grammars were applied for product family modelling in ERP systems in [Du et al. (2002)]. An automated manufacturing planning method based on graph grammars was proposed in [Fu et al. (2013)].

## 12.4   Analysis of Visual Events and Activities

The syntactic pattern recognition methods for the analysis of visual events and activities were developed on the basis of the And-Or graph model by S. C. Zhu and his collaborators. A method for goal inference and intent prediction in video events was presented in [Pei *et al.* (2011, 2013)]. The estimation of human attributes, parts and poses was made with And-Or graph grammars in [Rothrock *et al.* (2013); Park and Zhu (2015); Park *et al.* (2018)]. Spatial-temporal And-Or graphs were used for the prediction of human activities in [Qi *et al.* (2017)].

Complex semantic events in video sequences were recognized with event And-Or graphs in [Lin *et al.* (2009a)].

The *ETPL(k)/ETPR(k)* graph grammar model was used for the recognition of Polish Sign Language in [Flasiński and Myśliński (2010)].

## 12.5   Structure Analysis in Chemistry

The use of graph grammars for chemical graph transformations was proposed in [Rosselló and Valiente (2005)]. An inference algorithm for node replacement graph grammars was applied for the analysis of chemical structures in [Kukluk *et al.* (2007)]. The use of an inference algorithm for edge replacement graph grammars for the analysis of the G tetrad chemical structure[1] was proposed in [Kukluk *et al.* (2008)]. A method for the inferring of the probability distributions of graph size and node degree from stochastic graph grammars taken from the domain of AIDS research was presented in [Mukherjee and Oates (2008, 2010)]. Double-pushout graph grammars were used for the exploring of the chemical spaces of HCN (hydrogen cyanide) polymerization and hydrolysis in [Andersen *et al.* (2013)]. The Graph Grammar Library (GGL), which was implemented on the basis of double-pushout graph grammars for chemical studies, was described in [Mann *et al.* (2013)]. The use of an inference algorithm for $k$-testable graph languages for the analysis of mutagenicity data sets was proposed in [Gallego-Sánchez *et al.* (2018)].

## 12.6   Optical Character Recognition

Descriptive graph grammars and a distance measure between attributed graphs were used for the recognition of handwritten English characters in [Sanfeliu and Fu (1983a)]. Chinese characters were recognized with the help of expansive graph grammars in [Shi and Fu (1983)]. A graph grammar-based method for the recognition of vehicle identification numbers was presented in [Cowell (1995)]. Web grammars were applied for a handwritten digit recognition in [López and Sempere (1998)] and for the recognition of Arabic characters in [Cowell and Hussain (2007)]. Handwritten signatures were recognized with *ETPL(k)* graph grammars in [Ogiela and Piekarczyk (2012)]. A recognition method for isolated handwritten characters was

---

[1]Structures of this kind are analyzed in research into the HIV-1 virus.

constructed with the help of an inference algorithm for $k$-testable graph languages in [Gallego-Sánchez *et al.* (2018)].

## 12.7   Structure Analysis for Process Monitoring and Control

Graph rewriting was used for the modelling of distributed systems in [Degano and Montanari (1987)]. Programmed $ETPL(k)$ graph grammars were applied for software allocation in distributed systems in [Flasiński and Kotulski (1992)]. This model was also used in the real-time expert control system ZEX for a high-energy physics experiment in [Flasiński (1994); Behrens *et al.* (1994)]. The dynamic control of street lighting was performed with graph grammars in [Wojnicki and Kotulski (2018)].

## 12.8   Structure Analysis in Bioinformatics and Medicine

The inference method of node label controlled graph grammars was used for the analysis of protein sequence data in [Jonyer *et al.* (2004)]. Coronary arteries were analyzed with $ETPL(k)$ graph grammars in [Trzupek and Ogiela (2013)]. The application of an inference algorithm for $k$-testable graph languages for the analysis of hairpin RNA molecules data sets was presented in [Gallego-Sánchez *et al.* (2018)].

## 12.9   Summary

A summary of the applications of the graph syntactic pattern recognition methods presented in the previous sections is contained in Table 12.1.

Table 12.1    The applications of graph-based methods.

| Applications | Models | References |
|---|---|---|
| Scene analysis | *APGGs* , expansive graph grammars, *ATGGs*, *ETPL/ETPR* model, plex grammars, And-Or graph model | [Gips (1974)], [Bunke (1978)], [Bunke (1982a)], [Shi and Fu (1983)], [Lin and Fu (1984a)], [Lin and Fu (1984b)], [Sanfeliu (1984)], [Flasiński (1988)], [Flasiński (1989)], [Flasiński (1990)], [Flasiński (1991)], [Flasiński (1993)], [Flasiński (2018)], [Skomorowski (1999)], [Skomorowski (2007)], [Zhu and Mumford (2006)], [Han and Zhu (2009)], [Lin *et al.* (2009b)], [Zhao and Zhu (2011)], [Zarchi *et al.* (2016)], [Yu *et al.* (2017)] [Liu *et al.* (2018)] |
| Picture and diagram analysis | *APGGs, ATGGs, ETPL/ETPR* model, plex grammars, web grammars, $k$-testable graph languages | [Bunke (1978)], [Bunke (1982a)], [Bunke (1982b)], [Sanfeliu and Fu (1983b)], [Bunke and Haller (1990)], [Flasiński (1990)], [Peng *et al.* (1990)], [Min *et al.* (1993)], [Aizawa and Nakamura (1994)], [Collin and Colnet (1994)], [Sánchez *et al.* (2002)], [Gallego-Sánchez *et al.* (2018)] |

Table 12.1   (*Continued*)

| Applications | Models | References |
|---|---|---|
| Feature recognition for computer aided design and manufacturing | *APGGs*, *ETPL/ETPR* model, web grammars, bond graph grammars | [Finger and Rinderle (1989)], [Chuang and Henderson (1991)], [Finger *et al.* (1992)], [Jakubowski and Flasiński (1992)], [Heisserman and Woodbury (1993)], [Fu and Pennington de (1994)], [Klauck and Mauss (1994)], [Flasiński (1995b)], [Flasiński and Skomorowski (1998)], [Ben-Arieh (1999)], [Du *et al.* (2002)], [Fu *et al.* (2013)] |
| Analysis of visual events and activities | And-Or graph model, *ETPL/ETPR* model | [Lin *et al.* (2009a)], [Flasiński and Myśliński (2010)], [Pei *et al.* (2011)], [Pei *et al.* (2013)], [Rothrock *et al.* (2013)], [Park and Zhu (2015)], [Qi *et al.* (2017)], [Park *et al.* (2018)] |
| Structure analysis in chemistry | *NLC* graph grammars, edge replacement graph grammars, double-pushout graph grammars, *k*-testable graph languages | [Rosselló and Valiente (2005)], [Kukluk *et al.* (2007)], [Kukluk *et al.* (2008)], [Mukherjee and Oates (2008)], [Mukherjee and Oates (2010)], [Andersen *et al.* (2013)], [Mann *et al.* (2013)], [Gallego-Sánchez *et al.* (2018)] |
| Optical character recognition | Expansive graph grammars, *ETPL/ETPR* model, descriptive graph grammars, web grammars, *k*-testable graph languages | [Sanfeliu and Fu (1983a)], [Shi and Fu (1983)], [Cowell (1995)], [López and Sempere (1998)], [Cowell and Hussain (2007)], [Ogiela and Piekarczyk (2012)], [Gallego-Sánchez *et al.* (2018)] |
| Structure analysis for process monitoring and control | *ETPL/ETPR* model, programmed graph grammars | [Flasiński and Kotulski (1992)], [Flasiński (1994)], [Behrens *et al.* (1994)], [Wojnicki and Kotulski (2018)] |
| Structure analysis in bioinformatics and medicine | *NLC* graph grammars, *ETPL/ETPR* model, *k*-testable graph languages | [Jonyer *et al.* (2004)], [Trzupek and Ogiela (2013)], [Gallego-Sánchez *et al.* (2018)] |

PART 5

# FUTURE OF SYNTACTIC PATTERN RECOGNITION

# Chapter 13

# Summary of Results and Open Problems

Research into syntactic pattern recognition has over the course of almost 60 years delivered both the models of formal languages and automata theory as well as efficient methods for pattern recognition applications. A summary of the results of this research is presented in Sec. 13.1. However impressive these results may be, as we will see for ourselves, fundamental open problems still influence further progress within syntactic pattern recognition. These problems are discussed in Sec. 13.2.

## 13.1 Summary of Results

The research results obtained in syntactic pattern recognition can be divided into theoretical results and application results. These we shall present in the following sections.

### 13.1.1 *Theoretical Results*

Formal languages and automata theory[1] can be divided into three areas in an analogous way as syntactic pattern recognition. Thus, we distinguish the theories of: string languages and automata, tree languages and automata, and graph languages and automata.

First of all, the important classes of string grammars and languages, like, for example, *Picture Description Languages* (*PDLs*), shape grammars, array grammars, *Shape Feature Languages* (*SFLs*), combinatory categorial grammars, head grammars, *Augmented Regular Expressions* (*AREs*), dynamically programmed grammars and *DPLL(k)* grammars, linear indexed grammars, drawn picture languages, Wang systems, tiling systems, were defined in the context of application research conducted into syntactic pattern modelling and recognition (picture analysis, shape analysis, architectural object analysis, signal analysis for process monitoring and control, NLP). Stochastic grammars, developed in the late 1960s for the describing of patterns (see Sec. 3.3.1),[2] were an important contribution to the theory of string

---

[1]The theory of syntax analysis (parsing) is treated here as a part of formal languages and automata theory.

[2]Stochastic automata were defined earlier, i.e., in the early 1960s.

languages and automata as well. Although hidden Markov models were introduced within statistical inference, a variety of their formal extensions were developed in syntactic pattern recognition (speech recognition and NLP, structure analysis in bioinformatics and signal analysis for process monitoring and control).

As far as tree languages and automata theory is concerned, the following fundamental formal models were developed within research into syntactic pattern recognition (image analysis, OCR, texture analysis, pattern recognition in seismology, NLP): stochastic tree grammars, stochastic tree automata, fuzzy tree automata, error-correcting tree automata (all the models, i.e., minimum-distance SPECTA, maximum-likelihood SPECTA and GECTA), and Tree Adjoining Grammars.

The following parsing models of the theory of graph grammars were developed in the context of syntactic pattern recognition: Sanfeliu-Fu parser (tree-graph grammars), Shi-Fu parser (expansive graph grammars), $ETPL(k)$ and $ETPR(k)$ parsers (*edNLC* graph grammars), Bunke-Haller and Peng-Yamamoto-Aoki parsers (plex grammars). Attributed Programmed Graph Grammars were also defined for syntactic pattern recognition.

### 13.1.2  *Application Results*

In order to summarize the applications of syntactic pattern recognition we divide this area into those general subareas identified in Chap. 2. The applications are listed according to the bibliographical surveys carried out in Chaps. 6, 9 and 12.

Computer Vision (1961 – 2018)[3]

- earth resource satellite image analysis
- fingerprint recognition
- online/offline character recognition
- handwritten sentence recognition
- human gesture recognition
- human activity interpretation
- sign language recognition
- video surveillance
- abnormal event detection
- intent prediction in video events
- traffic monitoring
- airplane shape recognition
- EC diagram analysis
- engineering drawing analysis
- scene analysis for robotics
- outdoor scene analysis
- medical image analysis

Structure Analysis in Natural Sciences (1964 – 2018)

- chromosome analysis
- DNA/RNA sequence alignment
- DNA sequencing
- RNA secondary structure prediction
- protein secondary structure prediction
- gene prediction
- modelling sequencing errors

---

[3]Years in brackets relate to the year of the first publication and the year of the last publication in the surveys in Chaps. 6, 9 and 12.

- base calling
- analysis of chemical structures

- structure analysis in geology

Signal Analysis (1970 –2018)

- electrocardiogram interpretation
- electroencephalogram analysis
- carotid pulse waves recognition
- real-time monitoring and control
- accident identification in nuclear power plants
- fault diagnosis of discrete event systems
- wind power prediction
- tool wear condition monitoring

- air-traffic controlling
- anomaly detection in production plants
- supervisory process control
- radar surveillance and tracking
- radar target recognition
- seismic signal analysis for oil exploration
- analysis of earthquake/explosion data

Natural Language Processing and Speech Recognition (1972 – 2018)

- natural language interpretation
- machine translation
- spoken words/phrases recognition

- continuous speech recognition
- speech understanding
- question answering

Miscellaneous Applications

- reconstruction of architectural objects
- interpretation of building façades
- large-scale urban modelling
- control of street lighting
- feature recognition in CAD systems

- CAD/CAM integration
- technical analysis in portfolio trading
- technical analysis of price curves
- recognition of NASDAQ time-series patterns
- financial trend prediction

## 13.2 Open Problems

Firstly, let us note that pattern recognition problems in which the use of string-based models is sufficient are, in principle, easier to solve than those which require the application of tree-based models, whereas the development of graph-based models is the most difficult.[4] Secondly, the grammatical inference (induction) problem is, assuming the same class of grammars, more difficult to solve than the syntax analysis problem. These two facts have had a remarkable influence on the chronology of the development of syntactic pattern recognition methods, as is shown in Fig. 13.1.

Although a variety of effective grammatical inference algorithms have been proposed in past decades (see, e.g., [Higuera de la (2010); Heinz and Sempere (2016);

---

[4]Therefore, we shall formulate *Methodological Principle II* in Chap. 14.

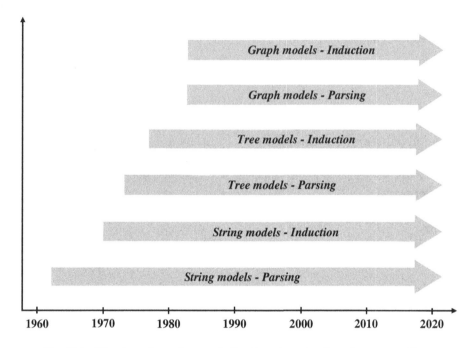

Fig. 13.1 The chronology of research directions in syntactic pattern recognition.

Wieczorek (2017)]), there still exists a need to develop new methods which could be applicable in syntactic pattern recognition. This concerns, especially, context-free string grammars, tree grammars and graph grammars. It seems that the developing of induction algorithms for the parsable classes of grammars used in syntactic pattern recognition would be most welcome in this area.

Some efficient syntactic pattern recognition models were defined in the "standard" version only.[5] Therefore, when one has to develop a pattern recognition system which should handle untypical, vague or distorted patterns, it is worth pausing to consider whether any "standard" known model can be used for this purpose by extending the said model to a stochastic, fuzzy or error-correcting version. The extension of a "standard" model may constitute an ambitious research project, especially if it concerns enhanced string grammars, tree grammars or graph grammars.

As we have seen in Chap. 4, many enhanced string grammars have been presented in order to generate certain pattern languages. Nevertheless, there is still a need for the developing of the new classes of such grammars, especially for computer vision.[6] Here matters concern both aspects of the grammar enhancement, i.e., the increasing of generative power and the increasing of descriptive power.

---

[5]By the term "standard model" we understand here a syntactic pattern recognition model which is not stochastic, fuzzy, error-correcting, etc.

[6]Let us notice that most enhanced *CF* string grammars were defined for applications in the NLP area.

Although the problem of graph grammar parsing has been investigated since 1972 and numerous syntax analyzers for graph languages have been proposed over the course of this time (see Sec. 10.7), only a few graph parsers have turned out to be useful in syntactic pattern recognition applications. Therefore, research into those parsable classes of graph grammars which are strong enough to generate real-world structural patterns should be continued.

Now, we shall consider three fundamental *methodological* open problems in syntactic pattern recognition.

In discussing enhanced models for syntactic pattern recognition in Chap. 4, we have introduced attributed grammars in Sec. 4.4.[7] Grammar attributes are used to specify structural primitives and (sub)structures in a more detailed way with the help of their (numeric) parameters. In syntactic pattern recognition we say that primitives/structures are characterized, then, additionally with *semantic information*. Semantic information can be used to compare structural elements in a more precise way, to define the predicates of production applicability as in the *APGGs* presented in Sec. 10.1, etc.

In the 1970s a novel, somewhat different, idea for the use of semantic information in syntactic pattern recognition was introduced, namely the concept of a combination of syntactic methods with decision-theoretic techniques [Kanal and Chandrasekaran (1972); Tang and Huang (1979); You and Fu (1979)]. Within this approach, called the *syntactic-semantic approach*, a hybrid pattern recognition system, firstly, performs the syntax analysis of a pattern structure, then uses decision-theoretic techniques to process feature vectors defined on the basis of the attributes of structural primitives and (sub)structures. Although a number of such hybrid syntactic-semantic models of pattern recognition based on attributed grammars have been developed [Tsai and Fu (1980); Thomason (1982); Fu (1983, 1985); Bunke and Sanfeliu (1992); Chang (1992); Bezdek (1995); Rangarajan (2014)], the constructing of such models is still an important open problem in the area of syntactic pattern recognition.

The second issue concerns the constructing of hybrid systems in which syntactic pattern recognition models and other Artificial Intelligence (AI) [Flasiński (2016a); Russell and Norvig (2009); Winston (1993)] methods are combined. The first of such systems were developed on the basis of rule-based models in the 1980s [Birman (1982); Ritchings and Colchester (1986); Wang *et al.* (1987)]. This approach was summarized in [Bunke (1988); Sanfeliu (1988); Bunke and Kandel (2002)]. The extension of this approach to probabilistic rule-based pattern recognition was proposed in [Tsatsoulis and Fu (1985); Kurzyński (2005)], whereas the hybrid system consisting of the rule-based module, the syntactic-semantic pattern recognition module and the semantic network (frame-based) module was presented in [Flasiński (1994); Behrens *et al.* (1994)]. The hybrid system developed on the basis of rules,

---

[7] As we have already seen in the book attributed string grammars can be extended to attributed tree and graph grammars.

heuristic search and syntax analysis was described in [Yang (1988, 1991, 1993)].

Heuristic search methods, neural networks and evolutionary algorithms have been used successfully for the inference of string grammars in syntactic pattern recognition [Watrous and Kuhn (1992); Dupont (1994); Zeng *et al.* (1994); Carrasco *et al.* (1996); Huang and Chao (2004); Bugalho and Oliveira (2005); Delgado and Pegalajar (2005); Keller and Lutz (2005); Lucas and Reynolds (2005); Won *et al.* (2007)]. Summing up, research into hybrid syntactic pattern recognition-AI models should be continued.

At the end of this section we shall consider the most important, in our opinion, fundamental methodological open problem, i.e., the problem of constructing holistic models in syntactic pattern recognition.[8] In Chap. 2 we have presented the basic methodological assumptions of syntactic pattern recognition, those formulated by K. S. Fu in his works in the late 1970s and which were summarized in his seminal monograph [Fu (1982)]. The general scheme of the syntactic pattern recognition system (see Fig. 2.5b) is an important element of this methodology. In this scheme two basic layers, i.e., the (numerical) layer of image (pre)processing and the (symbolic) layer of syntax analysis are distinguished. (The intermediate (numeric-symbolic) layer of structural pattern generation constitutes the third one.) On the one hand, such a definition of this scheme is consistent with the use of two strongly differing groups of algorithms/methods within syntactic pattern recognition systems. During the image (pre)processing stage, algorithms which process numerical data[9] are used, whereas during the syntax analysis stage, symbolic computation-based algorithms, originated in the theory of formal languages and automata, are applied. On the other hand, the separating of these stages and performing them in a strict sequential manner is disadvantageous, especially in the case of handling untypical/vague/distorted patterns.[10] The hybrid models discussed above were constructed also in order to neutralize the negative effects of the separation of the processing stages. However, it seems that the elaboration of a holistic model which integrates all the processing stages in a syntactic pattern recognition system is a *sine qua non* condition to solve this problem in a satisfactory manner. Important results concerning this issue were published in seminal monographs and papers [Grenander (1970); Montanari (1974); Grenander (1976, 1978, 1981); Muchnik (1972); Kanade (1977); Haralick (1978); Pavlidis (1992); Oommen and Kashyap (1998); Mumford (1996, 2002); Zhu (2003); Zhu and Mumford (2006)]. However, at the same time there arises the meta-methodological question as to whether we are able to elaborate such a *generic* holistic model or rather to develop methodological recommendations on how to construct models which better integrate the processing stages for specific

---

[8]Considerations on the problem of constructing holistic models concern mainly computer vision applications. They do not concern those application areas in which "*claire et distinct*" structural patterns are defined straightforwardly.

[9]These algorithms originated mainly from signal processing theory.

[10]From the methodological point of view, this situation is, somehow, analogous to the waterfall development model in software engineering.

pattern recognition problems.

Let us summarize our consideration. The list of important open problems in syntactic pattern recognition includes the following issues:

- the constructing of grammatical inference algorithms for context-free string grammars, tree grammars and graph grammars,
- the extension of syntactic pattern recognition models to stochastic, fuzzy and error-correcting versions,
- the defining of enhanced context-free string grammars,
- the defining of picture languages,
- the constructing of efficient parsers for graph grammars,
- the development of hybrid syntactic-semantic models of pattern recognition,
- the development of hybrid AI-syntactic pattern recognition systems,
- the elaboration of holistic models for syntactic pattern recognition.

# Chapter 14

# Methodological Issues

The methodological principles and recommendations for research into syntactic pattern recognition are presented in this chapter. General methodological principles are contained in Sec. 14.1, whereas those methodological issues which influence the further development of specific string-, tree-, and graph-based models are discussed in Sec. 14.2.[1]

## 14.1 General Methodological Principles

In syntactic pattern recognition, a language syntax is usually not given explicitly, contrary to "standard" applications in computer science such as, e.g., programming languages, compilers design, in which a syntax of an (artefactual) language is pre-defined. Instead, a pattern language is represented by a sample set of patterns (a learning set). Since this set is big, the constructing of the grammar "by hand" is impossible. Therefore, the constructing of a grammatical induction algorithm is necessary.[2] The lack of such an algorithm is a serious limitation to a syntactic pattern recognition model [Tanaka (1995); Jain *et al.* (2000); Goldfarb (2004); Flasiński (2016b)]. Let us formulate the first methodological principle:

**I.** *A complete syntactic pattern recognition model should consist of a syntax analysis method as well as a grammatical induction algorithm.*

As we know from the theory of formal languages and automata, the stronger the generative power of a grammar class is, the higher the computational complexity of the corresponding parsing algorithm. The same relates to grammatical inference algorithms, although in this case (any) polynomial complexity is sufficient.[3] Taking this into account, we can formulate the following principle.

**II.** *A syntactic pattern recognition model should be constructed according to the*

---

[1]The preliminary version of methodological recommendations for syntactic pattern recognition was presented in [Flasiński (2016b)].

[2]Except for application problems in which the syntax of a pattern language is pre-defined.

[3]Grammar induction is conducted in the off-line mode in pattern recognition systems.

*Ockham Razor principle with respect to the grammar generative power in order to obtain a computationally efficient parsing algorithm and a grammatical induction algorithm of a polynomial complexity.*

As we have discussed in Chap. 2 before a structural pattern is analyzed by a syntax analyzer it has to be constructed out of primitives obtained by the decomposition/segmentation of the processed image (cf. Fig. 2.5b). Primitives are usually pre-defined by specialists in a given application area in order to be semantically interpretable within this area. Therefore, decomposition/segmentation algorithms should be defined with the use of knowledge of this area. (The use of generic decomposition/segmentation methods may result in the decomposing of images into components which differ from semantically interpretable primitives.) The same concerns the earlier preprocessing operations (noise reduction, smoothing, etc.) which influence a correct segmentation. Therefore, the following principle is proposed:

**III.** *A decomposition/segmentation method for a syntactic pattern recognition system should be defined with the use of knowledge of a given application area in order to generate pre-defined structural primitives which have a semantic interpretation in this area.*[4] *Preprocessing techniques should be chosen so as to contribute towards the generating of such semantically interpretable primitives.*

As we have discussed in Sec. 3.3 structural patterns which are analyzed in practical applications are often vague/distorted and "standard" syntactic pattern recognition models can barely cope with such patterns. This problem can result from the following three reasons:

(1) There are typical and untypical patterns in a pattern recognition problem, i.e., some patterns occur more often than others in a learning set (a sample set of patterns). Then, we should try to estimate the probability distribution in the sample set and to extend both the grammar and the automaton (parser) to their probabilistic/stochastic versions (see Sec. 3.3.1).
(2) Objects/phenomena to be recognized are vague/fuzzy/ambiguous and statistical information is unavailable. (For example, information on patterns is based on subjective experience, expert opinions, etc.) Then, we should try to define a fuzzy grammar and a fuzzy automaton (parser) on the basis of a "standard" model developed (see Sec. 3.3.2).
(3) Distorted/deformed versions of patterns are considered in a pattern recognition problem. (For example, errors occurring at the image preprocessing stage are considered.). Then, a grammar should be expanded in order to include error productions and the corresponding error-correcting automaton (parser) should be defined (see Sec. 3.3.3).

---

[4]In the case this interpretation is essential.

Let us summarize our analysis with the following principle:

**IV.** *A syntactic pattern recognition model should be easily extendable to a stochastic, fuzzy or error-correcting version in order to cope with untypical/vague/distorted patterns.*

As we have discussed in Sec. 13.2, some problems encountered in the area of syntactic pattern recognition are so difficult that even the use of stochastic, fuzzy or error-correcting models is not successful. Then, attributed grammars should be used in order to describe structural primitives and (sub)structures with the help of parametric information. As a result the attributes/parameters can be used to support the syntax analysis with the methods of the decision-theoretic approach. Let us formulate the following principle:

**V.** *If the syntactic pattern recognition approach is too weak to handle structural patterns, it should be extended to the hybrid syntactic-semantic approach based on attributed grammars. The models of Artificial Intelligence, especially the rule-based system approach, can also enhance the functionality of syntactic pattern recognition systems.*

## 14.2 Model-Specific Methodological Recommendations

Let us begin with the consideration of methodological issues for string-based models. As we have stated in the previous section, a grammatical induction algorithm is the key element of a syntactic pattern recognition model.[5] In Chap. 4 we have presented enhanced context-free grammars which are very important from the point of view of syntactic pattern recognition applications. While the increasing of the *descriptive power* of *CF* grammars does not interfere with the formal definition of these grammars,[6] the increasing of the *generative power* does so. In Chap. 4 we have distinguished two main groups of *CF* grammars with an increased generative power: grammars with operator controlled derivations and grammars with programmed derivations, and, additionally, the model based on Augmented Regular Expressions (*AREs*). In the first group, special operators which control derivations (such as heads in head grammars, forward/backward operators in combinatory categorial grammars etc.) are "embedded" in the left- or right-hand sides of productions. In the second group and *AREs* the control mechanism is separated from the cores of productions. Grammatical inference algorithms, generally, consist in looking for similarities among sample strings. Let us note that the grammar alphabet contains only terminal symbols which occur in the language sample and nonterminals which are added as classes of abstractions for certain terminal substrings. In fact, the only

---

[5]Except for models in which one assumes that the syntax of a pattern language is pre-defined.

[6]This is achieved by the defining of a stronger representation scheme (representation mapping).

operator used is the "invisible" concatenation operator. Therefore, the use of auxiliary operators makes the induction process more difficult than in the case of the
applying of separated control mechanisms. Moreover, the parsing of programmed
grammars is even slightly more efficient than in the case of "pure" grammars because the programming mechanism narrows the scope of potential productions to be
applied. Let us summarize our considerations with the following recommendation:

**VI.** *The constructing of grammatical inference algorithms for (enhanced) context-
free grammars with increased generative power is, generally, easier, if the derivation
control mechanism is separated from the left- or right-hand sides of productions.*

In the case of tree-based models the problem of grammatical induction is one
of the key open problems. One can easily notice that the algorithms of grammatical inference for tree grammars presented in Chap. 8 have their analogues in the
induction algorithms for string grammars. So, the $k$-tail-based inference of tree
languages [Brayer and Fu (1977)] presented in Sec. 8.1 is the extension of the $k$-tail
inference algorithm of string languages [Biermann and Feldman (1972)] introduced
in Sec. 5.1.2, the inference algorithm of reversible tree languages [López *et al.*
(2004)] presented in Sec. 8.2 is based on the induction method of reversible regular
(string) languages [Angluin (1982)] introduced in Sec. 5.1.4, Brzozowski derivatives
for string languages introduced in Sec. 5.1.1 were extended for tree languages in the
tree-derivative-based inference method [Levine (1981)] presented in Sec. 8.3 etc. In
order to illustrate our considerations, let us compare, e.g., the (simple) inference
of canonical and derived grammars for regular string languages [Fu (1982)] and expansive tree languages [Barrero (1991a)]. The scheme of the induction of canonical
grammars is shown in Fig. 14.1a, whereas the scheme of the inference of derived
grammars on the basis of canonical grammars is shown in Fig. 14.1b. ($P_C$ denotes
the production set of the canonical grammar and $P_D$ denotes the production set of
the derived grammar.)

Summing up, we can formulate the following recommendation:

**VII.** *Schemes used for the inferring of string grammars and automata can be useful
for the defining of (analogous) induction algorithms for tree languages.*

Analyzing the research results and the open problems in syntactic pattern recognition, it seems that the most work is to be done in the area of graph-based models.
Firstly, let us consider the parsing problem. As we have discussed in Sec. 10.7,
there are two fundamental reasons for the intractability of this problem [Flasiński
(1998)]:

- the lack of any ordering in a graph structure and
- the (complex) form of a graph grammar production, especially the high computational complexity of the embedding transformation of a graph grammar.

**Regular String Grammar**

IF $a_1a_2a_3a_4a_5a_6 \in S^+$ THEN $A_1 \to a_1A_2$, $A_2 \to a_2A_3$, ... , $A_6 \to a_6 \in P_C$

**Expansive Tree Grammar**

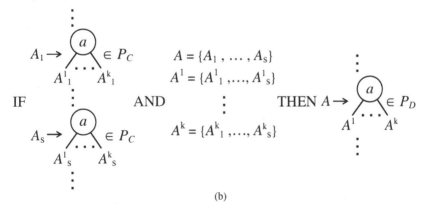

(a)

**Regular String Grammar**

$$\text{IF} \quad \begin{matrix} \vdots \\ A_1 \to a\bar{A}_1 \in P_C \\ \vdots \\ A_s \to a\bar{A}_s \in P_C \\ \vdots \end{matrix} \quad \text{AND} \quad \begin{matrix} \vdots \\ A = \{A_1,..., A_s\} \\ \bar{A} = \{\bar{A}_1,..., \bar{A}_s\} \\ \vdots \end{matrix} \quad \text{THEN} \quad \begin{matrix} \vdots \\ A \to a\bar{A} \in P_D \\ \vdots \end{matrix}$$

**Expansive Tree Grammar**

(b)

Fig. 14.1   The analogy between the induction of string and tree grammars.

The methodological suggestions concerning the first problem can be found in the last papers of K. S. Fu and his collaborators on the parsing of graph languages [Shi and Fu (1983); Sanfeliu and Fu (1983b)]. This is simply the imposing of linear ordering on the set of graph nodes. After the ordering of the nodes, the (string)

characteristic description of the graph (cf. Definition 10.8 in Sec. 10.2) is used
(see, e.g., [Shi and Fu (1983)]) and the ordering problem is solved effectively. This
methodological hint was used in the case of the defining of $ETPL(k)$ [Flasiński
(1988, 1993)] and $ETPR(k)$ [Flasiński (2018)] parsable graph languages, allowing
us to construct a variety of efficient syntactic pattern recognition systems (see Sec.
10.4). (Linear ordered graph grammars were also used in other areas of computer
science, e.g., in the area of distributed systems [Montanari and Ribeiro (2002);
Ribeiro and Dotti (2008)].)

In the models mentioned above, directed node- and edge-labelled, *EDG*, graphs
are used. However, the Fu-Shi graph characteristic description can be used for other
classes of graphs, as well. In the case of undirected node- and edge-labelled, *EG*,
graphs, the string of node indices $(i_1 \ldots i_r)$ (cf. Definition 10.8) should include the
indices of all the nodes which are adjacent to $v_k$ ($r$ is the valency of $v_k$ in this case).
Obviously, the string of edge labels $(e_1 \ldots e_r)$ should be redefined accordingly. In the
case of undirected node-labelled graphs, the string of edge labels $(e_1 \ldots e_r)$ should
be omitted.

Of course, one has to solve the problem of the unambiguous indexing of the set
of graph nodes in order to apply this methodological scheme. It appears that the
indexing *via* referring to the semantic properties of the represented objects (phenomena, processes, etc.), i.e., the use of *interpreted graphs*[7] is the successful strategy
which has been verified positively in many syntactic pattern recognition applications
(see Sec. 10.4). Let us introduce the following methodological recommendation:

**VIII.** *The use of the concept of interpreted graphs for the unambiguous indexing of
graph nodes and the Fu-Shi string characteristic description of graphs is an effective
methodological strategy for the constructing of efficient graph parsers for syntactic
pattern recognition.*

The second problem, which results from the complex form of graph grammar
production, especially its *embedding transformation* (see Sec. 10.7), seems to be
more troublesome. There are the following three strategies to handle this problem
in syntactic pattern recognition:

(1) *The defining of the subclasses of the (standard) grammars known in the theory
of graph grammars.* In this case the parsing schemes, which are analogous to
the parsing schemes for string languages, are constructed. For example, the
parsing for $ETPL(k)$ subclass [Flasiński (1988, 1993)] of classic *edNLC* graph
grammars is analogous to the parsing for $LL(k)$ string grammars (see Fig. 14.2),
whereas the parsing for $ETPR(k)$ subclass [Flasiński (2018)] of *edNLC* grammars is analogous to the parsing for $LR(k)$ string grammars. (Both parsable
subclasses belong to the connecting embedding approach in the theory of graph

---

[7]Let us remind ourselves that *interpreted graphs* which refer to the semantic aspect of represented
objects are formalized on the basis of Tarski's (semantic) model theory approach (see Sec. 10.4).

## LL(k) String Grammar

$$\alpha \beta \theta \underset{l(G)}{\overset{*}{\Rightarrow}} \overbrace{\alpha\, a_1 \ldots a_k\, a_{(k+1)} \ldots a_n}^{\text{terminal words}}$$

$$S \underset{l(G)}{\overset{*}{\Rightarrow}} \alpha A \theta \underset{l(G)}{\overset{\nearrow}{\underset{\Rightarrow}{}}}$$

$$\underset{l(G)}{\Rightarrow} \alpha \gamma \theta \underset{l(G)}{\overset{*}{\Rightarrow}} \alpha\, \underbrace{b_1 \ldots b_k}\, b_{(k+1)} \ldots b_m$$

$$\text{IF} \quad a_1 \ldots a_k = b_1 \ldots b_k \quad \text{THEN} \quad \beta = \gamma$$

## ETPL(k) Graph Grammar

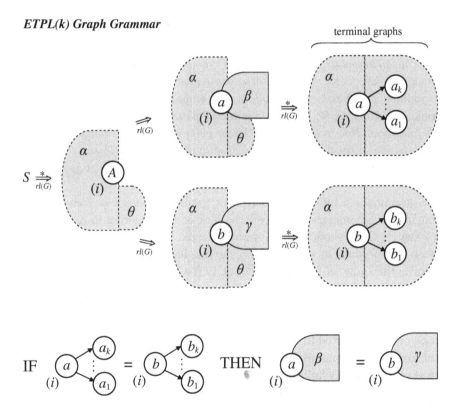

Fig. 14.2   The analogy between the parsing of $LL(k)$ string and $ETPL(k)$ graph grammars.

grammars.) In as far as the gluing embedding approach in the theory of graph grammars is concerned, the plex grammar parsers introduced in [Bunke and Haller (1990)] and [Peng *et al.* (1990)] are analogous to the Earley parser for *CF* string grammars.

(2) *The defining of the special classes of graph grammars.* In this approach, the form of productions of graph grammars is tree-like and the embedding mechanism is,

somehow, "hidden" in the right-hand sides of productions [Shi and Fu (1983); Sanfeliu and Fu (1983b)].[8]

(3) *The defining of the syntactic analysis schemes which are not based on standard parsing schemes.* Such an approach was used for Attributed Programmed Graph Grammars [Bunke (1982a)] and for And-Or graphs [Zhu and Mumford (2006)].

All three approaches listed above have turned out to be successful in syntactic pattern recognition. From the methodological point of view, all of them solve the problem of the handling of the embedding transformation during parsing. In the first approach, by limiting the power capabilities of the embedding transformation; in the second approach, by "hiding" the embedding transformation in the right-hand sides of productions; in the third approach, shall we say, by not using parsing. Summing up, we can formulate the following methodological principle:

**IX.** *The high computational complexity of the embedding transformation of a graph grammar is a key factor which influences the high computational complexity of the corresponding graph parser. Therefore, the embedding transformation of a graph grammar which is to be used for syntactic pattern recognition should be modified/defined according to the Ockham Razor principle, which usually means the need to limit its power capability. The use of graph-based syntactic pattern recognition models, which are not based on (standard) parsing schemes, is also worth studying.*

The grammatical inference problem for graph grammars is, somehow, similar to that for tree grammars. However, the lack of any ordering in a graph and the complexity of the embedding transformation are additional issues which have to be taken into account in this case. On the one hand, the solution to the ordering problem is the same as for graph grammars, i.e., the imposing of linear ordering on graphs. On the other hand, for the inducing of the embedding transformation, obviously, no analogies can be found in the areas of string and tree language induction. At the same time, certain generic concepts concerning the general scheme of induction can be adopted from the string and tree schemes. For example, the defining the graphs $G_i$ belonging to the succeeding rests $R_i$ in the induction of $ETPL(k)$ graph grammars (cf. Definition 11.1 in Sec. 11.2) is analogous to the defining of the Brzozowski derivatives in the induction of regular string grammars (cf. Definition 5.1 in Sec. 5.1.1). Let us introduce the following principle:

**X.** *Certain generic concepts of the standard induction schemes for string languages can be useful for the defining of analogous induction schemes for graph languages. The inference of the embedding transformation is the main problem in the induction of graph languages.*

---

[8]This methodological strategy is similar to the enhancing of *CF* grammars by "hiding" derivation control operators in the left- and right-hand sides of productions.

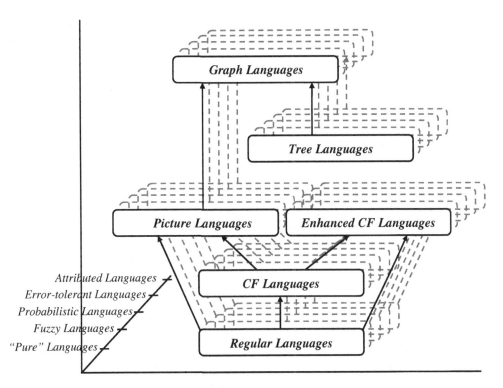

Fig. 14.3 The taxonomy of pattern recognition models according to the classes of formal languages.

## 14.3 Concluding Remarks

At the end of this book we can summarize our considerations by presenting a more detailed taxonomy of pattern recognition models according to the types of formal languages which is shown in Fig. 14.3. Firstly, we distinguish the basic classes of ("pure") languages used in syntactic pattern recognition. Secondly, for each class we can define its fuzzy, probabilistic, error-tolerant[9] and attributed extension. Graph languages can be treated as (strongly) "enhanced" picture languages.[10] In the book we have presented the models of syntactic pattern recognition according to this taxonomy.

Syntactic pattern recognition is an interesting research area. On the one hand, it is based on one of the most "classic" theory of computer science, namely the theory of formal languages and automata. Its theoretical basics, however, are not limited to this well-founded computer science theory, but include other fundamental

---

[9]Languages recognizable by error-correcting parsers are called here error-tolerant languages.

[10]For example, the structural primitives of Shaw's *Picture Description Languages* introduced in Sec. 4.8 can be treated as specific N attaching point entities (NAPEs) of plex languages, introduced in Sec. 10.5, for N = 2.

fields of computer science, such as computer vision, compiler design, computational complexity theory etc., as well as the important fields of applied mathematics, such as probability theory, fuzzy set theory, graph theory etc. On the other hand, it is also attractive due to the incredibly broad spectrum of its applications, let us mention just a few: computer vision, natural language processing, bioinformatics and computer aided manufacturing. Therefore, it seems to be especially appealing for young researchers, PhD students, post-doctoral students and the like. Indeed, research into syntactic pattern recognition may be an exciting journey into the world of structural entities and phenomena in order to comprehend their properties.

Textbooks and fundamental monographs on syntactic pattern recognition have been listed in Chap. 1. For surveys the reader is referred to [Thomason (1990b); Bunke (1993); Tanaka (1995); Majumdar and Ray (2001); Flasiński (2016b)]. Dedicated journals include *IEEE Transactions on Pattern Analysis and Machine Intelligence, Pattern Recognition, IEEE Transactions on Systems, Man, and Cybernetics, Computer Vision, Graphics and Image Processing* (formerly: *Computer Graphics and Image Processing*), *Pattern Recognition Letters, Computer Vision and Image Understanding, International Journal of Pattern Recognition and Artificial Intelligence* and *Pattern Analysis and Applications*. Research results relating to syntactic pattern recognition have been published in the proceedings of international pattern recognition conferences, including the IEEE Conference on Computer Vision and Pattern Recognition (CVPR), the IAPR International Conference on Pattern Recognition (ICPR), the IAPR Joint International Workshops on Statistical Techniques in Pattern Recognition and Structural and Syntactic Pattern Recognition (S+SSPR) and the IEEE International Conference on Computer Vision (ICCV). Theoretical models for syntactic pattern recognition have been also presented in *Information Sciences, Journal of Computer and System Sciences, Information and Computation* (formerly: *Information and Control*), *Theoretical Computer Science* and *Fundamenta Informaticae*.

# Appendix A

# Formal Languages and Automata - Selected Notions

The fundamental notions on the theory of formal languages and automata are introduced in this appendix. Chomsky's generative grammars are presented in the first section. The formal automata corresponding to Chomsky's grammars are introduced in the second section. These formalisms are basic for the string models presented in Chaps. 3 and 4. The last section contains definitions of *edNLC* graph grammars and languages. The *ETPL(k)/ETPR(k)* syntactic pattern recognition model presented in Sec. 10.4 is based on these graph grammars.

## A.1 Chomsky's String Grammars

Firstly, we shall introduce the basic notions concerning Chomsky's grammars.

An *alphabet* $\Sigma$ is a finite nonempty set of symbols.

A *string* over an alphabet $\Sigma$ is any string consisting of symbols of an alphabet $\Sigma$ that is of a finite length.

A string that does not include any symbol is called the *empty word* and it is denoted with $\lambda$.

A set of all the strings over an alphabet $\Sigma$ that are of a finite nonzero length is called the *Kleene plus* and it is denoted with $\Sigma^+$.

A set including all the strings over an alphabet $\Sigma$ that are of a finite length, including the empty word, is called the *Kleene star* and it is denoted with $\Sigma^*$. Thus, $\Sigma^* = \Sigma^+ \cup \{\lambda\}$.

$|x|$ denotes the length of a string $x \in \Sigma^*$.

$\Sigma^k$ denotes a set of strings of length $k$.

Let $A$ and $B$ be sets of strings. $AB$ denotes a set of strings: $AB = \{\alpha\beta : \alpha \in A, \beta \in B\}$, i.e. the set consisting of strings that are the *concatenation* of strings belonging to $A$ with strings belonging to $B$.

For example, if $A$, $B$, $C$ are sets of symbols, then defining a string $s$ as $s \in A^*BC^+$ means that $s$ is a concatenation of: a substring constructed of the symbols of $A$ (including the empty word), one symbol of $B$ and a substring of the symbols of $C$ (excluding the empty word).

The concept of *regular expressions* was introduced in [Kleene (1951)]. A regular expression $R$ over an alphabet $\Sigma$ and the language $L(R)$ it denotes are defined inductively in the following way [Hopcroft *et al.* (2006); Meduna (2014); Rozenberg and Salomaa (1997)].

(1) $R = \emptyset$ is a regular expression which denotes the language $L(R) = \emptyset$.
(2) $R = \lambda$ is a regular expression which denotes the language $L(R) = \lambda$.
(3) $R = a$, $a \in \Sigma$, is a regular expression which denotes the language $L(R) = \{a\}$.
    Let $R_1$ and $R_2$ be regular expressions, $L(R_1)$ and $L(R_2)$ be the languages they denote, respectively.
(4) $R = (R_1 + R_2)$ is a regular expression which denotes the language $L(R) = L(R_1) \cup L(R_2)$.
(5) $R = (R_1 R_2)$ is a regular expression which denotes the language $L(R) = L(R_1)L(R_2)$.
(6) $R = (R_1)^*$ is a regular expression which denotes the language $(L(R_1))^*$.

We assume that the Kleene star has higher precedence than concatenation and + (union), and concatenation has higher precedence than +.

Now, we can introduce grammars of the Chomsky model [Hopcroft *et al.* (2006); Meduna (2014); Rozenberg and Salomaa (1997)].

**Definition A.1 (Phrase-Structure Grammar):** A phrase-structure grammar (unrestricted grammar, type-0 grammar, *UNR*) is a quadruple

$$G = (\Sigma_N, \Sigma_T, P, S), \text{ where}$$

$\Sigma_N$ is a set of nonterminal symbols,
$\Sigma_T$ is a set of terminal symbols, $\Sigma = \Sigma_N \cup \Sigma_T$,
$P$ is a set of productions of the form: $\alpha \rightarrow \gamma$,
in which $\alpha \in \Sigma^* \Sigma_N \Sigma^*$ is called the left-hand side of the production, and $\gamma \in \Sigma^*$ is called the right-hand side of the production,
$S$ is the start symbol (axiom), $S \in \Sigma_N$.

We assume that $\Sigma_N \cap \Sigma_T = \emptyset$.

**Definition A.2 (Derivational Step):** Let $\beta, \theta \in \Sigma^*$. We denote

$$\beta \underset{G}{\Longrightarrow} \theta \quad (\text{or } \beta \Longrightarrow \theta, \text{ if } G \text{ is assumed})$$

iff $\beta = \eta_1 \alpha \eta_2$ , $\theta = \eta_1 \gamma \eta_2$ and $\alpha \rightarrow \gamma \in P$, where $P$ is a set of productions of the grammar $G$.
We say that $\beta$ directly derives $\theta$ in the grammar $G$, and we call such a direct deriving a derivational step in the grammar $G$. Any $\theta$ ($\beta$) which contains at least one nonterminal symbol is called a *sentential form*. Any $\theta$ which contains only terminal symbols is called a *sentence* or a *word*.
The reflexive and transitive closure of the relation $\underset{G}{\Longrightarrow}$ , denoted $\underset{G}{\overset{*}{\Longrightarrow}}$ ( $\overset{*}{\Longrightarrow}$ ) is

called a *derivation* in the grammar $G$. The transitive closure of the relation $\underset{G}{\Longrightarrow}$ is denoted with $\underset{G}{\overset{+}{\Longrightarrow}}$ ( $\overset{+}{\Longrightarrow}$ ).

**Definition A.3 (Language Generated by Grammar):** The language generated by the grammar $G = (\Sigma_N, \Sigma_T, P, S)$ is the set

$$L(G) = \{\phi \in \Sigma_T^* : S \underset{G}{\overset{*}{\Longrightarrow}} \phi\}.$$

**Definition A.4 (Context-Sensitive Grammar):** A context-sensitive grammar (type-1 grammar, *CSG*) is a quadruple

$$G = (\Sigma_N, \Sigma_T, P, S), \text{ where}$$

$\Sigma_N, \Sigma_T, S$ are defined as in Definition A.1,
$P$ is a set of productions of the form: $\eta_1 A \eta_2 \to \eta_1 \gamma \eta_2$,
in which $\eta_1, \eta_2 \in \Sigma^*$ , $A \in \Sigma_N$ , $\gamma \in \Sigma^+$. Additionally we assume that a production of the form $A \to \lambda$ is allowable, if $A$ does not occur in any production of $P$ in its right-hand side.

**Definition A.5 (Context-Free Grammar):** A context-free grammar (type-2 grammar, *CFG*) is a quadruple

$$G = (\Sigma_N, \Sigma_T, P, S), \text{ where}$$

$\Sigma_N, \Sigma_T, S$ are defined as in Definition A.1,
$P$ is a set of productions of the form: $A \to \gamma$,
in which $A \in \Sigma_N$ , $\gamma \in \Sigma^*$.

$G$ is a *$\lambda$-free grammar*, if it does not contain the production $A \to \lambda$.

A symbol $X \in \Sigma$ is *useful* for $G = (\Sigma_N, \Sigma_T, P, S)$ iff there is a derivation $S \underset{G}{\overset{*}{\Longrightarrow}} \alpha X \beta \underset{G}{\overset{*}{\Longrightarrow}} w, w \in \Sigma_T^*$.

$G = (\Sigma_N, \Sigma_T, P, S)$ is a *uniquely invertible grammar* iff it has no two productions $A \to \alpha$ , $B \to \alpha$ such that $A \neq B$.

**Definition A.6 (Regular Grammar):** A regular (right-regular) grammar (type-3 grammar, *REG*) is a quadruple

$$G = (\Sigma_N, \Sigma_T, P, S), \text{ where}$$

$\Sigma_N, \Sigma_T, S$ are defined as in Definition A.1,
$P$ is a set of productions of the form: $A \to \gamma$,
in which $A \in \Sigma_N$ , $\gamma \in \Sigma_T \cup \Sigma_T \Sigma_N \cup \{\lambda\}$.[1]

---

[1] In the book we assume that $G$ is a $\lambda$-free grammar, i.e. $\gamma \in \Sigma_T \cup \Sigma_T \Sigma_N$.

## A.2   String Automata

In this section we present definitions of the types of automata that correspond to types of Chomsky's grammars [Hopcroft *et al.* (2006); Meduna (2014); Rozenberg and Salomaa (1997)].

**Definition A.7 (Finite-State Automaton):** A (deterministic) finite-state automaton (*FSA*) is a quintuple

$$A = (Q, \Sigma_T, \delta, q_0, F), \text{ where}$$

$Q$ is a finite nonempty set of states,
$\Sigma_T$ is a finite set of input symbols,
$\delta : Q \times \Sigma_T \longrightarrow Q$ is the state-transition function[2],
$q_0 \in Q$ is the initial state,
$F \subseteq Q$ is a set of final states.

Let us introduce notions used for the description of a computation performed by *FSA*.

Let a current situation in an automaton be described with a pair $(q, \alpha) \in Q \times \Sigma_T^*$, called an *automaton instantaneous configuration*. The first element denotes a state of the automaton, the second a part of an input string which has not been analyzed till now. We denote a *direct step of an execution of an automaton*, called the *transition of an automaton*, with $\vdash$.

*FSA* processes an input string $\beta$ according to the following scheme. Firstly, the automaton is in the state $q_0$, and $\beta$ is at its input. Thus, $(q_0, \beta)$ is the *initial configuration* of the automaton. The automaton reads symbols of $\beta$ one by one, and it makes the succeeding steps as follows.

$$(q_i, a\gamma) \vdash (q_k, \gamma) \quad \Leftrightarrow \quad \delta(q_i, a) = q_k,$$

where $\delta$ is the state-transition function $q_i, q_k \in Q$, $a \in \Sigma_T$, $\gamma \in \Sigma_T^*$.
The automaton halts if it reaches the configuration $(q_m, \lambda)$ such that $q_m \in F$ ($\lambda$ is the empty word).

Let $\vdash^*$ denote the reflexive and transitive closure of the relation $\vdash$.

**Definition A.8 (Language Accepted by Finite-State Automaton):** The language accepted by the finite-state automaton $A = (Q, \Sigma_T, \delta, q_0, F)$ is the set

$$L(A) = \{\beta \in \Sigma_T^* : (q_0, \beta) \ \vdash^* (q_m, \lambda), \ q_m \in F\}.$$

Testing membership in the case of regular languages is efficient [Hopcroft *et al.* (2006)].

**Theorem A.1 (Time Complexity of Membership Problem for Regular Languages):** Testing whether a word $w \in L(A)$ with a (deterministic) finite-state

---

[2]For a non-deterministic automaton $\delta : Q \times \Sigma_T \longrightarrow 2^Q$.

automaton $A$ takes $\mathcal{O}(n)$ time, where $n$ is the length of $w$.

**Definition A.9 (Pushdown Automaton):** A (deterministic) pushdown automaton ($PDA$) is a seven-tuple

$$A = (Q, \Sigma_T, \Phi, \delta, q_0, Z_0, F), \text{ where}$$

$Q$ is a finite nonempty set of states,
$\Sigma_T$ is a finite set of input symbols,
$\Phi$ is a finite set of stack symbols,
$\delta : Q \times (\Sigma_T \cup \{\lambda\}) \times \Phi \longrightarrow Q \times \Phi^*$ is the transition function,
$q_0 \in Q$ is the initial state,
$Z_0 \in \Phi$ is the initial stack symbol,
$F \subseteq Q$ is a set of final states.

An instantaneous configuration of $PDA$ is described with $(q, \alpha, \phi) \in Q \times \Sigma_T^* \times \Phi^*$, where the first two elements are the same as for $FSA$, and the third element defines the content of the stack. (We assume that the first symbol is the topmost symbol of the stack.)

$PDA$ processes an input string $\beta$ in the following way. $(q_0, \beta, Z_0)$ is the initial configuration. The automaton reads the symbols of $\beta$ one by one, and it makes the succeeding steps as follows.

$$(q_i, a\gamma, Z\phi) \vdash (q_k, \gamma, \eta\phi) \quad \Leftrightarrow \quad \delta(q_i, a, Z) = (q_k, \eta),$$

where $\delta$ is the transition function, $q_i, q_k \in Q$, $a \in \Sigma_T \cup \{\lambda\}$, $\gamma \in \Sigma_T^*$, $\eta, \phi \in \Phi^*$.

Completing a computation can be defined in two (various) ways in the case of pushdown automata. In the case of an acceptance by the final state, $(q_m, \lambda, \xi)$, where $q_m \in F$ is the final configuration. In the case of an acceptance by an empty stack $(q_m, \lambda, \lambda)$ is the final configuration.

**Definition A.10 (Language Accepted by Pushdown Automaton):** The language accepted by the pushdown automaton $A = (Q, \Sigma_T, \Phi, \delta, q_0, Z_0, F)$ is the set

$$L(A) = \{\beta \in \Sigma_T^* : (q_0, \beta, Z_0) \vdash^* (q_m, \lambda, \xi), \ q_m \in F\} \text{ (by a final state), or}$$

$$L(A) = \{\beta \in \Sigma_T^* : (q_0, \beta, Z_0) \vdash^* (q_m, \lambda, \lambda), \ q_m \in Q\} \text{ (by an empty stack).}$$

Although linear-bounded automaton ($LBA$) is the next one in the hierarchy of string automata, we shall first introduce the Turing machine ($TM$), since $LBA$ can be defined as a kind of $TM$.

**Definition A.11 (Turing Machine):** A (one-tape) Turing machine ($TM$) is a seven-tuple

$$A = (Q, \Phi, B, \Sigma_T, \delta, q_0, F), \text{ where}$$

$Q$ is a finite nonempty set of states,

$\Phi$ is a finite nonempty set of tape symbols,

$B \in \Phi$ is the blank symbol,

$\Sigma_T \subseteq \Phi \setminus \{B\}$ is a set of input symbols,

$\delta : (Q \setminus F) \times \Phi \longrightarrow Q \times \Phi \times \{L, R\}$ is the transition function,

$q_0 \in Q$ is the initial state,

$F \subseteq Q$ is a set of final states.

*TM* consists of a finite control (described by the transition function) and an infinite tape divided into cells. An input word is put on the tape (one symbol into one cell) and all the remaining cells are marked with the blank symbol $B$. Firstly, the reading/writing head of the control is set over the cell which contains the first symbol of the word. This is described with the *initial configuration*: $q_0 X_1 X_2 \ldots X_n$, where $q_0$ is the initial state, $X_1 X_2 \ldots X_n$ denote the content of the cells.

An instantaneous configuration is of the form $X_1 X_2 \ldots X_{i-1} q X_i X_{i+1} \ldots X_n$, where the head is placed over the $i$-th cell, and $q$ is a state of *TM*.

*TM* processes an input word in the following way.

$$X_1 \ldots X_{i-1} q_k X_i X_{i+1} \ldots X_n \vdash X_1 \ldots X_{i-1} Y q_m X_{i+1} \ldots X_n \ ,$$

if $\delta(q_k, X_i) = (q_m, Y, R)$ (a change of a state from $q_k$ to $q_m$ a change of a symbol on the tape from $X_i$ to $Y$, and moving the head to the right), and

$$X_1 \ldots X_{i-1} q_k X_i X_{i+1} \ldots X_n \vdash X_1 \ldots X_{i-2} q_m X_{i-1} Y X_{i+1} \ldots X_n \ ,$$

if $\delta(q_k, X_i) = (q_m, Y, L)$.

The formal properties of *TM* are presented in [Hopcroft *et al.* (2006)].

Linear bounded automaton (*LBA*) can be viewed as a constrained form of *TM*. Instead of having an infinite tape, a computation of *LBA* is restricted to the part of the tape between the left end-marker and the right end-marker. We can define *LBA* in the following way.

**Definition A.12 (Linear-Bounded Automaton):** A linear-bounded automaton (*LBA*) is an eight-tuple

$$A = (Q, \Phi, M_L, M_R, \Sigma_T, \delta, q_0, F), \text{ where}$$

$Q$, $\Phi$, $\Sigma_T$, $q_0$, $F$ are defined as for the Turing machine,

$M_L \in \Phi \setminus \Sigma_T$ is the left end-marker,

$M_R \in \Phi \setminus \Sigma_T$ is the right end-marker $M_R \neq M_L$,

$\delta : (Q \setminus F) \times \Phi \longrightarrow Q \times \Phi \times \{L, R, S\}$ is the transition function.

The formal properties of *LBA* are presented in [Rozenberg and Salomaa (1997)].

## A.3   NLC Graph Grammars

Definitions of *edNLC* graph grammars and languages introduced in [Janssens and Rozenberg (1980a,b); Janssens *et al.* (1982)] are contained in this section. The classes of parsable *ETPL(k)* and *ETPR(k)* languages used for syntactic pattern recognition (see Sec. 10.4) are subclasses of *edNLC* graph languages.

**Definition A.13 (*EDG* Graph):** A directed node- and edge-labelled graph, *EDG* graph, over $\Sigma$ and $\Gamma$ is a quintuple

$$H = (V, E, \Sigma, \Gamma, \phi), \text{ where}$$

$V$ is a finite, non-empty set of nodes,
$\Sigma$ is a finite, non-empty set of node labels,
$\Gamma$ is a finite, non-empty set of edge labels,
$E$ is a set of edges of the form $(v, \gamma, w)$, in which $v, w \in V, \gamma \in \Gamma$, and
$\phi : V \to \Sigma$ is a node-labelling function.

The family of the *EDG* graphs over $\Sigma$ and $\Gamma$ is denoted by $EDG_{\Sigma,\Gamma}$. The components $V, E, \phi$ of a graph $H$ are sometimes denoted with $V_H, E_H, \phi_H$.

Let $A = (V_A, E_A, \Sigma, \Gamma, \phi_A)$, $B = (V_B, E_B, \Sigma, \Gamma, \phi_B)$ and $C = (V_C, E_C, \Sigma, \Gamma, \phi_C)$ be *EDG* graphs. An isomorphism from $A$ onto $B$ is a bijective function $h$ from $V_A$ onto $V_B$ such that

$$\phi_B \circ h = \phi_A \quad and \quad E_B = \{(h(v), \gamma, h(w)) : (v, \gamma, w) \in E_A\}.$$

We say that $A$ is *isomorphic to $B$*, and denote this with $A \cong B$.
A graph $C$ is a (full) *subgraph of $B$* iff $V_C \subseteq V_B, E_C = \{(v, \gamma, w) \in E_B : v, w \in V_C\}$ and $\phi_C$ is the restriction to $V_C$ of $\phi_B$. We also say that $C$ is the *subgraph spanned by $V_C$* in $B$.
By $B \setminus C$ we denote the subgraph spanned by $V_B \setminus V_C$ in $B$.
A graph $C$ is a *partial graph of $B$* iff $V_C = V_B$ and $E_C \subseteq E_B$.
A (directed) *path* in $A$ is a sequence of its edges of the following form:
$(v_{k_1}, \gamma_{k_1}, v_{k_2}), (v_{k_2}, \gamma_{k_2}, v_{k_3}), \ldots, (v_{k_{(m-2)}}, \gamma_{k_{(m-2)}}, v_{k_{(m-1)}}), (v_{k_{(m-1)}}, \gamma_{k_{(m-1)}}, v_{k_m})$.
A path such that $v_{k_1} = v_{k_m}$ is called a *cycle*.
We say that $A$ is *acyclic* iff no path of $A$ is a cycle.
$v \in V_A$ is called a *predecessor of $v' \in V_A$* ($v' \in V_A$ is called a *successor of $v \in V_A$*) iff there exits a path from $v$ to $v'$ in $A$.

An undirected node- and edge-labelled graph, *EG* graph, over $\Sigma$ and $\Gamma$ is a quintuple $H = (V, E, \Sigma, \Gamma, \phi)$, where $V, \Sigma, \Gamma, \phi$ are defined as in Definition A.13, but the edges are of the form $(\{v, w\}, \gamma)$, $v, w \in V, v \neq w, \gamma \in \Gamma$. The family of the *EG* graphs over $\Sigma$ and $\Gamma$ is denoted by $EG_{\Sigma,\Gamma}$.

An undirected node-labelled graph, $G$ graph, $G$ *graph* over $\Sigma$ is a quadruple $H = (V, E, \Sigma, \phi)$, where $V, \Sigma, \phi$ are defined as in Definition A.13, but the edges are of the form $\{v, w\}$, $v, w \in V, v \neq w$. The family of the $G$ graphs over $\Sigma$ is denoted by $G_\Sigma$.

**Definition A.14 (*edNLC* Graph Grammar):** An edge-labelled directed Node Label Controlled, *edNLC*, graph grammar is a quintuple

$$G = (\Sigma, \Sigma_T, \Gamma, P, Z), \text{ where}$$

$\Sigma$ is a finite, non-empty set of node labels,
$\Sigma_T \subseteq \Sigma$ is a set of terminal node labels,
$\Gamma$ is a finite, non-empty set of edge labels,
$P$ is a finite set of productions of the form $(l, D, C)$, in which
$l \in \Sigma \setminus \Sigma_T$, $D \in EDG_{\Sigma,\Gamma}$,
$C : \Gamma \times \{in, out\} \to 2^{\Sigma \times \Sigma \times \Gamma \times \{in, out\}}$ is the embedding transformation,
$Z \in EDG_{\Sigma,\Gamma}$ is the start graph called the axiom.

**Definition A.15 (*edNLC* Graph Language):** Let $G = (\Sigma, \Sigma_T, \Gamma, P, Z)$ be an *edNLC* graph grammar.
(1) Let $H, \overline{H} \in EDG_{\Sigma,\Gamma}$. Then $H$ directly derives $\overline{H}$ in $G$, denoted by $H \underset{G}{\Longrightarrow} \overline{H}$, if there exists a node $v \in V_H$ and a production $(l, D, C)$ in $P$ such that the following holds.
   (a) $l = \phi_H(v)$.
   (b) There exists an isomorphism from $\overline{H}$ onto the graph $X$ in $EDG_{\Sigma,\Gamma}$ constructed as follows. Let $\overline{D}$ be a graph isomorphic to $D$ such that $V_H \cap V_{\overline{D}} = \emptyset$ and let $h$ be an isomorphism from $D$ onto $\overline{D}$. Then

$$X = (V_X, E_X, \Sigma, \Gamma, \phi_X),$$

where

$$V_X = (V_H \setminus \{v\}) \cup V_{\overline{D}},$$

$$\phi_X(y) = \begin{cases} \phi_H(y) \text{ if } y \in V_H \setminus \{v\} \\ \phi_{\overline{D}}(y) \text{ if } y \in V_{\overline{D}}, \end{cases}$$

$$E_X = (E_H \setminus \{(n, \gamma, m) : n = v \text{ or } m = v\}) \cup E_{\overline{D}}$$
$$\cup \{(n, \gamma, m) : n \in V_{\overline{D}}, m \in V_{X \setminus \overline{D}} \text{ and there exists an edge } (m, \beta, v) \in E_H \text{ such that}$$
$$(\phi_X(n), \phi_X(m), \gamma, out) \in C(\beta, in)\} \cup$$
$$\cup \{(m, \gamma, n) : n \in V_{\overline{D}}, m \in V_{X \setminus \overline{D}} \text{ and there exists an edge } (m, \beta, v) \in E_H \text{ such that}$$
$$(\phi_X(n), \phi_X(m), \gamma, in) \in C(\beta, in)\} \cup$$
$$\cup \{(n, \gamma, m) : n \in V_{\overline{D}}, m \in V_{X \setminus \overline{D}} \text{ and there exists an edge } (v, \beta, m) \in E_H \text{ such that}$$
$$(\phi_X(n), \phi_X(m), \gamma, out) \in C(\beta, out)\} \cup$$

$\cup \{(m, \gamma, n) : n \in V_{\overline{D}} \,, m \in V_{X \setminus \overline{D}}$ and there exists an edge $(v, \beta, m) \in E_H$ such that
$$(\phi_X(n), \phi_X(m), \gamma, in) \in C(\beta, out)\}.$$

(2) By $\xrightarrow[G]{*}$ we denote the transitive and reflexive closure of $\xrightarrow[G]{}$ .

(3) The language of $G$, denoted $L(G)$, is the set

$$L(G) = \{H : Z \xrightarrow[G]{*} H \quad \text{and} \quad H \in EDG_{\Sigma_T, \Gamma}\}.$$

An example of a derivation step of an *edNLC* grammar is presented in Chap. 10.

# Bibliography

Abe, N. and Mamitsuka, H. (1997). Predicting protein secondary structure using stochastic tree grammars, *Machine Learning* **29**, pp. 275–301.

Abe, N., Mizumoto, M., Toyoda, J. I., and Tanaka, K. (1973). Web grammars and several graphs, *Journal of Computer and System Sciences* **7**, pp. 37–65.

Ábrahám, S. (1965). Some questions of phrase structure grammars, *Computational Linguistics* **4**, pp. 61–70.

Agarwal, S., Vaz, C., Bhattacharya, A., and Srinivasan, A. (2010). Prediction of novel precursor miRNAs using a context-sensitive hidden Markov model (CSHMM), *BMC Bioinformatics* **11** (Suppl 1): S29.

Aggarwal, J. K. and Cai, Q. (1999). Human motion analysis: A review, *Computer Vision and Image Understanding* **73**, pp. 428–440.

Agui, T. and Nagahashi, H. (1979). A coding method of Chinese characters, *IEEE Trans. Pattern Analysis and Machine Intelligence* **1**, pp. 333–341.

Agui, T., Nakajima, M., Kim, T. K., and Takahashi, E. T. (1979). A coding method of Chinese characters, *IEEE Trans. Pattern Analysis and Machine Intelligence* **1**, pp. 245–251.

Aho, A. V. (1968). Indexed grammars - an extension of context-free grammars, *Journal of the Association for Computing Machinery* **15**, pp. 647–671.

Aho, A. V., Lam, M. S., Sethi, R., and Ullman, J. D. (2007). *Compilers: Principles, Techniques, and Tools* (Pearson Education, Boston, MA).

Aho, A. V. and Peterson, T. G. (1972). A minimum distance error-correcting parser for context-free languages, *SIAM Journal on Computing* **1**, pp. 305–312.

Ahola, V., Aittokallio, T., Uusipaikka, E., and Vihinen, M. (2003). Efficient estimation of emission probabilities in profile hidden Markov models, *Bioinformatics* **19**, pp. 2359–2368.

Aizawa, K. and Nakamura, A. (1994). Path-controlled graph grammars for syntactic pattern recognition, *International Journal of Pattern Recognition and Artificial Intelligence* **8**, pp. 485–500.

Aizawa, K. and Nakamura, A. (1999a). Parsing of two-dimensional images represented by quadtree adjoining grammars, *Pattern Recognition* **32**, pp. 277–294.

Aizawa, K. and Nakamura, A. (1999b). Quadtree adjoining grammar, *International Journal of Pattern Recognition and Artificial Intelligence* **13**, pp. 573–588.

Ajdukiewicz, K. (1935). Die syntaktische Konnexität, *Studia Philosophica (English transl. in: McCall, S. (ed.), Polish Logic 1920-1939, Oxford University Press, 1967, pp. 207–231)* **1**, pp. 1–27.

Albus, J. E. (1977). Electrocardiogram interpretation using stochastic finite state model, in K. S. Fu (ed.), *Syntactic Pattern Recognition Applications* (Springer, Berlin - Heidelberg - New York).

Alegre, F. and Dellaert, F. (2004). A probabilistic approach to the semantic interpretation of building facades, in *Proc. Int. Workshop on Vision Techniques Applied to the Rehabilitation of City Centres* (Lisbon, Portugal), pp. 25–37.

Alonso Pardo, M. A., Nederhof, M. J., and Villemonte de la Clergerie, E. (2000). Tabulation of automata for tree-adjoining languages, *Grammars* **3**, pp. 89–110.

Alquézar, R. and Sanfeliu, A. (1996). Learning of context-sensitive languages described by Augmented Regular Expressions, in *Proc. 13th IAPR Int. Conf. on Pattern Recognition* (Vienna, Austria), pp. 745–749.

Alquézar, R. and Sanfeliu, A. (1997). Recognition and learning of a class of context-sensitive languages described by Augmented Regular Expressions, *Pattern Recognition* **30**, pp. 163–182.

Alshawi, H., Douglas, S., and Bangalore, S. (2000). Learning dependency translation models as collections of finite-state head transducers, *Computational Linguistics* **26**, pp. 45–60.

Alur, R. and Dill, D. L. (1994). A theory of timed automata, *Theoretical Computer Science* **126**, pp. 183–235.

Álvaro, F., Sánchez, J. A., and Benedí, J. M. (2014). Recognition of on-line handwritten mathematical expressions using 2D stochastic context-free grammars and hidden Markov models, *Pattern Recognition Letters* **35**, pp. 58–67.

Álvaro, F., Sánchez, J. A., and Benedí, J. M. (2016). An integrated grammar-based approach for mathematical expression recognition, *Pattern Recognition* **51**, pp. 135–147.

Amengual, J. C. and Vidal, E. (1996). Two different approaches for cost-efficient Viterbi parsing with error correction, *Lecture Notes in Computer Science* **1121**, pp. 30–39.

Amengual, J. C. and Vidal, E. (1998). Efficient error-correcting Viterbi parsing, *IEEE Trans. Pattern Analysis and Machine Intelligence* **20**, pp. 1109–1116.

Andersen, J. L., Andersen, T., Flamm, C., Hanczyc, M. M., Merkle, D., and Stadler, P. F. (2013). Navigating the chemical space of HCN polymerization and hydrolysis: guiding graph grammars by mass spectrometry data, *Entropy* **15**, pp. 4066–4083.

Anderson, J. W. J., Tataru, P., Staines, J., Hein, J., and Lyngso, R. (2012). Evolving stochastic context-free grammars for RNA secondary structure prediction, *BMC Bioinformatics* **13**:78.

Anderson, K. R. (1982). Syntactic analysis of seismic waveforms using augmented transition network grammars, *Geoexploration* **20**, pp. 161–182.

Anderson, R. H. (1968). *Syntax-Directed Recognition of Hand-Printed Two-dimensional Mathematics*, Ph.D. thesis, Harvard University, Cambridge, MA, USA.

Angluin, D. (1978). On the complexity of minimum inference of regular sets, *Information and Control* **39**, pp. 337–350.

Angluin, D. (1980a). Finding patterns common to a set of strings, *Journal of Computer and System Sciences* **21**, pp. 46–62.

Angluin, D. (1980b). Inductive inference of formal languages from positive data, *Information and Control* **45**, pp. 117–135.

Angluin, D. (1982). Inference of reversible languages, *Journal of the Association for Computing Machinery* **29**, pp. 741–765.

Angluin, D. (1987). Learning regular sets from queries and counter-examples, *Information and Computation* **75**, pp. 87–106.

Anselmo, M., Giammarresi, D., and Madonia, M. (2009). A computational model for tiling recognizable two-dimensional languages, *Theoretical Computer Science* **410**, pp. 3520–3529.

Arivazhagan, A., Mehta, N. K., and Jain, P. K. (2008). Development of a feature recognition module for tapered and curved base features, *The International Journal of Advanced Manufacturing Technology* **39**, pp. 319–332.

Ash, S., Cline, M. A., Homer, R. W., Hurst, T., and Smith, G. B. (1997). SYBYL line notation (SLN): A versatile language for chemical structure representation, *Journal of Chemical Information and Computer Sciences* **37**, pp. 71–79.

Asveld, P. R. J. (2005a). Fuzzy context-free languages - Part 1: fuzzy context-free grammars, *Theoretical Computer Science* **347**, pp. 167–190.

Asveld, P. R. J. (2005b). Fuzzy context-free languages - Part 2: recognition and parsing algorithms, *Theoretical Computer Science* **347**, pp. 191–213.

Bahl, L. R., Jelinek, F., and Mercer, R. L. (1983). A maximum likelihood approach to continuous speech recognition, *IEEE Trans. Pattern Analysis and Machine Intelligence* **5**, pp. 179–190.

Bailador, G. and Triviño, G. (2010). Pattern recognition using temporal fuzzy automata, *Fuzzy Sets and Systems* **161**, pp. 37–55.

Baker, B. S. (1978). Tree transducers and tree languages, *Information and Control* **37**, pp. 241–266.

Baker, B. S. (1979). Composition of top-down and bottom-up tree transductions, *Information and Control* **41**, pp. 186–213.

Baldi, P. and Brunak, S. (2001). *Bioinformatics: The Machine Learning Approach* (MIT Press, Cambridge, MA).

Baldi, P., Chauvin, Y., Hunkapillar, T., and McClure, M. (1994). Hidden Markov models of biological primary sequence information, *Proceedings of the National Academy of Sciences of the USA* **91**, pp. 1059–1063.

Balemi, S., Hoffmann, G. J., Gyugyi, P., Wong-Toi, H., and Franklin, G. F. (1993). Supervisory control of a Rapid Thermal Multiprocessor, *IEEE Trans. Automatic Control* **38**, pp. 1040–1059.

Ballard, D. H. and Brown, C. M. (1982). *Computer Vision* (Prentice Hall, Englewood Cliffs).

Banerjee, S. and Rosenfeld, A. (1992). MAP estimation of context-free grammars, *Pattern Recognition Letters* **13**, pp. 95–101.

Bar-Hillel, Y. (1953). A quasi-arithmetic notation for syntactic description, *Language* **29**, pp. 47–58.

Bar-Hillel, Y., Perles, M., and Shamir, E. (1961). On formal properties of simple phrase structure grammars, *Zeitschrift für Phonetik, Sprachwissenschaft und Kommunikationsforschung* **14**, pp. 143–172.

Barnard, J. M., Lynch, M. F., and Welford, S. M. (1981). Computer storage and retrieval of generic chemical structures in patents, 2. GENSAL, a formal language for the description of generic chemical structures, *Journal of Chemical Information and Computer Sciences* **21**, pp. 151–161.

Barnard, J. M., Lynch, M. F., and Welford, S. M. (1984). Computer storage and retrieval of generic chemical structures in patents, 6. An interpreter program for the generic structure description language GENSAL, *Journal of Chemical Information and Computer Sciences* **24**, pp. 66–71.

Barnard, M. E. (1989). Detection of airborne compact sources in infra-red scenes using syntactic pattern recognition, *Pattern Recognition Letters* **10**, pp. 123–126.

Barrero, A. (1991a). Inference of tree grammars using negative samples, *Pattern Recognition* **24**, pp. 1–8.

Barrero, A. (1991b). Unranked tree languages, *Pattern Recognition* **24**, pp. 9–18.

Barrero, A., Gonzalez, R. C., and Thomason, M. G. (1981). Equivalence and reduction of expansive tree grammars, *IEEE Trans. Pattern Analysis and Machine Intelligence* **3**, pp. 204–206.

Bartsch-Spörl, B. (1983). Grammatical inference of graph grammars for syntactic pattern recognition, *Lecture Notes in Computer Science* **153**, pp. 1–7.

Basu, S. and Fu, K. S. (1987). Image segmentation by syntactic method, *Pattern Recognition* **20**, pp. 33–44.

Batyrshin, I., Sheremetov, L., and Herrera-Avelar, R. (2007). Perception based patterns in time series data mining, in I. Batyrshin, J. Kacprzyk, L. Sheremetov, and L. A. Zadeh (eds.), *Perception-based Data Mining and Decision Making in Economics and Finance* (Springer, Berlin - Heidelberg).

Bauderon, M. and Courcelle, B. (1987). Graph expressions and graph rewritings, *Mathematical Systems Theory* **20**, pp. 83–127.

Bauer, B. and Kraiss, K. F. (2002). Video-based sign recognition using self-organizing subunits, in *Proc. 16th Int. Conf. on Pattern Recognition* (Quebec City, Quebec, Canada), pp. 434–437.

Baum, L. E. and Petrie, T. (1966). Statistical inference for probabilistic functions of finite state Markov chains, *The Annals of Mathematical Statistics* **37**, pp. 1554–1563.

Baum, L. E., Petrie, T., Soules, G., and Weiss, N. (1970). A maximization technique occurring in the statistical analysis of probabilistic functions of Markov chains, *The Annals of Mathematical Statistics* **41**, pp. 164–171.

Becker, S. and Haala, N. (2009). Grammar supported facade reconstruction from mobile LiDAR mapping, in *Proc. Workshop on City Models, Roads and Traffic, vol. XXXVIII* (Paris, France), pp. 229–234.

Behrens, U., Flasiński, M., Hagge, L., and Ohrenberg, K. (1994). ZEX - An expert system for ZEUS, *IEEE Trans. Nuclear Science* **41**, pp. 152–156.

Belaid, A. and Haton, J. P. (1984). A syntactic approach for handwritten mathematical formula recognition, *IEEE Trans. Pattern Analysis and Machine Intelligence* **6**, pp. 105–111.

Belforte, G., Mori De, R., and Ferraris, F. (1979). A contribution to the automatic processing of electrocardiograms using syntactic methods, *IEEE Trans. Biomedical Engineering* **26**, pp. 125–136.

Ben-Arieh, D. (1999). Geometrical reasoning based on attributed graph grammar for prismatic parts, *IIE Transactions* **31**, pp. 61–74.

Bernardes, J. S., Dávila, A. M., Costa, V. S., and Zaverucha, G. (2007). Improving model construction of profile HMMs for remote homology detection through structural alignment, *BMC Bioinformatics* **8**:435.

Berthod, M. and Maroy, J. P. (1979). Learning in syntactic recognition of symbols drawn on a graphic tablet, *Computer Graphics and Image Processing* **9**, pp. 166–182.

Bertolami, R. and Bunke, H. (2008). Hidden Markov model based ensemble methods for offline handwritten text line recognition, *Pattern Recognition* **41**, pp. 3452–3460.

Besombes, J. and Marion, J. Y. (2007). Learning tree languages from positive examples and membership queries, *Theoretical Computer Science* **382**, pp. 183–197.

Bezdek, J. C. (1995). Hybrid modeling in pattern recognition and control, *Knowledge-Based Systems* **8**, pp. 359–371.

Bhargava, B. K. and Fu, K. (1974a). Stochastic tree systems for syntactic pattern recognition, in *Proc. Twelfth Annual Allerton Conference on Circuit and System Theory* (Monticello, IL), pp. 278–287.

Bhargava, B. K. and Fu, K. (1974b). Transformation and inference of tree grammars for syntactic pattern recognition, in *Proc. IEEE Int. Conf. on Systems, Man, and Cybernetics* (Dallas, TX), pp. 330–333.

Bhatnagar, R. K., Williams, R. L., and Tennety, V. (2000). Syntactic pattern recognition for HRR signatures, *Proceedings of the SPIE* **4053**, pp. 452–466.

Bhuyan, M. K., Bora, P. K., and Ghosh, D. (2011). An integrated approach to the recognition of a wide class of continuous hand gestures, *International Journal of Pattern Recognition and Artificial Intelligence* **25**, pp. 227–252.

Bicego, M., Grosso, E., and Otranto, E. (2008). A hidden Markov model approach to classify and predict the sign of financial local trends, *Lecture Notes in Computer Science* **5342**, pp. 852–861.

Bielecka, M., Bielecki, A., Korkosz, M., and Zieliński, B. (2011). Modified Jakubowski shape transducer for detecting osteophytes and erosions in finger joints, *Lecture Notes in Computer Science* **6594**, pp. 147–155.

Biermann, A. W. and Feldman, J. A. (1972). On the synthesis of finite-state machines from samples of their behavior, *IEEE Trans. Computers* **21**, pp. 592–597.

Birman, K. P. (1982). Rule-based learning for more accurate ECG analysis, *IEEE Trans. Pattern Analysis and Machine Intelligence* **4**, pp. 369–380.

Bishop, C. M. (1995). *Neural Networks for Pattern Recognition* (Clarendon Press, Oxford).

Bishop, C. M. (2006). *Pattern Recognition and Machine Learning* (Springer, New York).

Björklund, J. and Fernau, H. (2016). Learning tree languages, in J. Heinz and J. M. Sempere (eds.), *Topics in Grammatical Inference* (Springer, Berlin - Heidelberg), pp. 174–213.

Blanco, A., Delgado, M., and Pegalajar, M. C. (2001). Fuzzy automaton induction using neural network, *International Journal of Approximate Reasoning* **27**, pp. 1–26.

Blum, M. and Hewitt, C. (1967). Automata on a two-dimensional tape, in *Proc. 8th IEEE Annual Symposium Switching and Automata Theory* (Austin, TX, USA), pp. 155–160.

Bobick, A. F. and Wilson, A. D. (1997). A state-based approach to the representation and recognition of gesture, *IEEE Trans. Pattern Analysis and Machine Intelligence* **19**, pp. 1325–1337.

Booth, T. L. and Thompson, R. A. (1973). Applying probability measures to abstract languages, *IEEE Trans. Computers* **22**, pp. 442–450.

Boulch, A., Houllier, S., Marlet, R., and Tournaire, O. (2013). Semantizing complex 3D scenes using constrained attribute grammars, *Computer Graphics Forum* **32**, pp. 33–42.

Boullier, P. and Sagot, B. (2011). Multi-component tree insertion grammars, *Lecture Notes in Artificial Intelligence* **5591**, pp. 31–46.

Bouyer, P., Chevalier, F., and D'Souza, D. (2005). Fault diagnosis using timed automata, *Lecture Notes in Computer Science* **3441**, pp. 219–233.

Bouyer, P., D'Souza, D., Madhusudan, P., and Petit, A. (2003). Timed control with partial observability, *Lecture Notes in Computer Science* **2725**, pp. 180–192.

Brainerd, W. S. (1968). The minimalization of tree automata, *Information and Control* **13**, pp. 484–491.

Brainerd, W. S. (1969). Tree generating regular systems, *Information and Control* **14**, pp. 217–239.

Bralley, P. (1996). An introduction to molecular linguistics, *Bioscience* **46**, pp. 146–153.

Brandenburg, F. J. (1983). On the complexity of the membership problem of graph grammars, in *Proc. Int. Workshop on Graphtheoretic Concepts in Computer Science* (Osnabrück, Germany), pp. 40–49.

Brandenburg, F. J. (1988). On polynomial time graph grammars, *Lecture Notes in Computer Science* **294**, pp. 227–236.

Brandenburg, F. J. and Chytil, M. (1991). Cycle chain code picture languages, *Lecture Notes in Computer Science* **532**, pp. 157–173.

Brandenburg, F. J. and Skodinis, K. (2005). Finite graph automata for linear and boundary graph languages, *Theoretical Computer Science* **332**, pp. 199–232.

Brayer, J. M. (1977). Parsing of web grammars, in *Proc. IEEE Workshop Picture Data Description and Management* (Chicago, IL, USA).

Brayer, J. M. and Fu, K. S. (1977). A note on $k$-tail method of tree grammar inference, *IEEE Trans. Systems, Man, and Cybernetics* **7**, pp. 293–299.

Brejová, B., Brown, D. G., and Vinař, T. (2007). The most probable annotation problem in HMMs and its application to bioinformatics, *Journal of Computer and System Sciences* **73**, pp. 1060–1077.

Brendel, V. and Busse, H. G. (1984). Genome structure described by formal languages, *Nucleic Acids Research* **12**, pp. 2561–2568.

Briscoe, T. and Carroll, J. (1993). Generalized probabilistic LR parsing of natural language (corpora) with unification-based grammars, *Computational Linguistics* **19**, pp. 25–59.

Brown, K. N., McMahon, C. A., and Sims Williams, J. H. (1995). Features, aka the semantics of a formal language of manufacturing, *Research in Engineering Design* **7**, pp. 151–172.

Brown, M. and Wilson, C. (1996). RNA pseudoknot modeling using intersections of stochastic context free grammars with applications to database search, in *Proc. 1996 Pacific Symposium on Biocomputing* (Hawaii), pp. 109–125.

Brown, M. P. (2000). Small subunit ribosomal RNA modeling using stochastic context-free grammars, in *Proc. 8th Int. Conf. on Intelligent Systems for Molecular Biology* (San Diego, CA, USA), pp. 57–66.

Brzozowski, J. A. (1964). Derivatives of regular expressions, *Journal of the Association for Computing Machinery* **11**, pp. 481–494.

Bucurescu, I. and Pascu, A. (1981). Fuzzy pushdown automata, *International Journal of Computer Mathematics* **10**, pp. 109–119.

Bugalho, M. and Oliveira, A. L. (2005). Inference of regular languages using state merging algorithms with search, *Pattern Recognition* **38**, pp. 1457–1467.

Bunke, H. (1978). Programmed graph grammars. in *Proc. Int. Workshop on Graph Grammars and Their Application to Computer Science and Biology* (Bad Honnef, Germany), pp. 155–166.

Bunke, H. (1982a). Attributed programmed graph grammars and their application to schematic diagram interpretation, *IEEE Trans. Pattern Analysis and Machine Intelligence* **4**, pp. 574–582.

Bunke, H. (1982b). On the generative power of sequential and parallel graph grammars, *Computing* **29**, pp. 89–112.

Bunke, H. (1988). Hybrid approaches, in G. Ferrate, T. Pavlidis, A. Sanfeliu, and H. Bunke (eds.), *Syntactic and Structural Pattern Recognition* (Springer, Berlin - Heidelberg), pp. 335–361.

Bunke, H. (1993). Structural and syntactic pattern recognition, in C. H. Chen, L. F. Pau, and P. S. P. Wang (eds.), *Handbook of Pattern Recognition and Computer Vision* (World Scientific, Singapore), pp. 163–209.

Bunke, H. and Caelli, T. M. (eds.) (2001). *Hidden Markov Models: Applications in Computer Vision* (World Scientific, Singapore).

Bunke, H. and Haller, B. (1990). A parser for context free plex grammars, *Lecture Notes in Computer Science* **411**, pp. 136–150.

Bunke, H. and Kandel, A. (eds.) (2002). *Hybrid Methods in Pattern Recognition* (World Scientific, Singapore).

Bunke, H. and Pasche, D. (1990). Parsing multivalued strings and its application to image and waveform recognition, in R. Mohr, T. Pavlidis, and A. Sanfeliu (eds.), *Structural Pattern Analysis* (World Scientific, Singapore), pp. 1–15.

Bunke, H., Roth, and Schukat-Talamazzini, E. G. (1995). Off-line handwriting recognition using hidden Markov models, *Pattern Recognition* **28**, pp. 1399–1413.

Bunke, H. and Sanfeliu, A. (eds.) (1990). *Syntactic and Structural Pattern Recognition - Theory and Applications* (World Scientific, Singapore).

Bunke, H. and Sanfeliu, A. (1992). Statistical and syntactic models and pattern recognition techniques, in C. Torras (ed.), *Computer Vision: Theory and Industrial Applications* (Springer, Berlin - Heidelberg), pp. 215–266.

Cai, L., Malmberg, R. L., and Wu, Y. (2003). Stochastic modeling of RNA pseudoknotted structures: A grammatical approach, *Bioinformatics* **19**, pp. 66–73.

Carlucci, L. (1972). A formal system for texture languages, *Pattern Recognition* **4**, pp. 53–72.

Carrasco, R. C., Daciuk, J., and Forcada, M. L. (2009). Incremental construction of minimal tree automata, *Algorithmica* **55**, pp. 95–110.

Carrasco, R. C., Forcada, M. L., and Santamaria, L. (1996). Inferring stochastic regular grammars with recurrent neural networks, *Lecture Notes in Computer Science* **1147**, pp. 274–281.

Carrasco, R. C. and Oncina, J. (1999). Learning deterministic regular grammars from stochastic samples in polynomial time, *RAIRO - Theoretical Informatics and Applications* **33**, pp. 1–20.

Carrasco, R. C., Oncina, J., and Calera-Rubio, J. (2001). Stochastic inference of regular tree languages, *Machine Learning* **44**, pp. 185–197.

Casacuberta, F. (1990). Some relations among stochastic finite state networks used in automatic speech recognition, *IEEE Trans. Pattern Analysis and Machine Intelligence* **12**, pp. 691–695.

Casacuberta, F. (1995). Statistical estimation of stochastic context-free grammars, *Pattern Recognition Letters* **16**, pp. 565–573.

Casacuberta, F. and Vidal, E. (2007). Learning finite-state models for machine translation, *Machine Learning* **66**, pp. 69–91.

Casacuberta, F., Vidal, E., and Picó, D. (2005). Inference of finite-state transducers from regular languages, *Pattern Recognition* **38**, pp. 1431–1443.

Cassandras, C. G. and Lafortune, S. (eds.) (2010). *Introduction to Discrete Event Systems* (Springer, New York).

Castaño, J. M. (2004). Global Index Grammars and descriptive power, *Journal of Logic, Language and Information* **13**, pp. 403–419.

Castro, J. M. and Casacuberta, F. (1996). The morphic generator grammatical inference methodology and multilayer perceptrons: A hybrid approach to acoustic modeling, *Lecture Notes in Computer Science* **1121**, pp. 21–29.

Ceterchi, R., Mutyam, M., Păun, G., and Subramanian, K. G. (2003). Array-rewriting P systems, *Natural Computing* **2**, pp. 229–249.

Chan, K. F. and Yeung, D. Y. (2000). An efficient syntactic approach to structural analysis of on-line handwritten mathematical expressions, *Pattern Recognition* **33**, pp 375–384.

Chan, K. F. and Yeung, D. Y. (2001). Error detection, error correction and performance evaluation in on-line mathematical expression recognition, *Pattern Recognition* **34**, pp. 1671–1684.

Chang, J. H. and Fan, K. C. (2002). A new model for fingerprint classification by ridge distribution sequences, *Pattern Recognition* **35**, pp. 1209–1223.

Chang, K. P. (1992). Application of guarded fuzzy-attribute context free grammar to syntactic pattern recognition, *International Journal of Pattern Recognition and Artificial Intelligence* **6**, pp. 777–797.

Chang, N. S. and Fu, K. S. (1979). Parallel parsing of tree languages for syntactic pattern recognition, *Pattern Recognition* **11**, pp. 213–222.

Chang, S. K. (1970). A method for the structural analysis of two-dimensional mathematical expressions, *Information Sciences* **2**, pp. 253–272.

Chang, S. K. (1971). Picture processing grammar and its applications, *Information Sciences* **3**, pp. 121–148.

Chang, S. K. (ed.) (1986). *Visual Languages* (Springer, New York).

Chang, S. K. (1990). A visual language compiler for information retrieval by visual reasoning, *IEEE Trans. Software Engineering* **16**, pp. 1136–1149.

Chang, S. K. and Liu, S. H. (1984). Picture indexing and abstraction techniques for pictorial databases, *IEEE Trans. Pattern Analysis and Machine Intelligence* **6**, pp. 475–484.

Chang, S. K., Shi, Q. Y., and Yan, C. W. (1987). Iconic indexing by 2-D strings, *IEEE Trans. Pattern Analysis and Machine Intelligence* **9**, pp. 413–428.

Charbonnier, F., Alla, H., and David, R. (1999). The supervised control of discrete-event dynamic systems, *IEEE Trans. Control Systems Technology* **7**, pp. 175–187.

Chen, C. H. (ed.) (2010). *Handbook of Pattern Recognition and Computer Vision - IV* (World Scientific, Singapore).

Chen, C. H. (ed.) (2011). *Emerging Topics in Computer Vision and its Applications* (World Scientific, Singapore).

Chen, C. H. (ed.) (2016). *Handbook of Pattern Recognition and Computer Vision - V* (World Scientific, Singapore).

Chen, C. H., Pau, L. F., and Wang, P. S. P. (eds.) (1993). *Handbook of Pattern Recognition and Computer Vision - I* (World Scientific, Singapore).

Chen, C. H., Pau, L. F., and Wang, P. S. P. (eds.) (1999). *Handbook of Pattern Recognition and Computer Vision - II* (World Scientific, Singapore).

Chen, C. H. and Wang, P. S. P. (eds.) (2005). *Handbook of Pattern Recognition and Computer Vision - III* (World Scientific, Singapore).

Chen, Q., Georganas, N. D., and Petriu, E. M. (2008). Hand gesture recognition using Haar-like features and a stochastic context-free grammar, *IEEE Trans. Instrumentation and Measurement* **57**, pp. 1562–1571.

Cherubini, A., Crespi Reghizzi, S., Pradella, M., and San Pietro, P. (2006). Picture languages: tiling systems versus tile rewriting grammars, *Theoretical Computer Science* **356**, pp. 90–103.

Chi, Z. and Geman, S. (1998). Estimation of probabilistic context-free grammars, *Computational Linguistics* **24**, pp. 299–305.

Chiang, D. (2007). Hierarchical phrase-based translation, *Computational Linguistics* **33**, pp. 201–228.

Chiang, D., Joshi, A. K., and Searls, D. B. (2006). Grammatical representations of macromolecular structure, *Journal of Computational Biology* **13**, pp. 1077–1100.

Cho, K., Cho, H., and Um, K. (2004). Human action recognition by inference of stochastic regular grammars, *Lecture Notes in Computer Science* **3138**, pp. 388–396.

Choi, B. K., Barash, M. M., and Anderson, D. C. (1984). Automatic recognition of machined surfaces from a 3D solid model, *Computer-Aided Design* **16**, pp. 81–86.

Chomsky, N. (1956). Three models for the description of language, *IRE Trans. Information Theory* **2**, pp. 113–124.

Chomsky, N. (1959). On certain formal properties of grammars, *Information and Control* **2**, pp. 137–167.

Chomsky, N. (1962). Context-free grammars and pushdown storage, Tech. Rep. 65, MIT Research Laboratory of Electronics, Cambridge, MA.

Chomsky, N. (1965). *Aspects of the Theory of Syntax* (MIT Press, Cambridge, MA).

Chomsky, N. and Miller, G. A. (1958). Finite state languages, *Information and Control* **1**, pp. 91–112.

Chuang, S. H. and Henderson, M. R. (1991). Compound feature recognition by web grammar parsing, *Research in Engineering Design* **2**, pp. 147–158.

Chuong, B. D., Daniel, A. W., and Serafim, B. (2006). CONTRAfold: RNA secondary structure prediction without physics-based models, *Bioinformatics* **22**, pp. e90–e98.

Cieslak, R., Desclaux, C., Fawaz, A. S., and Varaiya, P. (1988). Supervisory control of discrete-event processes with partial observations, *IEEE Trans. Automatic Control* **33**, pp. 249–260.

Civera, J., Vilar, J. M., Cubel, E., Lagarda, A. L., Barrachina, S., Casacuberta, F., Vidal, E., Picó, D., and González, J. (2004). A syntactic pattern recognition approach to computer assisted translation, *Lecture Notes in Computer Science* **3138**, pp. 207–215.

Clark, A. and Eyraud, R. (2007). Polynomial identification in the limit of substitutable context-free languages, *Journal of Machine Learning Research* **8**, pp. 1725–1745.

Clark, A., Fox, C., and Lappin, S. (eds.) (2010). *The Handbook of Computational Linguistics and Natural Language Processing* (Wiley - Blackwell, Chichester, UK).

Clark, A. and Thollard, F. (2004). PAC-learnability of probabilistic deterministic finite state automata, *Journal of Machine Learning Research* **5**, pp. 473–497.

Clark, A. and Yoshinaka, R. (2014). Distributional learning of parallel multiple context-free grammars, *Machine Learning* **96**, pp. 5–31.

Clark, A. N. (1994). Pattern recognition of noisy sequences of behavioural events using functional combinators, *The Computer Journal* **37**, pp. 385–398.

Clowes, M. B. (1971). On seeing things, *Artificial Intelligence* **2**, pp. 79–116.

Cocke, J. and Schwartz, J. T. (1970). Programming languages and their compilers, Tech. rep., Courant Institute of Mathematical Science, New York.

Collado-Vides, J. (1989). A transformational-grammar approach to the study of the regulation of gene expression, *Journal of Theoretical Biology* **136**, pp. 403–425.

Collado-Vides, J. (1992). Grammatical model of the regulation of gene expression, *Proceedings of the National Academy of Sciences of the United States of America* **89**, pp. 9405–9409.

Collin, S. and Colnet, D. (1994). Syntactic analysis of technical drawing dimensions, *Journal of Pattern Recognition and Artificial Intelligence* **8**, pp. 1131–1148.

Comon, H., Dauchet, M., Gilleron, R., Löding, C., Jacquemard, F., Lugiez, D., Tison, S., and Tommasi, M. (2007). Tree Automata Techniques and Applications, `http://www.grappa.univ-lille3.fr/tata`.

Cooper, K. D. and Torczon, L. (2011). *Engineering a Compiler* (Morgan Kaufmann, Amsterdam).

Corazza, A., Mori De, R., Gretter, R., and Satta, G. (1991). Computation of probabilities for an island-driven parser, *IEEE Trans. Pattern Analysis and Machine Intelligence* **13**, pp. 936–950.

Corazza, A., Mori De, R., Gretter, R., and Satta, G. (1994). Optimal probabilistic evaluation functions for search controlled by stochastic context-free grammars, *IEEE Trans. Pattern Analysis and Machine Intelligence* **16**, pp. 1018–1027.

Corazza, A. and Satta, G. (2007). Probabilistic context-free grammars estimated from infinite distributions, *IEEE Trans. Pattern Analysis and Machine Intelligence* **29**, pp. 1379–1393.

Costagliola, G. and Chang, S. K. (1990). DR PARSERS: a generalization of LR parsers, in *Proc. IEEE Workshop on Visual Languages* (Skokie, IL, USA), pp. 174–180.

Costagliola, G. and Chang, S. K. (1999). Using linear positional grammars for the LR parsing of 2-D symbolic languages, *Grammars* **2**, pp. 1–34.

Costagliola, G., Deufemia, V., Ferrucci, F., and Gravino, C. (2003). On regular drawn symbolic picture languages, *Information and Computation* **187**, pp. 209–245.

Costagliola, G., Ferrucci, F., and Gravino, C. (2005). Adding symbols to picture languages: definitions and properties, *Theoretical Computer Science* **337**, pp. 51–104.

Costagliola, G., Lucia De, A., Orefice, S., and Tortora, G. (1997). A parsing methodology for the implementation of visual systems, *IEEE Trans. Software Engineering* **23**, pp. 777–799.

Cowell, J. (1995). Syntactic pattern recognizer for vehicle identification numbers, *Image and Vision Computing* **13**, pp. 13–19.

Cowell, J. and Hussain, F. (2007). A syntactic recognizer for Arabic characters, *Machine Graphics and Vision* **16**, pp. 57–83.

Crespi-Reghizzi, S. (1970). *The Mechanical Acquisition of Precedence Grammars*, Ph.D. thesis, University of California, Los Angeles, Los Angeles.

Crespi-Reghizzi, S. and Mandrioli, D. (1976). Commutative grammars, *Calcolo* **13**, pp. 173–189.

Crespi-Reghizzi, S., Melkanoff, M. A., and Lichten, L. (1973). The use of grammatical inference for designing programming languages, *Communications of the Association for Computing Machinery* **16**, pp. 83–90.

Crespi-Reghizzi, S. and Pradella, M. (2005). Tile rewriting grammars and picture languages, *Theoretical Computer Science* **340**, pp. 257–272.

Crespi-Reghizzi, S. and Pradella, M. (2008). A CKY parser for picture grammars, *Information Processing Letters* **105**, pp. 213–217.

Crimi, C., Guercio, A., Nota, G., Pacini, G., Tortora, G., and Tucci, M. (1991). Relation grammars and their application to multi-dimensional languages, *Journal of Visual Languages and Computing* **2**, pp. 333–346.

Crimi, C., Guercio, A., Pacini, G., Tortora, G., and Tucci, M. (1990). Grammatical inference algorithms for the generation of visual languages, *Journal of Visual Languages and Computing* **1**, pp. 355–368.

Daciuk, J. and Noord van, G. (2004). Finite automata for compact representation of tuple dictionaries, *Theoretical Computer Science* **313**, pp. 45–56.

Daciuk, J. and Weiss, D. (2012). Smaller representation of finite-state automata, *Theoretical Computer Science* **450**, pp. 10–21.

Damen, D. and Hogg, D. (2012). Explaining activities as consistent groups of events: A Bayesian framework using attribute multiset grammars, *International Journal of Computer Vision* **98**, pp. 83–102.

Dassow, J. (2004). Grammars with regulated rewriting, in V. M. C. Martin-Vide and G. Păun (eds.), *Formal Languages and Applications* (Springer, Berlin).

Dassow, J. and Păun, G. (1990). *Regulated Rewriting in Formal Language Theory* (Springer, New York).

Dassow, J., Păun, G., and Salomaa, A. (1997). Grammars with controlled derivations, in G. Rozenberg and A. Salomaa (eds.), *Handbook of Formal Languages, vol. II* (Springer, Berlin-Heidelberg), pp. 101–154.

Davis, E. R. (2012). *Computer and Machine Vision: Theory, Algorithms, Practicalities* (Elsevier - Academic Press, Amsterdam).

Davis, M. D. (1958). *Computability and Unsolvability* (McGraw-Hill, New York).

Degano, P. and Montanari, U. (1987). A model for distributed systems based on graph rewriting, *Journal of the Association for Computing Machinery* **34**, pp. 411–449.

Delgado, M. and Pegalajar, M. C. (2005). A multiobjective genetic algorithm for obtaining the optimal size of a recurrent neural network for grammatical inference, *Pattern Recognition* **38**, pp. 1444–1456.

Della Vigna, P. and Ghezzi, C. (1978). Context-free graph grammars, *Information and Control* **37**, pp. 207–233.

Dempster, A. P., Laird, N. M., and Rubin, D. B. (1977). Maximum likelihood from incomplete data via the EM algorithm, *Journal of the Royal Statistical Society, Series B* **39**, pp. 1–38.

Denis, F., Lemay, A., and Terlutte, A. (2004). Learning regular languages using RFSA, *Theoretical Computer Science* **313**, pp. 267–294.

DePalma, G. F. and Yau, S. S. (1975). Fractionally fuzzy grammars with application to pattern recognition, in L. A. Zadeh, K. S. Fu, K. Tanaka, and M. Shimura (eds.), *Fuzzy Sets and their Applications to Cognitive and Decision Processes* (Academic Press, New York), pp. 329–352.

Dill, K. E., Lucas, A., Hockenmaier, J., Huang, L., Chiang, D., and Joshi, A. K. (2007). Computational linguistics: A new tool for exploring biopolymer structures and statistical mechanics, *Polymer* **48**, pp. 4289–4300.

Dima, C. (2001). Real-time automata, *Journal of Automata, Languages and Combinatorics* **6**, pp. 2–23.

Ding, L., Samad, A., Xue, X., Huang, X., Malmberg, R. L., and Cai, L. (2014). Stochastic k-tree grammar and its application in biomolecular structure modeling, *Lecture Notes in Computer Science* **8370**, pp. 308–322.

Do, C. B., Mahabhashyam, M. S., Brudno, M., and Batzoglou, S. (2005). ProbCons: Probabilistic consistency-based multiple sequence alignment, *Genome Research* **15**, pp. 330–340.

Don, H. S. (1992). A syntactic approach to time-varying pattern analysis, *Information Sciences* **61**, pp. 67–101.

Don, H. S. and Fu, K. S. (1986). A parallel algorithm for stochastic image segmentation, *IEEE Trans. Pattern Analysis and Machine Intelligence* **8**, pp. 594–603.

Doner, J. E. (1965). Decidability of the weak second-order theory of two successors, *Notices American Mathematic Society* **12**, pp. 365–468.

Doner, J. E. (1970). Tree acceptors and some of their applications, *Journal of Computer and System Sciences* **4**, pp. 406–451.

Dong, S. and Searls, D. B. (1994). Gene structure prediction by linguistic methods, *Genomics* **23**, pp. 540–551.

Dori, D. (1989). A syntactic/geometric approach to recognition of dimensions in engineering machine drawings, *Computer Vision, Graphics and Image Processing* **47**, pp. 271–291.

Dori, D. and Pnueli, A. (1988). The grammar of dimensions in machine drawings, *Computer Vision, Graphics and Image Processing* **42**, pp. 1–18.

Doshi, S., Huang, F., and Oates, T. (2002). Inferring the structure of graph grammars from data, in *Proc. Int. Conf. on Knowledge-Based Computer Systems* (Mumbai, India).

Dowell, R. D. and Eddy, S. R. (2004). Evaluation of several lightweight stochastic context-free grammars for RNA secondary structure prediction, *BMC Bioinformatics* **5**:71.

Downing, F. and Flemming, U. (1981). The bungalows of Buffalo, *Environment and Planning B* **8**, pp. 269–293.

Drewes, F. (1996). Language theoretic and algorithmic properties of d-dimensional collages and patterns in a grid, *Journal of Computer and System Sciences* **53**, pp. 33–66.

Drewes, F. (2000). Tree-based picture generation, *Theoretical Computer Science* **246**, pp. 1–51.

Drewes, F. (2009). MAT learners for recognizable tree languages and tree series, *Acta Cybernetica* **19**, pp. 249–274.

Drewes, F., Hoffmann, B., and Minas, M. (2015). Predictive top-down parsing for hyper-edge replacement grammars, *Lecture Notes in Computer Science* **9151**, pp. 19–34.

Drewes, F., Hoffmann, B., and Minas, M. (2017). Predictive shift-reduce parsing for hyper-edge replacement grammars, *Lecture Notes in Computer Science* **10373**, pp. 106–122.

D'Souza, D. and Madhusudan, P. (2002). Timed control synthesis for external specifications, *Lecture Notes in Computer Science* **2285**, pp. 571–582.

Du, X., Jiao, J., and Tseng, M. M. (2002). Graph grammar based product family modeling, *Concurrent Engineering: Research and Applications* **10**, pp. 113–128.

Duan, T., Griffiths, C. M., and Johnsen, S. O. (1996). Syntactic simulation of 1-D sedimentary sequences in a coal bearing succession using a stochastic context-free grammar, *Journal of Sedimentary Research* **66**, pp. 1091–1101.

Duan, T., Griffiths, C. M., and Johnsen, S. O. (1999). A new approach to reservoir heterogeneity modelling: conditional simulation of 2-D parasequences in shallow marine depositional sequences using an attributed controlled grammar, *Computers and Geosciences* **25**, pp. 667–681.

Duarte, J. P. (2005). Towards the mass customization of housing: the grammar of Siza's houses at Malagueira, *Environment and Planning B* **32**, pp. 347–380.

Duda, R. O., Hart, P. E., and Stork, D. G. (2001). *Pattern Classification* (Wiley, New York).

Dupont, P. (1994). Regular grammatical inference from positive and negative samples by genetic search: the GIG method, in C. Carrasco and J. Oncina (eds.), *Grammatical Inference and Applications* (Springer, Berlin-Heidelberg), pp. 236–245.

Dupont, P., Denis, F., and Esposito, Y. (2005). Links between probabilistic automata and hidden Markov models: probability distributions, learning models and induction algorithms, *Pattern Recognition* **38**, pp. 1026–1039.

Durbin, R., Eddy, S. R., Krogh, A., and Mitchison, G. (2002). *Biological Sequence Analysis: Probabilistic Models of Proteins and Nucleic Acids* (Cambridge University Press, Cambridge, UK).

Dyer, R. D., Rosenfeld, A., and Samet, H. (1979). Region representation: boundary code from quadtrees, *Communications of the Association for Computing Machinery* **23**, pp. 171–179.

Dyrka, W. and Nebel, J. C. (2009). A stochastic context free grammar based framework for analysis of protein sequences, *BMC Bioinformatics* **10**:323.

Dyrka, W., Nebel, J. C., and Kotulska, M. (2013). Probabilistic grammatical model of protein language and its application to helix-helix contact site classification, *Algorithms for Molecular Biology* **8**:31.

Earley, J. (1970). An efficient context-free parsing algorithm, *Communications of the Association for Computing Machinery* **13**, pp. 94–102.

Eddy, S. R. (1998). Profile hidden Markov models, *Bioinformatics* **14**, pp. 755–763.

Ehrig, H., Engels, G., Kreowski, H. J., and Rozenberg, G. (eds.) (1999). *Handbook of Graph Grammars and Computing by Graph Transformation, Vol. 2: Applications, Languages and Tools* (World Scientific, Singapore).

Eijck van, J. (2008). Sequentially indexed grammars, *Journal of Logic and Computation* **18**, pp. 205–228.

Engelfriet, J. and Schmidt, E. M. (1977). IO and OI. Part I, *Journal of Computer and System Sciences* **15**, pp. 328–353.

Engelfriet, J. and Schmidt, E. M. (1978). IO and OI. Part II, *Journal of Computer and System Sciences* **16**, pp. 67–99.

Ertunc, H. M., Loparo, K. A., and Ocak, H. (2001). Tool wear condition monitoring in drilling operations using hidden Markov models (HMM), *International Journal of Machine Tools and Manufacture* **141**, pp. 1363–1384.

España Boquera, S., Castro Bleda, M. J., Gorbe-Moya, J., and Zamora-Martinez, F. (2011). Improving offline handwritten text recognition with hybrid HMM/ANN models, *IEEE Trans. Pattern Analysis and Machine Intelligence* **33**, pp. 767–779.

Fan, T. I. and Fu, K. S. (1979). A syntactic approach to time-varying image analysis, *Computer Graphics and Image Processing* **11**, pp. 138–149.

Fanaswala, M. and Krishnamurthy, V. (2013). Detection of anomalous trajectory patterns in target tracking via stochastic context-free grammars and reciprocal process models, *IEEE Journal of Selected Topics in Signal Processing* **7**, pp. 76–90.

Fanaswala, M. and Krishnamurthy, V. (2014). Syntactic models for trajectory constrained track-before-detect, *IEEE Trans. Signal Processing* **62**, pp. 6130–6142.

Fang, G., Gao, W., and Zhao, D. (2007). Large-vocabulary continuous sign language recognition based on transition-movement models, *IEEE Trans. Systems, Man, and Cybernetics - Part A: Systems and Humans* **37**, pp. 1–9.

Feder, J. (1968). Languages of encoded line patterns, *Information and Control* **13**, pp. 230–244.

Feder, J. (1971). Plex languages, *Information Sciences* **3**, pp. 225–241.

Fehder, P. F. and Barnett, M. P. (1965). Syntactic scanning of chemical information, *Journal of Chemical Documentation* **5**, pp. 8–13.

Feldman, J. (1967). First thoughts on grammatical inference, Tech. Rep. Artificial Intelligence Memo no. 55, Computer Science Dept. Stanford University, Stanford, CA.

Feldman, J. (1972). Some decidability results on grammatical inference and complexity, *Information and Control* **20**, pp. 244–262.

Ferber, G. (1986). Classifying and validating intermittent EEG patterns with syntactic methods, *Pattern Recognition* **19**, pp. 289–295.

Fernau, H. (2003). Identification of function distiguishable languages, *Theoretical Computer Science* **290**, pp. 1679–1711.

Fernau, H. (2007). Learning tree languages from text, *RAIRO - Theoretical Informatics and Applications* **41**, pp. 351–374.

Fernau, H. and Freund, R. (1996). Bounded parallelism in array grammars used for character recognition, *Lecture Notes in Computer Science* **1121**, pp. 40–49.

Fernau, H., Freund, R., and Holzer, M. (1998). Character recognition with k-head finite array automata, *Lecture Notes in Computer Science* **1451**, pp. 282–291.

Fernau, H., Freund, R., Markus, L., Subramanian, K. G., and Wiederhold, P. (2015). Contextual array grammars and array P systems, *Annals of Mathematics and Artificial Intelligence* **75**, pp. 5–26.

Fernau, H., Paramasivan, M., Thomas, D. G., Schmid, M. L., and Thomas, D. G. (2018). Simple picture processing based on finite automata and regular grammars, *Journal of Computer and System Sciences* **95**, pp. 232–258.

Ferruci, F., Pacini, G., Satta, G., Sessa, M. I., Tortora, G., Tucci, M., and Vitiello, G. (1996). Symbol-Relation grammars: A formalism for graphical languages, *Information and Computation* **131**, pp. 1–46.

Filipski, A. J. (1980). A least mean-squared error approach to syntactic classification, *IEEE Trans. Pattern Analysis and Machine Intelligence* **2**, pp. 252–255.

Finger, S., Fox, M. S., Prinz, F. B., and Rinderle, J. R. (1992). Concurrent design, *Applied Artificial Intelligence* **6**, pp. 257–283.

Finger, S. and Rinderle, J. R. (1989). A transformational approach to mechanical design using bond graph grammars, in *Proc. Proc. 1st ASME Conf. on Design Theory and Methodology* (Montreal, Canada), pp. 107–116.

Finkel, R. and Bentley, J. L. (1974). Quad trees: a data structure for retrieval on composite keys, *Acta Informatica* **4**, pp. 1–9.

Flasiński, M. (1988). Parsing of edNLC-graph grammars for scene analysis, *Pattern Recognition* **21**, pp. 623–629.

Flasiński, M. (1989). Characteristics of edNLC-graph grammars for syntactic pattern recognition, *Computer Vision, Graphics and Image Processing* **47**, pp. 1–21.

Flasiński, M. (1990). Distorted pattern analysis with the help of Node Label Controlled graph languages, *Pattern Recognition* **23**, pp. 765–774.

Flasiński, M. (1991). Some notes on a problem of constructing the best matched graph, *Pattern Recognition* **24**, pp. 1223–1224.

Flasiński, M. (1993). On the parsing of deterministic graph languages for syntactic pattern recognition, *Pattern Recognition* **26**, pp. 1–16.

Flasiński, M. (1994). Further development of the ZEUS Expert System: Computer science foundations of design, Tech. Rep. 94-048, Deutsches Elektronen-Synchrotron, Hamburg, Germany.

Flasiński, M. (1995a). Towards quasi context sensitive structure grammars model for inference support in hybrid expert systems, *Schedae Informaticae* (Series: *Universitas Iagellonica Acta Scientiarum Litterarumque*) **6**, pp. 161–173.

Flasiński, M. (1995b). Use of graph grammars for the description of mechanical parts, *Computer-Aided Design* **27**, pp. 403–433.

Flasiński, M. (1998). Power properties of NLC graph grammars with a polynomial membership problem, *Theoretical Computer Science* **201**, pp. 189–231.

Flasiński, M. (2007). Inference of parsable graph grammars for syntactic pattern recognition, *Fundamenta Informaticae* **80**, pp. 379–413.

Flasiński, M. (2016a). *Introduction to Artificial Intelligence* (Springer International, Switzerland).

Flasiński, M. (2016b). Syntactic pattern recognition: paradigm issues and open problems, in C. H. Chen (ed.), *Handbook of Pattern Recognition and Computer Vision* (World Scientific, New Jersey-London-Singapore), pp. 3–25.

Flasiński, M. (2018). Generative power of reduction-based parsable ETPR(k) graph grammars for syntactic pattern recognition, *Journal of Automation, Mobile Robotics and Intelligent Systems* **12**, pp. 61–81.

Flasiński, M. and Jurek, J. (1999). Dynamically programmed automata for quasi context sensitive languages as a tool for inference support in pattern recognition-based real-time control expert systems, *Pattern Recognition* **32**, pp. 671–690.

Flasiński, M. and Kotulski, L. (1992). On the use of graph grammars for the control of a distributed software allocation, *The Computer Journal* **35**, pp. A165–A175.

Flasiński, M. and Lewicki, G. (1991). The convergent method of constructing polynomial discriminant functions for pattern recognition, *Pattern Recognition* **24**, pp. 1009–1015.

Flasiński, M. and Myśliński, S. (2010). On the use of graph parsing for recognition of isolated hand postures of Polish Sign Language, *Pattern Recognition* **43**, pp. 2249–2264.

Flasiński, M. and Skomorowski, M. (1998). Parsing of random graph languages for automated inspection in statistical-based quality assurance systems, *Machine Graphics and Vision* **7**, pp. 565–623.

Flemming, U. (1981). More than the sum of its parts: the grammar of Queen Anne houses, *Environment and Planning B* **14**, pp. 323–350.

Fletcher, P. (2001). Connectionist learning of regular graph grammars, *Connection Science* **13**, pp. 127–188.

Floyd, R. W. (1963). Syntactic analysis and operator precedence, *Journal of the Association for Computing Machinery* **10**, pp. 316–333.

Forsyth, D. A. and Ponce, J. (2012). *Computer Vision: A Modern Approach* (Pearson, Boston).

Franck, R. (1978). A class of linearly parsable graph grammars, *Acta Informatica* **10**, pp. 175–201.

Fred, A. L. N. and Leitao, J. M. N. (1992). Use of stochastic grammars for hypnogram analysis, in *Proc. 11th IAPR Int. Conf. on Pattern Recognition* (Los Alamitos, CA, USA), pp. 242–245.

Freeman, H. (1961). On the encoding of arbitrary geometric configurations, *IRE Trans. Electronic Computers* **10**, pp. 260–268.

Freund, R., Păun, G., and Rozenberg, G. (2007). Contextual array grammars, in K. G. Subramanian, K. Rangarajan, and M. Mukund (eds.), *Formal Models, Languages and Applications* (World Scientific, Singapore - New Jersey - London), pp. 112–136.

Fu, K. S. (1970). Learning control systems - review and outlook, *IEEE Trans. Automatic Control* **15**, pp. 210–221.

Fu, K. S. (1971). Stochastic automata, stochastic languages and pattern recognition, *Journal of Cybernetics* **1**, pp. 31–49.

Fu, K. S. (1973). Stochastic languages for picture analysis, *Computer Graphics and Image Processing* **2**, pp. 433–453.

Fu, K. S. (1974). *Syntactic Methods in Pattern Recognition* (Academic Press, New York).

Fu, K. S. (1976a). Pattern recognition in remote sensing of the earth's resources, *IEEE Trans. Geoscience Electronics* **14**, pp. 10–18.

Fu, K. S. (1976b). Tree languages and syntactic pattern recognition, in C. H. Chen (ed.), *Pattern Recognition and Artificial Intelligence* (Academic Press, New York).

Fu, K. S. (ed.) (1977). *Syntactic Pattern Recognition Applications* (Springer, Berlin - Heidelberg - New York).

Fu, K. S. (1980a). Stochastic tree languages and their application to picture processing, in P. R. Krishnaiah (ed.), *Multivariate Analysis V* (North-Holland, Amsterdam).

Fu, K. S. (1980b). Syntactic image modeling using stochastic tree grammars, *Computer Graphics and Image Processing* **12**, pp. 136–152.

Fu, K. S. (1982). *Syntactic Pattern Recognition and Applications* (Prentice Hall, Englewood Cliffs).

Fu, K. S. (1983). A step towards unification of syntactic and statistical pattern recognition, *IEEE Trans. Pattern Analysis and Machine Intelligence* **5**, pp. 200–205.

Fu, K. S. (1985). A semantic-syntactic approach to image analysis, *Journal of Information Science and Engineering* **1**, pp. 1–20.

Fu, K. S. and Bhargava, B. K. (1973). Tree systems for syntactic pattern recognition, *IEEE Trans. Computers* **22**, pp. 1087–1099.

Fu, K. S. and Booth, T. L. (1975a). Grammatical inference: introduction and survey - Part I, *IEEE Trans. Systems, Man, and Cybernetics* **5**, pp. 95–111.

Fu, K. S. and Booth, T. L. (1975b). Grammatical inference: introduction and survey - Part II, *IEEE Trans. Systems, Man, and Cybernetics* **5**, pp. 409–423.

Fu, K. S. and Booth, T. L. (1986a). Grammatical inference: introduction and survey - Part I, *IEEE Trans. Pattern Analysis and Machine Intelligence* **8**, pp. 343–359.

Fu, K. S. and Booth, T. L. (1986b). Grammatical inference: introduction and survey - Part II, *IEEE Trans. Pattern Analysis and Machine Intelligence* **8**, pp. 360–375.

Fu, K. S. and Fan, T. I. (1982). Tree translation and its application to a time-varying image analysis problem, *IEEE Trans. Systems, Man, and Cybernetics* **12**, pp. 856–867.

Fu, K. S. and Huang, T. (1972). Stochastic grammars and languages, *International Journal of Computer and Information Sciences* **1**, pp. 135–170.

Fu, K. S. and Li, T. (1969). On stochastic automata and languages, *Information Sciences* **1**, pp. 403–419.

Fu, K. S. and Rosenfeld, A. (1976). Pattern recognition and image processing, *IEEE Trans. Computers* **25**, pp. 1336–1346.

Fu, W., Eftekharian, A. A., and Campbell, M. I. (2013). Automated manufacturing planning approach based on volume decomposition and graph-grammars, *Journal of Computing and Information Science in Engineering* **13** : 021010.

Fu, Z. and Pennington de, A. (1994). Geometric reasoning based on graph grammars parsing, *Journal of Mechanical Design* **116**, pp. 763–769.

Fujisaki, T., Jelinek, E., Cocke, J., Black, E., and Nishino, T. (1989). A probabilistic method for sentence disambiguation, in *Proc. 1st Int. Workshop on Parsing Technologies* (Pittsburgh, PA, USA), pp. 105–114.

Fujiyoshi, A., Suzuki, M., and Uchida, S. (2000). Verification of mathematical formulae based on a combination of context-free grammar and tree grammar, *Lecture Notes in Computer Science* **5144**, pp. 415–429.

Fukuda, H. and Kamata, K. (1984). Inference of tree automata from sample set of trees, *International Journal of Computer and Information Sciences* **13**, pp. 177–196.

Fukunaga, K. (1990). *Introduction to Statistical Pattern Recognition* (Academic Press, Boston).

Fung, L. W. and Fu, K. S. (1975). Stochastic syntactic decoding for pattern classification, *IEEE Trans. Computers* **24**, pp. 662–669.

Fürst, L., Mernik, M., and Mahnič, V. (2011). Improving the graph grammar parser of Rekers and Schürr, *IET Software* **5**, pp. 246–261.

Gadde, R., Marlet, R., and Paragios, N. (2016). Learning grammars for architecture-specific facade parsing, *International Journal of Computer Vision* **117**, pp. 290–316.

Gallego-Sánchez, López, D., and Calera-Rubio, J. (2018). Grammatical inference of directed acyclic graph languages with polynomial time complexity, *Journal of Computer and System Sciences* **95**, pp. 19–34.

Gao, W., Fang, G. L., Zhao, D. B., and Chen, Y. Q. A. (2004). A Chinese sign language recognition system based on SOFM/SRN/HMM, *Pattern Recognition* **37**, pp. 2389–2402.

Garain, U. and Chaudhuri, B. B. (2000). A syntactic approach for processing mathematical expressions in printed documents, in *Proc. 15th IAPR Int. Conf. on Pattern Recognition* (Barcelona, Spain), pp. 523–526.

García, P., Segarra, E., Vidal, E., and Galiano, I. (1990a). On the use of the morphic generator grammatical inference (MGGI) methodology in automatic speech recognition, *International Journal of Pattern Recognition and Artificial Intelligence* **4**, pp. 667–685.

García, P. and Vidal, E. (1990). Inference of k-testable languages in the strict sense and applications to syntactic pattern recognition, *IEEE Trans. Pattern Analysis and Machine Intelligence* **12**, pp. 920–925.

García, P., Vidal, E., and Casacuberta, F. (1987). Local languages, the successor method and a step towards a general methodology for the inference of regular grammars, *IEEE Trans. Pattern Analysis and Machine Intelligence* **6**, pp. 841–845.

García, P., Vidal, E., and Oncina, J. (1990b). Learning locally testable languages in the strict sense, in *Proc. Int. Workshop on Algorithmic Learning Theory* (Tokyo, Japan), pp. 325–338.

Garey, M. R. and Johnson, D. S. (eds.) (1979). *Computers and Intractability: A Guide to the Theory of NP-Completeness* (W. H. Freeman and Co, San Francisco, CA).

Gath, I. and Schwartz, L. (1989). Syntactic pattern recognition applied to sleep EEG staging, *Pattern Recognition Letters* **10**, pp. 265–272.

Gazdar, G. (1988). Applicability of indexed grammars to natural languages, in U. Reyle and C. Rohrer (eds.), *Natural Language Parsing and Linguistic Theories* (D. Reidel Publ. Comp., Englewood Cliffs).

Gécseg, F. and Steinby, M. (1984). *Tree Automata* (Akadémiai Kiadó, Budapest).

Geyik, S. C., Bulut, E., and Szymanski, B. K. (2013). Grammatical inference for modeling mobility patterns in networks, *IEEE Trans. Mobile Computing* **12**, pp. 2119–2131.

Giammarresi, D. and Restivo, A. (1992). Recognizable picture languages, *International Journal of Pattern Recognition and Artificial Intelligence* **6**, pp. 241–256.

Giammarresi, D. and Restivo, A. (1997). Two-dimensional languages, in G. Rozenberg and A. Salomaa (eds.), *Handbook of Formal Languages - III* (Springer, New York, NY), pp. 215–267.

Giammarresi, D., Restivo, A., Seibert, S., and Thomas, W. (1996). Monadic second-order logic over rectangular pictures and recognizability by tiling systems, *Information and Computation* **125**, pp. 32–45.

Gianotti, C. (1993). Analysis of economic and business information, in C. H. Chen, L. F. Pau, and P. S. P. Wang (eds.), *Handbook of Pattern Recognition and Computer Vision* (World Scientific, Singapore), pp. 569–594.

Giese, D. A., Bourne, J. R., and Ward, J. W. (1979). Syntax analysis of electroencephalogram, *IEEE Trans. Systems, Man, and Cybernetics* **9**, pp. 429–435.

Gildea, D. and Jurafsky, D. (1995). Automatic induction of finite state transducers for simple phonological rules, in *Proc. 33rd Meeting of the Association for Computational Linguistics* (Cambridge, MA, USA), pp. 9–15.

Gips, J. (1974). A syntax-directed program that performs a three-dimensional perceptual task, *Pattern Recognition* **6**, pp. 189–200.

Gips, J. (1975). *Shape Grammars and their Uses* (Birkhäuser Verlag, Basel - Stuttgart).

Golab, T., Ledley, R. S., and Rotolo, L. S. (1971). FIDAC: Film input to digital automatic computer, *Pattern Recognition* **3**, pp. 123–156.

Gold, E. M. (1967). Language identification in the limit, *Information and Control* **10**, pp. 447–474.

Gold, E. M. (1978). Complexity of automaton identification from given data, *Information and Control* **37**, pp. 302–320.

Goldfarb, L. (2004). Pattern representation and the future of pattern recognition, in *Proc. International Conference on Pattern Recognition* (Cambridge, UK).

Golin, E. J. (1991a). *A Method for the Specification and Parsing of Visual Languages*, Ph.D. thesis, Brown University, Providence, RI, USA.

Golin, E. J. (1991b). Parsing visual languages with picture layout grammars, *Journal of Visual Languages and Computing* **2**, pp. 371–394.

Golin, E. J. and Reiss, S. P. (1990). The specification of visual language syntax, *Journal of Visual Languages and Computing* **1**, pp. 141–157.

Gollery, M. (ed.) (2008). *Handbook of Hidden Markov Models in Bioinformatics* (Chapman and Hall / CRC, Boca Raton, FL).

Gonzales, R. C., Edwards, J. J., and Thomason, M. G. (1976). An algorithm for the inference of tree grammars, *International Journal of Computer and Information Science* **5**, pp. 145–164.

Gonzales, R. C. and Thomason, M. G. (1974). On the inference of tree grammars for syntactic pattern recognition, in *Proc. IEEE Int. Conf. on Systems, Man, and Cybernetics* (Dallas, TX), pp. 311–315.

Gonzales, R. C. and Thomason, M. G. (1978). *Syntactic Pattern Recognition: An Introduction* (Addison-Wesley, Reading).

Gonzales, R. C. and Woods, R. E. (2008). *Digital Image Processing* (Prentice-Hall, Upper Saddle River, NJ).

González-Villanueva, L., Alvarez-Alvarez, A., Ascari, L., and Triviño, G. (2013). Computational model of human body motion performing a complex exercise by means of fuzzy finite state machine, in *Proc. Int. Conf. on Medical Imaging using Bio-Inspired and Soft Computing* (Brussels, Belgium), pp. 245–251.

Gorn, S. (1967). Explicit definitions and linguistics dominoes, in J. F. Hart and S. Takasu (eds.), *Systems and Computer Science* (University of Toronto Press, Toronto).

Grenander, U. (1967). Syntax-controlled probabilities, Tech. rep., Brown University, Providence, R.I.

Grenander, U. (1970). A unified approach to pattern analysis, *Advances in Computers* **10**, pp. 175–188.

Grenander, U. (1976). *Pattern Synthesis. Lectures in Pattern Theory - Volume I* (Springer, New York - Heidelberg - Berlin).

Grenander, U. (1978). *Pattern Analysis. Lectures in Pattern Theory - Volume II* (Springer, New York - Heidelberg - Berlin).

Grenander, U. (1981). *Regular Structures. Lectures in Pattern Theory - Volume III* (Springer, New York - Heidelberg - Berlin).

Griffiths, C. M. (1990). The language of rocks - an example of the use of syntactic analysis in the interpretation of sedimentary environments from wireline logs, in A. Hurst, M. A. Lovell, and A. C. Morton (eds.), *Geological Applications of Wireline Logs* (The Geological Society, London).

Grinchtein, O., Jonsson, B., and Leucker, M. (2005). Inference of timed transition systems, *Electronic Notes in Theoretical Computer Science* **138**, pp. 87–99.

Grinchtein, O., Jonsson, B., and Pettersson, P. (2006). Inference of event-recording automata using decision trees, *Lecture Notes in Computer Science* **4137**, pp. 435–449.

Grobel, K. and Assan, M. (1997). Isolated sign language recognition using hidden Markov models, in *Proc. IEEE Int. Conf. on Systems, Man, and Cybernetics* (Orlando, FL, USA), pp. 162–167.

Grune, D., Reeuwijk, K., Bal, H. E., Jacobs, C. J. H., and Langendoen, K. (2012). *Modern Compilers Design* (Springer, New York).

Gruska, J. (1971). A characterization of context-free languages, *Journal of Computer and System Sciences* **5**, pp. 353–364.

Guessarian, I. (1983). Pushdown tree automata, *Mathematical Systems Theory* **16**, pp. 237–263.

Guiducci, A., Melen, R., Nardi, D., Neri, F., Nesti, F., and Quaglia, G. (1983). Automatic scaling of ionograms by the method of structural description, *Pattern Recognition* **16**, pp. 489–499.

Guo, D., Zhou, W., Li, H., and Wang, M. (2018). Online early-late fusion based on adaptive HMM for sign language recognition, *ACM Trans. on Multimedia Computing, Communications, and Applications* **14**:8.

Guzman, A. (1968). Decomposition of a visual scene into three-dimensional bodies, in *Proc. AFIPS Fall Joint Computer Conference* (San Francisco, CA), pp. 291–304.

Habel, A. and Kreowski, H. J. (1987). May we introduce to you: hyperedge replacement, *Lecture Notes in Computer Science* **291**, pp. 15–26.

Han, F. and Zhu, S. C. (2009). Bottom-up/top-down image parsing with attribute grammar, *IEEE Trans. Pattern Analysis and Machine Intelligence* **31**, pp. 59–73.

Haralick, R. M. (1978). Structural pattern recognition, homomorphisms, and arrangements, *Pattern Recognition* **10**, pp. 223–236.

Haralick, R. M. (1980). Using perspective transformations in scene analysis, *Computer Graphics and Image Processing* **13**, pp. 191–221.

Haralick, R. M. and Shapiro, L. G. (1979a). The consistent labeling problem: Part I, *IEEE Trans. Pattern Analysis and Machine Intelligence* **1**, pp. 173–184.

Haralick, R. M. and Shapiro, L. G. (1979b). The consistent labeling problem: Part II, *IEEE Trans. Pattern Analysis and Machine Intelligence* **1**, pp. 193–203.

Harmanci, A. O., Sharma, G., and Mathews, D. H. (2007). Efficient pairwise RNA structure prediction using probabilistic alignment constraints in *Dynalign, BMC Bioinformatics* **8**:357.

Harris, Z. S. (1957). Co-occurrence and transformation in linguistic structure, *Language* **33**, pp. 283–340.

Harris, Z. S. (1962). *String Analysis of Language Structure* (Mouton and Co., The Hague).

Harris, Z. S. (1964). Transformations in linguistic structure, *Proceedings of the American Philosophical Society* **108**, pp. 418–422.

Harris, Z. S. (1968). *Mathematical Structures of Language* (Interscience, New York).

Harrison, M. A. (1978). *Introduction to Formal Language Theory* (Addison-Wesley, Reading).

Hart, J. M. (1973). An infinite hierarchy of linear local adjunct languages, *Information and Control* **23**, pp. 245–259.

Hart, J. M. (1974). Ambiguity and decision problems for local adjunct languages, *Journal of Computer and System Sciences* **8**, pp. 8–21.

Hartmanis, J. (1960). Symbolic analysis of a decomposition of information processing machines, *Information and Control* **3**, pp. 154–178.

Hartmanis, J. and Stearns, R. E. (1964). Pair algebra and its application to automata theory, *Information and Control* **7**, pp. 485–507.

Hartmanis, J. and Stearns, R. E. (1966). *Algebraic Theory of Sequential Machines* (Prentice Hall, Englewood Cliffs).

Hashtrudi Zad, S., Kwong, R., and Wonham, W. (2003). Fault diagnosis in discrete-event systems: framework and model reduction, *IEEE Trans. Automatic Control* **48**, pp. 1199–1212.

Head, T. (1987). Formal language theory and DNA: an analysis of the generative capacity of specific recombinant behaviors, *Bulletin of Mathematical Biology* **49**, pp. 737–759.

Heinz, J. and Sempere, J. M. (eds.) (2016). *Topics in Grammatical Inference* (Springer, Berlin Heidelberg).

Heisserman, J. and Woodbury, R. (1993). Generating languages of solid models, in *Proc. 2nd ACM Symp. on Solid Modelling and Applications* (Montreal, Canada), pp. 103–112.

Heller, S. R., McNaught, A., Pletnev, I., Stein, S., and Tchekhovskoi, D. (2015). InChI, the IUPAC International Chemical Identifier, *Journal of Cheminformatics* **7**:23.

Helm, R., Marriott, K., and Oderski, M. (1991). Building visual language parsers, in *Proc. SIGCHI Conference on Human Factors in Computing Systems* (New Orleans, LA, USA), pp. 105–112.

Henderson, T. C. and Davis, L. (1981). Hierarchical models and analysis of shape, *Pattern Recognition* **14**, pp. 197–204.

Henderson, T. C. and Samal, A. (1986). Shape grammar compilers, *Pattern Recognition* **19**, pp. 279–288.

Herman, M. and Kanade, T. (1986). Incremental reconstruction of 3D scenes from multiple, complex images, *Artificial Intelligence* **30**, pp. 289–341.

Higuera de la, C. (1997). Characteristic sets for polynomial grammatical inference, *Machine Learning* **27**, pp. 125–138.

Higuera de la, C. (2005). A bibliographical study of grammatical inference, *Pattern Recognition* **38**, pp. 1332–1348.

Higuera de la, C. (2010). *Grammatical Inference* (Cambridge University Press, Cambridge).

Higuera de la, C. and Oncina, J. (2002). Learning deterministic linear languages, in *Proc. 15th Conference on Computational Learning Theory*, pp. 45–52.

Higuera de la, C. and Thollard, F. (2000). Identification in the limit with probability one of stochastic deterministic finite automata, *Lecture Notes in Artificial Intelligence* **1891**, pp. 141–156.

Hill, E. J. and Griffiths, C. M. (2007). Simulating sedimentary successions using syntactic pattern recognition techniques, *Mathematical Geology* **39**, pp. 141–157.

Hill, E. J. and Griffiths, C. M. (2008). Formal description of sedimentary architecture of analogue models for use in 2D reservoir simulation, *Marine and Petroleum Geology* **25**, pp. 131–141.

Hill, E. J. and Griffiths, C. M. (2009). Describing and generating facies models for reservoir characterisation: 2D map view, *Marine and Petroleum Geology* **26**, pp. 1554–1563.

Höchsmann, M., Töller, T., Giegerich, R., and Kurtz, S. (2003). Local similarity in RNA secondary structures, in *Proc. Computational Systems Bioinformatics Conference* (Stanford, USA), pp. 155–168.

Hockenmaier, J., Bierner, G., and Baldridge, J. (2004). Extending the coverage of a CCG system, *Journal of Logic and Computation* **2**, pp. 165–208.

Hockenmaier, J. and Steedman, M. (2007). CCGbank: A corpus of CCG derivations and dependency structures extracted from the Penn Treebank, *Computational Linguistics* **33**, pp. 355–396.

Hogenhout, W. R. and Matsumoto, Y. (1998). A fast method for statistical grammar induction, *Natural Language Processing* **4**, pp. 191–209.

Hohmann, B., Havemann, S., Krispel, U., and Fellner, D. W. (2010). A GML shape grammar for semantically enriched 3D building models, *Computers and Graphics* **34**, pp. 322–334.

Holmes, I. and Rubin, G. M. (2002). Pairwise RNA structure comparison with stochastic context-free grammars, in *Proc. 2002 Pacific Symposium on Biocomputing* (Hawaii), pp. 163–174.

Homer, R. W., Swanson, J., Jilek, R. J., Hurst, T., and Clark, R. D. (2008). SYBYL line notation (SLN): A single notation to represent chemical structures, queries, reactions, and virtual libraries, *Journal of Chemical Information and Modeling* **48**, pp. 2294–2307.

Hong, P., Turk, M., and Huang, T. S. (2000). Gesture modeling and recognition using finite state machines, in *Proc. 4th IEEE International Conference on Automatic Face and Gesture Recognition* (Grenoble, France), pp. 410–415.

Hopcroft, J. E., Motwani, R., and Ullman, J. D. (2006). *Introduction to Automata Theory, Languages, and Computation* (Addison-Wesley, Reading, MA).

Horning, J. J. (1969). *A Study of Grammatical Inference*, Ph.D. thesis, Stanford University, Stanford, USA.

Horowitz, S. L. (1975). A syntactic algorithm for peak detection in waveforms with applications to cardiography, *Communications of the Association for Computing Machinery* **18**, pp. 281–285.

Horowitz, S. L. (1977). Peak recognition in waveforms, in K. S. Fu (ed.), *Syntactic Pattern Recognition Applications* (Springer, Berlin - Heidelberg - New York).

Hsu, B. Y., Wong, T. K. F., Hon, W. K., Liu, X., Lam, T. W., and Yiu, S. M. (2013). A local structural prediction algorithm for RNA triple helix structure, *Lecture Notes in Computer Science* **7968**, pp. 102–113.

Huang, K. Y. (1992). Pattern recognition to seismic exploration, in I. Palaz and S. K. Sengupta (eds.), *Automated Pattern Analysis in Petroleum Exploration* (Springer, New York), pp. 121–154.

Huang, K. Y. (2002). *Syntactic Pattern Recognition for Seismic Oil Exploration* (World Scientific, New Jersey - Singapore - London - Hong Kong).

Huang, K. Y. and Chao, Y. H. (2004). Seismic pattern recognition using neural network and tree automaton, in *Proc. 2004 IEEE Int. Symposium on Geoscience and Remote Sensing* (Anchorage, AK, USA), pp. 3080–3083.

Huang, K. Y. and Fu, K. S. (1984). Detection of bright spots in seismic signal using tree classifiers, *Geoexploration* **23**, pp. 121–145.

Huang, K. Y. and Fu, K. S. (1985a). Syntactic pattern recognition for the classification of Ricker wavelets, *Geophysics* **50**, pp. 1548–1555.

Huang, K. Y. and Fu, K. S. (1985b). Syntactic pattern recognition for the recognition of bright spots, *Pattern Recognition* **18**, pp. 421–428.

Huang, K. Y. and Leu, D. R. (1992). Modified Earley parsing and MPM method for attributed grammar and seismic pattern recognition, *Journal of Information Science and Engineering* **8**, pp. 541–565.

Huang, K. Y. and Leu, D. R. (1995). Recognition of Ricker wavelets by syntactic analysis, *Geophysics* **60**, pp. 1541–1549.

Huang, K. Y. and Sheen, T. H. (1986). A tree automaton system of syntactic pattern recognition for the recognition of seismic patterns, in *Proc. 1986 Annual Int. Meeting of Society of Exploration Geophysicists* (Houston, TX, USA), pp. 183–187.

Huang, T. and Fu, K. S. (1971). On stochastic context-free languages, *Information Sciences* **3**, pp. 201–224.

Huang, T. and Fu, K. S. (1972). Stochastic syntactic analysis for programmed grammars and syntactic pattern recognition, *Computer Graphics and Image Processing* **1**, pp. 257–283.

Huffman, D. A. (1971). Impossible objects as nonsense sentences, in B. Melzer and D. Michie (eds.), *Machine Intelligence 6* (Edinburgh University Press, Edinburgh), pp. 295–323.

Humenik, K. and Pinkham, R. S. (1990). Production probability estimators for context-free grammars, *Journal of Systems and Software* **12**, pp. 43–53.

Husen, M. N., Lee, S., and Q., K. M. (2017). Syntactic pattern recognition of car driving behavior detection, in *Proc. 11th Int. Conf. Ubiquitous Information Management and Communication* (Beppu, Japan).

Huynh, D. T. (1983). Commutative grammars: the complexity of uniform word problems, *Information and Control* **57**, pp. 21–39.

Huynh, D. T. (1985). The complexity of equivalence problems for commutative grammars, *Information and Control* **66**, pp. 103–121.

Inoue, K. and Nakamura, A. (1977). Some properties of two-dimensional on-line tessellation acceptors, *Information Sciences* **13**, pp. 95–121.

Inoue, K. and Takanami, I. (1991). A survey of two-dimensional automata theory, *Information Sciences* **55**, pp. 99–121.

Itoga, S. (1981). A new heuristic for inferring regular grammars, *IEEE Trans. Pattern Analysis and Machine Intelligence* **3**, pp. 191–197.

Ivanov, Y. A. and Bobick, A. F. (2000). Recognition of visual activities and interactions by stochastic parsing, *IEEE Trans. Pattern Analysis and Machine Intelligence* **22**, pp. 852–872.

Jain, A. K. (1989). *Fundamentals of Digital Image Processing* (Prentice-Hall, Upper Saddle River, NJ).

Jain, A. K., Duin, R. P. W., and Mao, J. (2000). Statistical pattern recognition: a review, *IEEE Trans. Pattern Analysis and Machine Intelligence* **22**, pp. 4–37.

Jain, R., Kasturi, R., and Schunck, B. G. (1995). *Machine Vision* (McGraw-Hill, New York).

Jakubowski, R. (1982). Syntactic characterization of machine parts shapes, *Cybernetics and Systems* **13**, pp. 1–24.

Jakubowski, R. (1985). Extraction of shape features for syntactic recognition of mechanical parts, *IEEE Trans. Systems, Man, and Cybernetics* **15**, pp. 642–651.

Jakubowski, R. (1986). A structural representation of shape and its features, *Information Sciences* **39**, pp. 129–151.

Jakubowski, R. (1990). Decomposition of complex shapes for their structural recognition, *Information Sciences* **50**, pp. 35–71.

Jakubowski, R. and Flasiński, M. (1992). Towards generalized sweeping model for designing with extraction and recognition of 3D solid features, *Journal of Design and Manufacturing* **2**, pp. 239–258.

Jakubowski, R. and Kasprzak, A. (1977). Syntactic description and recognition of rotary machine elements, *IEEE Trans. Computers* **26**, pp. 1039–1043.

Janssens, D. and Rozenberg, G. (1980a). On the structure of node-label-controlled graph languages, *Information Sciences* **20**, pp. 191–216.

Janssens, D. and Rozenberg, G. (1980b). Restrictions, extensions, and variations of NLC grammars, *Information Sciences* **20**, pp. 217–244.

Janssens, D. and Rozenberg, G. (1982). Graph grammars with neighbourhood-controlled embedding, *Theoretical Computer Science* **21**, pp. 55–74.

Janssens, D., Rozenberg, G., and Verraedt, R. (1982). On sequential and parallel node-rewriting graph grammars, *Computer Graphics and Image Processing* **18**, pp. 279–304.

Jelinek, F. (1985). Markov source modeling of text generation, in J. K. Skwirzynski (ed.), *The Impact of Processing Techniques on Communications* (Martinus Nijhoff Publishers, Dordrecht), pp. 569–598.

Jelinek, F. (1997). *Statistical Methods for Speech Recognition* (MIT Press, Cambridge, MA).

Jelinek, F. and Lafferty, J. D. (1991). Computation of the probability of initial substring generation by stochastic context-free grammars, *Computational Linguistics* **17**, pp. 315–323.

Jeltsch, E. and Kreowski, H. J. (1991). Grammatical inference based on hyperedge replacement, *Lecture Notes in Computer Science* **531**, pp. 461–474.

Jonyer, I., Holder, L. B., and Cook, D. J. (2004). MDL-based context free graph grammar induction and applications, *International Journal on Artificial Intelligence Tools* **13**, pp. 65–79.

Joo, S. W. and Chellappa, R. (2006a). Attribute grammar-based event recognition and anomaly detection, in *Proc. 2006 IEEE Conf. on Computer Vision and Pattern Recognition* (New York, NY, USA), pp. 107–114.

Joo, S. W. and Chellappa, R. (2006b). Recognition of multi-object events using attribute grammars, in *Proc. 2006 IEEE Int. Conf. on Image Processing* (Atlanta, GA, USA), pp. 2897–2990.

Jorge, J. A. P. and Glinert, E. P. (1995). Online parsing of visual languages using adjacency grammars, in *Proc. 1995 IEEE Symposium on Visual Languages* (Darmstadt, Germany), pp. 250–257.

Joshi, A. K. (1962). A procedure for a transformational decomposition of English sentences, *Transformations and Discourse Analysis Papers, University of Pennsylvania* **42**.

Joshi, A. K. (1966). Transformational analysis by computer, in *Proc. NIH Seminar on Computational Linguistics* (U.S. Dept. HEW, Bethesda, MD).

Joshi, A. K. (1985). How much context-sensitivity is necessary for characterizing structural descriptions – Tree Adjoining Grammars, in D. Dowty et al. (ed.), *Natural Language Processing – Theoretical, Computational and Psychological Perspective* (Cambridge University Press, New York, NY).

Joshi, A. K., Kosaraju, S. R., and Yamada, H. M. (1972a). String adjunct grammars: I. Local and distributed adjunction, *Information and Control* **21**, pp. 93–116.

Joshi, A. K., Kosaraju, S. R., and Yamada, H. M. (1972b). String adjunct grammars: II. Equational representation, null symbols, and linguistic relevance, *Information and Control* **21**, pp. 235–260.

Joshi, A. K., Levy, L. S., and Takahashi, M. (1975). Tree adjunct grammars, *Journal of Computer and System Sciences* **10**, pp. 136–163.

Joshi, A. K. and Schabes, Y. (1992). Tree-adjoining grammars and lexicalized grammars, in M. Nivat and A. Podelski (eds.), *Tree Automata and Languages* (North Holland, Amsterdam), pp. 409–431.

Joshi, A. K. and Schabes, Y. (1997). Tree adjoining grammars, in G. Rozenberg and A. Salomaa (eds.), *Handbook of Formal Languages - III* (Springer, New York, NY), pp. 69–123.

Joshi, A. K., Vijay-Shanker, K., and Weir, D. (1991). The convergence of mildly context-sensitive grammar formalisms, in P. Sells, S. Shieber, and T. Wasow (eds.), *Foundational Issues in Natural Language Processing* (MIT Press, Cambridge, MA), pp. 31–81.

Joshi, S. and Chang, T. C. (1990). Feature extraction and feature based design approaches in the development of design interface for process planning, *Journal of Intelligent Manufacturing* **1**, pp. 1–15.

Juhola, M. (1986). A syntactic method for analysis of saccadic eye movements, *Pattern Recognition* **19**, pp. 353–359.

Jurafsky, D. (1996). A probabilistic model of lexical and syntactic access and disambiguation, *Cognitive Science* **20**, pp. 137–194.

Jurafsky, D. and Martin, J. H. (2008). *Speech and Language Processing* (Prentice Hall, Englewood Cliffs).

Jurafsky, D., Wooters, C., Segal, J., Stolcke, A., Fosler, E., Tajchman, G., and Morgan, N. (1995). Using a stochastic context-free grammar as a language model for speech recognition, in *Proc. IEEE Conference on Acoustics, Speech and Signal Processing* (Detroit, MI, USA), pp. 189–192.

Jurek, J. (2000). On the linear computational complexity of the parser for quasi context sensitive languages, *Pattern Recognition Letters* **21**, pp. 179–187.

Jurek, J. (2004). Towards grammatical inferencing of GDPLL(k) grammars for applications in syntactic pattern recognition-based expert systems, *Lecture Notes in Computer Science* **3070**, pp. 604–609.

Jurek, J. (2005). Recent developments of the syntactic pattern recognition model based on quasi-context sensitive languages, *Pattern Recognition Letters* **26**, pp. 1011–1018.

Kallmeyer, L. (2010). *Parsing Beyond Context-Free Grammars* (Springer, Berlin-Heidelberg).

Kamata, K., Watanabe, A., Satoh, T., and Sase, M. (1988). A structural recognition algorithm for handwritten numerals, in *Proc. 1988 IEEE Int. Conf. on Systems, Man, and Cybernetics* (Beijing, China), pp. 365–368.

Kanade, T. (1977). Model representations and control structures in image understanding, in *Proc. 5th Int. Joint Conf. Artificial Intelligence* (Cambridge, MA), pp. 1074–1082.

Kanade, T. (1980). A theory of Origami world, *Artificial Intelligence* **13**, pp. 279–311.

Kanade, T. (1981). Recovery of the three-dimensional shape of an object from a single view, *Artificial Intelligence* **17**, pp. 409–460.

Kanal, L. and Chandrasekaran, B. (1972). On linguistic, statistical and mixed models for pattern recognition, in S. Watanabe (ed.), *Frontiers of Pattern Recognition* (Academic Press, New York), pp. 163–192.

Karplus, K., Barrett, C., and Hughey, R. (1998). Hidden Markov models for detecting remote protein homologies, *Bioinformatics* **14**, pp. 846–856.

Kasami, T. (1965). An efficient recognition and syntax-analysis algorithm for context-free languages, Tech. Rep. 65-758, US Air Force, Cambridge, MA.

Kashyap, R. L. (1979). Syntactic decision rules for recognition of spoken words and phrases using a stochastic automaton, *IEEE Trans. Pattern Analysis and Machine Intelligence* **1**, pp. 154–163.

Kato, Y., Akutsu, T., and Seki, H. (2009). A grammatical approach to RNA-RNA interaction prediction, *Pattern Recognition* **42**, pp. 531–538.

Kato, Y., Seki, H., and Kasami, T. (2004). Subclasses of tree adjoining grammars for RNA secondary structure, in *Proc. 7th Int. Workshop on Tree Adjoining Grammar and Related Formalisms* (Vancouver, Canada), pp. 48–55.

Kaufmann, G. and Bunke, H. (1998). Amount translation and error localization in check processing using syntax-directed translation, in *Proc. 14th IAPR Int. Conf. on Pattern Recognition* (Brisbane, Australia), pp. 1530–1534.

Kaul, M. (1983). Parsing of graphs in linear time, *Lecture Notes in Computer Science* **153**, pp. 206–218.

Keller, B. and Lutz, R. (2005). Evolutionary induction of stochastic context free grammars, *Pattern Recognition* **38**, pp. 1393–1406.

Kepser, S. and Rogers, J. (2011). The equivalence of tree adjoining grammars and monadic linear context-free tree grammars, *Journal of Logic, Language and Information* **20**, pp. 361–384.

Kermorvant, C., Higuera de la, C., and Dupont, P. (2004). Improving probabilistic automata learning with additional knowledge, *Lecture Notes in Computer Science* **3138**, pp. 260–268.

Kickert, W. J. M. and Koppelaar, H. (1976). Applications of fuzzy set theory to syntactic pattern recognition of handwritten capitals, *IEEE Trans. Systems, Man, and Cybernetics* **6**, pp. 148–151.

Kim, C. and Sudborough, I. H. (1987). The membership and equivalence problems for picture languages, *Theoretical Computer Science* **52**, pp. 177–191.

Kirousis, L. M. and Papadimitriou, C. H. (1988). The complexity of recognizing polyhedral scenes, *Journal of Computer and System Sciences* **37**, pp. 14–38.

Kirsch, R. A. (1963). The application of automata theory to problems in information retrieval, Tech. Rep. 7882, National Bureau of Standards - U.S. Department of Commerce, Washington, D.C.

Kirsch, R. A. (1964). Computer interpretation of English text and picture patterns, *IEEE Trans. Electronic Computers* **13**, pp. 363–376.

Kirsch, R. A. (1971). Computer determination of the constituent structure of biological images, *Computers and Biomedical Research* **4**, pp. 315–328.

Klauck, C. and Mauss, J. (1994). Feature recognition in Computer-Integrated Manufacturing, *Journal of Integrated Computer-Aided Engineering* **1**, pp. 359–373.

Kleene, S. C. (1951). Representation of events in nerve nets and finite automata, Tech. Rep. RM–704, RAND Corporation, Santa Monica, CA.

Kleene, S. C. (1956). Representation of events in nerve nets and finite automata, in C. E. Shannon and J. McCarthy (eds.), *Automata Studies* (Princeton University Press, Princeton), pp. 3–42.

Klein, D. and Manning, C. D. (2005). Natural language grammar induction with a generative constituent-context model, *Pattern Recognition* **38**, pp. 1407–1419.

Klerx, T., Anderka, M., Büning, H. K., and Priesterjahn, S. (2014). Model-based anomaly detection for discrete event systems, in *Proc. 26th Int. Conf. on Tools with Artificial Intelligence* (Limassol, Cyprus), pp. 665–672.

Klette, R. (2014). *Concise Computer Vision* (Springer, London).

Knight, K. and Graehl, J. (2005). An overview of probabilistic tree transducers for natural language processing, *Lecture Notes in Computer Science* **3406**, pp. 1–24.

Knight, K. and May, J. (2009). Applications of weighted automata in natural language processing, in M. Droste, W. Kuich, and H. Vogler (eds.), *Handbook of Weighted Automata* (Springer, Heidelberg), pp. 571–596.

Knight, T. (1981). Languages of designs: from known to new, *Environment and Planning B* **8**, pp. 213–238.

Knudsen, B. and Heyn, J. (1999). RNA secondary structure prediction using stochastic context-free grammars and evolutionary history, *Bioinformatics* **15**, pp. 446–454.

Knudsen, B. and Heyn, J. (2003). Pfold: RNA secondary structure prediction using stochastic context-free grammars, *Nucleic Acids Research* **31**, pp. 3423–3428.

Knudsen, B. and Miyamoto, M. M. (2003). Sequence alignments and pair hidden Markov models using evolutionary history, *Journal of Molecular Biology* **333**, pp. 453–460.

Knuth, D. (1965). On the translation of languages from left to right, *Information and Control* **8**, pp. 607–639.

Knuth, D. (1968). Semantics of context-free languages, *Mathematical Systems Theory* **2**, pp. 127–145.

Knuutila, T. and Steinby, M. (1994). Inference of tree languages from a finite sample: an algebraic approach, *Theoretical Computer Science* **129**, pp. 337–367.

Kobayashi, H., Ikeda, M., and Tanaka, E. (1986). A top-down error-correcting parser for a context-sensitive language, *Systems and Computers in Japan* **17**, pp. 84–91.

Komenda, J., Masopust, T., and Schuppen van, J. H. (2012). Supervisory control synthesis of discrete event systems using a coordination scheme, *Automatica* **48**, pp. 247–254.

Komenda, J., Masopust, T., and Schuppen van, J. H. (2015). Coordination control of discrete-event systems revisited, *Discrete Event Dynamic Systems* **25**, pp. 65–94.

Koning, H. and Eizenberg, J. (1981). The language of the prairie: Frank Lloyd Wright's prairie houses, *Environment and Planning B* **8**, pp. 295–323.

Koshiba, T., Mäkinen, E., and Takada, Y. (1997). Learning deterministic even linear languages from positive examples, *Theoretical Computer Science* **185**, pp. 63–79.

Koski, A. (1996). Primitive coding of structural ECG features, *Pattern Recognition Letters* **17**, pp. 1215–1222.

Koski, A. (1998). Modelling ECG signals with hidden Markov models, *Artificial Intelligence in Medicine* **8**, pp. 453–471.

Koski, A., Juhola, M., and Meriste, M. (1995). Syntactic recognition of ECG signals by attributed finite automata, *Pattern Recognition* **28**, pp. 1927–1940.

Koutroumbas, K. and Theodoridis, S. (2008). *Pattern Recognition* (Academic Press, Boston).

Koutsourakis, P., Simon, L., Teboul, O., Tziritas, G., and Paragios, N. (2009). Single view reconstruction using shape grammars for urban environments, in *Proc. IEEE 12th Int. Conf. on Computer Vision* (Kyoto, Japan), pp. 1795–1802.

Krishnamoorthy, M., Nagy, G., Seth, S., and Viswanathan, M. (1993). Syntactic segmentation and labeling of digitized pages from technical journals, *IEEE Trans. Pattern Analysis and Machine Intelligence* **15**, pp. 737–747.

Krishnamurthy, E. V. and Lynch, M. F. (1981). Analysis and coding of generic chemical formulae in chemical patents, *Journal of Information Science* **3**, pp. 75–79.

Kroch, A. (1987). Unbounded dependencies and subjacency in a tree adjoining grammar, in A. Manaster-Ramer (ed.), *Mathematics of Language* (John Benjamins, Amsterdam), pp. 143–172.

Krogh, A., Brown, M., Mian, I. S., Sjöander, K., and Haussler, D. (1994a). Hidden Markov models in computational biology: Applications to protein modeling, *Journal of Molecular Biology* **235**, pp. 1501–1531.

Krogh, A., Mian, I. S., and Haussler, D. (1994b). A hidden Markov model that finds genes in E.coli DNA, *Nucleic Acids Research* **22**, pp. 4768–4778.

Kudo, M. and Shimbo, M. (1988). Efficient regular grammatical inference techniques by the use of partial similarities and their logical relationships, *Pattern Recognition* **21**, pp. 401–409.

Kuhlmann, M. and Satta, G. (2012). Tree-adjoining grammars are not closed under strong lexicalization, *Computational Linguistics* **38**, pp. 617–629.

Kukluk, J., Holder, L. B., and Cook, D. J. (2007). Inference of node replacement graph grammars, *Intelligent Data Analysis* **11**, pp. 377–400.

Kukluk, J., Holder, L. B., and Cook, D. J. (2008). Inference of edge replacement graph grammars, *International Journal on Artificial Intelligence Tools* **17**, pp. 539–554.

Kulkarni, V. S. and Pande, S. S. (1995). A system for automatic extraction of 3D part features using syntactic pattern recognition techniques, *International Journal of Production Research* **33**, pp. 1569–1586.

Kulp, D., Haussler, D., Reese, M. G., and Eeckman, F. H. (1996). A generalized hidden Markov model for the recognition of human genes in DNA, in *Proc. 4th Int. Conf. on Intelligent Systems for Molecular Biology* (St. Louis, MO, USA), pp. 134–142.

Kumar, P., Gauba, H., Roy, P. P., and Dogra, D. P. (2017). Coupled HMM-based multi-sensor data fusion for sign language recognition, *Pattern Recognition Letters* **86**, pp. 1–8.

Kuroda, K., Harada, K., and Hagiwara, M. (1997). Large scale on-line handwritten Chinese character recognition using improved syntactic pattern recognition, in *Proc. 1997 IEEE Conf. Systems, Man, and Cybernetics* (Orlando, USA), pp. 4530–4535.

Kuroda, K., Harada, K., and Hagiwara, M. (1999). Large scale on-line handwritten Chinese character recognition using successor method based on stochastic regular grammar, *Pattern Recognition* **32**, pp. 1307–1315.

Kuroda, S. (1964). Classes of languages and linear bounded automata, *Information and Control* **7**, pp. 207–223.

Kurzyński, M. (2005). Combining rule-based and sample-based classifiers - probabilistic approach, *Lecture Notes in Computer Science* **3704**, pp. 298–307.

Kwon, K. C. and Kim, J. H. (1999). Accident identification in nuclear power plants using hidden Markov models, *Engineering Applications of Artificial Intelligence* **12**, pp. 491–501.

Kyprianou, L. K. (1980). *Shape Classification in Computer-Aided Design*, Ph.D. thesis, University of Cambridge, Cambridge, United Kingdom.

Lam, K. P. and Fletcher, P. (2009). Concurrent grammar inference machines for 2-D pattern recognition: a comparison with the level set approach, *Proceedings of the SPIE* **7245** : 724515.

Landweber, P. S. (1963). Three theorems on phrase structure grammars of type 1, *Information and Control* **6**, pp. 131–137.

Lang, K. (1992). Random DFA's can be approximately learned from sparse uniform examples, in *Proc. Fifth Annual Workshop Computational Learning Theory*, pp. 45–52.

Lang, K., Pearlmutter, B. A., and Price, R. A. (1998). Results of the Abbadingo One DFA learning competition and a new evidence-driven state merging algorithm, in *Proc. Fourth Int. Colloquium Grammatical Inference* (Ames, USA), pp. 1–12.

Laroche, P., Nivat, M., and Saoudi, A. (1994). Context-sensitivity of puzzle grammars, *International Journal of Pattern Recognition and Artificial Intelligence* **8**, pp. 525–542.

Lautemann, C. (1988). Efficient algorithms on context-free graph languages, *Lecture Notes in Computer Science* **317**, pp. 362–378.

Ledley, R. S. (1964). High-speed automatic analysis of biomedical pictures, *Science* **146**, pp. 216–223.

Ledley, R. S., Rotolo, L. S., Golab, T. J., Jacobsen, J. D., Ginsberg, M. D., and Wilson, J. B. (1965). FIDAC: Film input to digital automatic computer and associated syntax-directed pattern-recognition programming system, in J. T. Tippet, D. Beckovitz, L. Clapp, C. Koester, and A. Vanderburgh Jr. (eds.), *Optical and Electro-optical Information Processing* (MIT Press, Cambridge, MA), pp. 591–613.

Lee, E. T. (1982). Fuzzy tree automata and syntactic pattern recognition, *IEEE Trans. Pattern Analysis and Machine Intelligence* **4**, pp. 445–449.

Lee, E. T. and Zadeh, L. A. (1969). Note on fuzzy languages, *Information Sciences* **1**, pp. 421–434.

Lee, H. C. and Fu, K. S. (1972). A stochastic syntax analysis procedure and its application to pattern classification, *IEEE Trans. Computers* **21**, pp. 660–666.

Lee, K. H., Eom, K. B., and Kashyap, R. L. (1992). Character recognition based on attribute-dependent programmed grammar, *IEEE Trans. Pattern Analysis and Machine Intelligence* **14**, pp. 1122–1128.

Lefebvre, F. (1996). A grammar-based unification of several alignment and folding algorithms, in *Proc. 4th Int. Conf. on Intelligent Systems for Molecular Biology* (St. Louis, MO, USA), pp. 143–154.

Leung, S. W., Mellish, C., and Robertson, D. (2001). Basic Gene Grammars and DNA-Chart Parser for language processing of *Escherichia coli* promoter DNA sequences, *Bioinformatics* **17**, pp. 226–236.

Levenshtein, V. I. (1966). Binary codes capable of correcting deletions, insertions and reversals, *Soviet Physics Doklady* **10**, pp. 707–710.

Levine, B. (1981). Derivatives of tree sets with applications to grammatical inference, *IEEE Trans. Pattern Analysis and Machine Intelligence* **3**, pp. 285–293.

Levine, B. (1982). The use of tree derivatives and a sample support parameter for inferring tree systems, *IEEE Trans. Pattern Analysis and Machine Intelligence* **4**, pp. 25–34.

Levy, L. S. (1973). Structural aspects of local adjunct languages, *Information and Control* **23**, pp. 260–287.

Levy, L. S. and Joshi, A. K. (1978). Skeletal structural descriptions, *Information and Control* **39**, pp. 192–211.

Lewis II, P. M. and Stearns, R. E. (1968). Syntax-directed transduction, *Journal of the Association for Computing Machinery* **15**, pp. 465–488.

Li, R. Y. and Fu, K. S. (1976). Tree system approach for LANDSAT data interpretation, in *Symp. Machine Processing of Remotely Sensed Data* (West Lafayette, IN, USA), pp. 10–17.

Liang, K. C., Wang, X., and Anastassiou, D. (2007). Bayesian basecalling for DNA sequence analysis using hidden Markov models, *IEEE/ACM Trans. Computational Biology and Bioinformatics* **4**, pp. 430–440.

Lin, L., Gong, H., Li, L., and Wang, L. (2009a). Semantic event representation and recognition using syntactic attribute graph grammar, *Pattern Recognition Letters* **30**, pp. 180–186.

Lin, L., Wu, T., Porway, J., and Xu, Z. (2009b). A stochastic graph grammar for compositional object representation and recognition, *Pattern Recognition* **42**, pp. 1297–1307.

Lin, Q., Adepu, S., Verver, S., and Mathur, A. (2018). TABOR: A graphical model-based approach for anomaly detection in industrial control systems, in *Proc. Asia Conf. on Computer and Communications Security*, pp. 525–536.

Lin, Q., Hammerschmidt, C., Pellegrino, G., and Verver, S. (2016). Short-term time series forecasting with regression automata, in *Proc. 22nd ACM SIGKDD Conf. Knowledge Discovery and Data Mining*.

Lin, W. C. and Fu, K. S. (1982). Conversion and parsing of tree transducers for syntactic pattern analysis, *International Journal of Computer and Information Sciences* **11**, pp. 417–458.

Lin, W. C. and Fu, K. S. (1984a). 3D-plex grammars, *Information Sciences* **34**, pp. 1–24.

Lin, W. C. and Fu, K. S. (1984b). A syntactic approach to 3-D object representation, *IEEE Trans. Pattern Analysis and Machine Intelligence* **6**, pp. 351–364.

Lin, W. C. and Fu, K. S. (1986). A syntactic approach to three-dimensional object recognition, *IEEE Trans. Systems, Man, and Cybernetics* **16**, pp. 405–422.

Liu, H. H. and Fu, K. S. (1982). A syntactic approach to seismic pattern recognition, *IEEE Trans. Pattern Analysis and Machine Intelligence* **4**, pp. 136–140.

Liu, H. H. and Fu, K. S. (1983). An application of syntactic pattern recognition to seismic discrimination, *IEEE Trans. Geoscience and Remote Sensing* **21**, pp. 125–132.

Liu, T., Chaudhuri, S., Kim, V. G., Huang, Q., Mitra, N. J., and Funkhouser, T. (2014). Creating consistent scene graphs using a probabilistic grammar, *ACM Trans. on Graphics* **33**:211.

Liu, X., Zhao, Y., and Zhu, S. C. (2018). Single-view 3D scene reconstruction and parsing by attribute grammar, *IEEE Trans. Pattern Analysis and Machine Intelligence* **40**, pp. 710–725.

Lonati, V. and Pradella, M. (2010). Deterministic recognizability of picture languages with Wang automata, *Discrete Mathematics and Theoretical Computer Science* **12**, pp. 73–94.

López, D., Calera-Rubio, J., and Gallego-Sánchez (2012). Inference of k-testable directed acyclic graph languages, in *Proc. 11th Int. Conf. on Grammatical Inference* (Washington, D.C., USA), pp. 149–163.

López, D. and España, S. (2002). Error-correcting tree language inference, *Pattern Recognition Letters* **23**, pp. 1–12.

López, D. and Piñaga, I. (2000). Syntactic pattern recognition by error correcting analysis on tree automata, *Lecture Notes in Computer Science* **1876**, pp. 133–142.

López, D. and Sempere, J. M. (1998). Handwritten digit recognition through inferring graph grammars. A first approach, *Lecture Notes in Computer Science* **1451**, pp. 483–491.

López, D., Sempere, J. M., and García, P. (2000). Error correcting analysis for tree languages, *International Journal of Pattern Recognition and Artificial Intelligence* **14**, pp. 357–368.

López, D., Sempere, J. M., and García, P. (2004). Inference of reversible tree languages, *IEEE Trans. Systems, Man, and Cybernetics – Part B: Cybernetics* **34**, pp. 1658–1665.

Lottaz, C., Iseli, C., Jongeneel, C. V., and Bucher, P. (2003). Modeling sequencing errors by combining hidden Markov models, *Bioinformatics* **19** (Suppl. 2), pp. i103–i112.

Lu, H. R. and Fu, K. S. (1984a). A general approach to inference of context-free programmed grammars, *IEEE Trans. Systems, Man, and Cybernetics* **14**, pp. 191–202.

Lu, H. R. and Fu, K. S. (1984b). Inferability of context-free programmed grammars, *International Journal of Computer and Information Sciences* **13**, pp. 33–58.

Lu, S. Y. and Fu, K. S. (1976). Structure-preserved error-correcting tree automata for syntactic pattern recognition, in *Proc. IEEE Conf. on Decision and Control* (Clearwater, FL, USA), pp. 413–419.

Lu, S. Y. and Fu, K. S. (1977). Stochastic error-correcting syntax analysis for recognition of noisy patterns, *IEEE Trans. Computers* **26**, pp. 1268–1276.

Lu, S. Y. and Fu, K. S. (1978). Error-correcting tree automata for syntactic pattern recognition, *IEEE Trans. Computers* **27**, pp. 1040–1053.

Lu, S. Y. and Fu, K. S. (1979). Stochastic tree grammar inference for texture synthesis and discrimination, *Computer Graphics and Image Processing* **9**, pp. 234–245.

Lucas, S. M. and Reynolds, T. J. (2005). Learning deterministic finite automata with a smart state labeling evolutionary algorithm, *IEEE Trans. Pattern Analysis and Machine Intelligence* **27**, pp. 1063–1074.

Luh, R., Schramm, G., Wagner, M., Janicke, H., and Schrittwieser, S. (2018). SEQUIN: a grammar inference framework for analyzing malicious system behavior, *Journal of Computer Virology and Hacking Techniques* **14**.

Lunze, J. and Schröder, J. (2001). State observation and diagnosis of discrete-event systems described by stochastic automata, *Discrete Event Dynamic Systems* **11**, pp. 319–369.

Lunze, J. and Supavatanakul, P. (2002). Diagnosis of discrete-event system described by timed automata, in *Proc. 15th IFAC World Congress* (Barcelona, Spain), pp. 77–82.

Luo, S. and Zhou, G. (1992). Attribute grammar for analysis of ECG arrhythmias, in *Proc. 14th IEEE Int. Conf. of IEEE Engineering in Medicine and Biology Society* (Paris, France), pp. 787–788.

Lynch, M. F., Barnard, J. M., and Welford, S. M. (1981). Computer storage and retrieval of generic chemical structures in patents, 1. Introduction and general strategy, *Journal of Chemical Information and Computer Sciences* **21**, pp. 148–150.

Lyngso, R. B. and Pedersen, C. N. (2000). RNA pseudoknot prediction in energy-based models, *Journal of Computational Biology* **7**, pp. 409–427.

Maier, A., Niggemann, O., Just, R., Jäger, M., and Vodenčarević, A. (2011). Anomaly detection in production plants using timed automata, in *Proc. 8th International Conference on Informatics in Control, Automation and Robotics* (Noordwijkerhout, The Netherlands), pp. 363–369.

Majoros, W. H., Pertea, M., Delcher, A. L., and Salzberg, S. L. (2005). Efficient decoding algorithms for generalized hidden Markov model gene finders, *BMC Bioinformatics* **6**:16.

Majumdar, A. K. and Ray, A. K. (2001). Syntactic pattern recognition, in S. K. Pal and A. Pal (eds.), *Pattern Recognition: From Classical to Modern Approaches* (World Scientific, New Jersey - London - Singapore), pp. 185–229.

Majumdar, A. K. and Roy, A. K. (1983). Inference of fuzzy regular pattern grammar, *Pattern Recognition Letters* **2**, pp. 27–32.

Mak, R. (2009). *Writing Compilers and Interpreters* (Wiley, Indianapolis).

Malaviya, A. and Peters, L. (2000). Fuzzy handwriting description language: FOHDEL, *Pattern Recognition* **33**, pp. 119–131.

Malik, D. S. and Mordeson, J. N. (1996). On fuzzy regular languages, *Information Sciences* **88**, pp. 263–273.

Mamitsuka, H. and Abe, N. (1994). Predicting location and structure of beta-sheet regions using stochastic tree grammars, in *Proc. 2nd Int. Conf. on Intelligent Systems for Molecular Biology* (Stanford, CA, USA), pp. 276–284.

Mandorli, F., Otto, H. E., and Kimura, F. (1993). A reference kernel model for feature-based CAD systems supported by conditional attribute rewrite systems, in *Proc. 2nd ACM Symp. on Solid Modelling and Applications* (Montreal, Canada), pp. 343–354.

Mann, M., Ekker, H., and Flamm, C. (2013). The graph grammar library - a generic framework for chemical graph rewrite systems, *Lecture Notes in Computer Science* **7909**, pp. 52–53.

Manning, C. D. and Schütze, H. (2003). *Foundations of Statistical Natural Language Processing* (MIT Press, Cambridge, MA).

Marcus, S. (1969). Contextual grammars, *Rev. Roum. Math. Pures Appl.* **14**, pp. 1525–1534.

Markov, A. A. (1913). Essai d'une recherche statistique sur le texte du roman *Eugene Onegin* illustrant la liaison des epreuve en chain, *Bulletin de l'Académie Impériale des Sciences de St.-Pétersbourg* **7**, pp. 153–162.

Marques de Sá, J. P. (2001). *Pattern Recognition. Concepts, Methods and Applications* (Springer-Verlag, Berlin-Heidelberg-New York).

Marr, D. (1982). *Vision: A Computational Investigation into the Human Representation and Processing of Visual Information* (W.H. Freeman, San Francisco).

Marriott, K. (1994). Constraint multiset grammars, in *Proc. 10th IEEE Symposium on Visual Languages* (St. Louis, MO, USA), pp. 118–127.

Marriott, K. (1995). Parsing visual languages with constraint multiset grammars, *Lecture Notes in Computer Science* **982**, pp. 24–25.

Marriott, K. and Meyer, B. (1997). On the classification of visual languages by grammar hierarchies, *Journal of Visual Languages and Computing* **8**, pp. 375–402.

Marriott, K. and Meyer, B. (eds.) (1998). *Visual Language Theory* (Springer, New York).

Marti, U. V. and Bunke, H. (2001). Using a statistical language model to improve the performance of an HMM-based cursive handwriting recognition system, *International Journal of Pattern Recognition and Artificial Intelligence* **15**, pp. 65–90.

Martinović, A. and Gool Van, L. (2013). Bayesian grammar learning for inverse procedural modeling, in *Proc. 2013 IEEE Conf. on Computer Vision and Pattern Recognition* (Portland, OR, USA), pp. 201–208.

Maryanski, F. J. and Booth, T. L. (1977). Inference of finite-state probabilistic grammars, *IEEE Trans. Computers* **26**, pp. 521–536.

Mas, J., Jorge, J. A. P., Sánchez, G., and Lladós, J. (2008). Representing and parsing sketched symbols using Adjacency Grammars and a grid-directed parser, *Lecture Notes in Computer Science* **5046**, pp. 169–180.

Mas, J., Lladós, J., Sánchez, G., and Jorge, J. A. P. (2010). A syntactic approach based on distortion-tolerant Adjacency Grammars and a spatial-directed parser to interpret sketched diagrams, *Pattern Recognition* **43**, pp. 4148–4164.

Masini, G. and Mohr, R. (1983). Mirabelle, a system for structural analysis of drawings, *Pattern Recognition* **16**, pp. 363–372.

Mathias, M., Martinović, A., Weissenberg, J., and Gool Van, L. (2011). Procedural 3D building reconstruction using shape grammars and detectors, in *Proc. 2011 International Conference on 3D Imaging, Modeling, Processing, Visualization and Transmission* (Hangzhou, China), pp. 304–311.

Matsui, H., Sato, K., and Sakakibara, Y. (2005). Pair stochastic tree adjoining grammars for aligning and predicting pseudoknot RNA structures, *Bioinformatics* **21**, pp. 2611–2617.

Matz, O. (1997). Regular expressions and context-free grammars for picture languages, *Lecture Notes in Computer Science* **1200**, pp. 283–294.

Matz, O. (2002). Dot-depth, monadic quantifier alternation, and first-order closure over grids and pictures, *Theoretical Computer Science* **270**, pp. 1–70.

Maurer, H. A., Rozenberg, G., and Welzl, E. (1982). Using string languages to describe picture languages, *Information and Control* **54**, pp. 155–185.

Maurer, H. A., Rozenberg, G., and Welzl, E. (1983). Chain-code picture languages, *Lecture Notes in Computer Science* **153**, pp. 232–244.

Maurer, H. A., Salomaa, A., and Wood, D. (1980). Pure grammars, *Information and Control* **44**, pp. 47–72.

Mäurer, I. (2007). Characterizations of recognizable picture series, *Theoretical Computer Science* **374**, pp. 214–228.

May, J. and Knight, K. (2006). Tiburon: A weighted tree automata toolkit, *Lecture Notes in Computer Science* **4094**, pp. 102–113.

Mazanek, S. and Minas, M. (2008). Functional-logic graph parser combinators, *Lecture Notes in Computer Science* **5117**, pp. 261–275.

Meduna, A. (2014). *Formal Languages and Computation: Models and Their Applications* (CRC Press, Boca Raton, FL).

Miao, Q. and Makis, V. (2007). Condition monitoring and classification of rotating machinery using wavelets and hidden Markov models, *Mechanical Systems and Signal Processing* **21**, pp. 840–855.

Mickunas, M. D., Lancaster, R. L., and Schneider, V. B. (1976). Transforming LR(k) grammars to LR(1), SLR(1), and (1,1) bounded right-context grammars, *Journal of the Association for Computing Machinery* **23**, pp. 511–533.

Miclet, L. (1980). Regular inference with a tail-clustering method, *IEEE Trans. Systems, Man, and Cybernetics* **10**, pp. 737–743.

Milgram, D. L. and Rosenfeld, A. (1971). Array automata and array grammars, in *Proc. IFIP Congress on Information Processing* (North-Holland, Ljubljana, Yugoslavia), pp. 69–74.

Miller, L. G. and Levinson, S. E. (1988). Syntactic analysis for large vocabulary speech recognition using a context-free covering grammar, in *Proc. 1988 Int. Conf. on Acoustics, Speech, and Signal Processing* (New York, NY), pp. 271–274.

Min, W., Tang, Z., and Tang, L. (1993). Using web grammar to recognize dimensions in engineering drawings, *Pattern Recognition* **26**, pp. 1407–1416.

Minnen, D., Essa, I., and Starner, T. (2003). Expectation grammars: leveraging high-level expectations for activity recognition, in *Proc. 2003 IEEE Conf. on Computer Vision and Pattern Recognition* (Madison, WI, USA), pp. 626–632.

Mizumoto, M., Toyoda, J., and Tanaka, K. (1969). Some considerations on fuzzy automata, *Journal of Computer and System Sciences* **3**, pp. 409–422.

Mizumoto, M., Toyoda, J., and Tanaka, K. (1972). General formulation of formal grammars, *Information Sciences* **4**, pp. 87–100.

Mizumoto, M., Toyoda, J., and Tanaka, K. (1975). Various kinds of automata with weights, *Journal of Computer and System Sciences* **10**, pp. 219–236.

Moayer, B. and Fu, K. S. (1975). A syntactic approach to fingerprint pattern recognition, *Pattern Recognition* **7**, pp. 1–23.

Moayer, B. and Fu, K. S. (1976a). An application of stochastic languages to fingerprint pattern recognition, *Pattern Recognition* **8**, pp. 173–179.

Moayer, B. and Fu, K. S. (1976b). A tree system approach for fingerprint pattern recognition, *IEEE Trans. Computers* **25**, pp. 262–274.

Mohandes, M., Deriche, M., Johar, U., and Ilyas, S. (2012). A signer-independent Arabic Sign Language recognition system using face detection, geometric features, and a Hidden Markov Model, *Computers and Electrical Engineering* **38**, pp. 422–433.

Mohri, M. (1997). Finite-state transducers in language and speech processing, *Computational Linguistics* **23**, pp. 269–312.

Mohri, M., Pereira, F., and Riley, M. (1996). Weighted automata in text and speech processing, in *Proc. 12th Biennial European Conf. on Artificial Intelligence* (Budapest, Hungary), pp. 559–584.

Mohri, M., Pereira, F., and Riley, M. (2008). Speech recognition with weighted finite-state transducers, in J. Benesty, M. M. Sondhi, and Y. Huang (eds.), *Handbook on Speech Processing* (Springer, Heidelberg).

Montanari, U. (1970). Separable graphs, planar graphs and web grammars, *Information and Control* **16**, pp. 243–267.

Montanari, U. (1974). Networks of constraints: fundamental properties and applications to picture processing, *Information Sciences* **17**, pp. 95–132.

Montanari, U. and Ribeiro, L. (2002). Linear ordered graph grammars and their algebraic foundations, *Lecture Notes in Computer Science* **2505**, pp. 317–333.

Moore, D. and Essa, I. (20032). Recognizing multitasked activities from video using stochastic context-free grammar, in *Proc. 18th AAAI National Conference on Artificial Intelligence* (Edmonton, Alberta, Canada), pp. 770–776.

Mordeson, J. N. and Malik, D. S. (2002). *Fuzzy Automata and Languages, Theory and Applications* (Chapman and Hall/CRC, London/Boca Raton).

Mori De, R. (1972). A descriptive technique for automatic speech recognition, *IEEE Trans. Audio and Electroacoustic* **21**, pp. 89–100.

Mori De, R., Laface, P., Makhonine, V. A., and Mezzalama, M. (1977). A syntactic procedure for the recognition of glottal pulses in continuous speech, *Pattern Recognition* **9**, pp. 181–189.

Muchnick, S. (1997). *Advanced Compiler Design and Implementation* (Morgan Kaufmann, San Francisco).

Muchnik, I. B. (1972). Simulation of process of forming the language for description and analysis of the forms of images, *Pattern Recognition* **4**, pp. 101–140.

Mude Van Der, A. and Walker, A. (1978). On the inference of stochastic regular grammars, *Information and Control* **38**, pp. 310–329.

Muggleton, S., Bryant, C., Srinivasan, A., Whittaker, A., Topp, S., and Rawlings, C. (2001). Are grammatical representations useful for learning from biological sequence data? *Journal of Computational Biology* **8**, pp. 493–522.

Mukherjee, S. and Oates, T. (2008). Estimating graph parameters using graph grammars, *Lecture Notes in Computer Science* **5278**, pp. 292–294.

Mukherjee, S. and Oates, T. (2010). Inferring probability distributions of graph size and node degree from stochastic graph grammars, in *Proc. SIAM Int. Conf. on Data Mining* (Columbus, OH, USA), pp. 490–501.

Müller, P., Zeng, G., Wonka, P., and Gool Van, L. (2007). Image-based procedural modeling of facades, *ACM Trans. on Graphics* **26**:85.

Mullins, S. and Rinderle, J. R. (1991). Grammatical approaches to engineering design, Part I: An introduction and commentary, *Research in Engineering Design* **2**, pp. 121–135.

Mumford, D. (1996). Pattern theory: A unifying perspective, in D. Knill and W. Richards (eds.), *Perception as Bayesian Inference* (Cambridge University Press, Cambridge).

Mumford, D. (2002). Pattern theory: the mathematics of perception, in *Proc. Int. Congress of Mathematicians* (Beijing, China), pp. 401–422.

Munch, K. and Krogh, A. (2006). Automatic generation of gene finders for eukaryotic species, *BMC Bioinformatics* **7**:263.

Muñoz-Salinas, R., Medina-Carnicer, R., Madrid-Cuevas, F. J., and Carmona-Poyato, A. (2008). Depth silhouettes for gesture recognition, *Pattern Recognition Letters* **29**, pp. 319–329.

Murgue, T. and Higuera de la, C. (2004). Distances between distributions: comparing language models, *Lecture Notes in Computer Science* **3138**, pp. 269–277.

Musialski, P., Wonka, P., Aliaga, D. G., Wimmer, M., Gool Van, L., and Purgathofer, W. (2013). A survey of urban reconstruction, *Computer Graphics Forum* **32**, pp. 146–177.

Myers, D. G. and DeWall, C. N. (2018). *Psychology* (Worth Publishers, New York).

Myhill, J. (1960). Linear bounded automata, Tech. Rep. WADD 60–165, Wright-Patterson Air Force Base, Ohio.

Mylopoulos, J. (1972a). On the application of formal language and automata theory to pattern recognition, *Pattern Recognition* **4**, pp. 37–51.

Mylopoulos, J. (1972b). On the recognition of topological invariants by 4-way finite automata, *Computer Graphics and Image Processing* **1**, pp. 71–88.

Nagahashi, H. and Kakatsuyama, M. (1986). A pattern description and generation method of structural characters, *IEEE Trans. Pattern Analysis and Machine Intelligence* **8**, pp. 112–118.

Nakamura, A. (2001). Picture languages, in L. S. Davis (ed.), *Foundations of Image Understanding* (Springer, Boston, MA), pp. 127–155.

Nakamura, K. and Matsumoto, M. (2005). Incremental learning of context free grammars based on bottom-up parsing and search, *Pattern Recognition* **38**, pp. 1384–1392.

Narasimhan, R. N. (1964). Labeling schemata and syntactic descriptions of pictures, *Information and Control* **7**, pp. 151–179.

Narasimhan, R. N. (1966). Syntax-directed interpretation of classes of pictures, *Communications of the Association for Computing Machinery* **9**, pp. 166–173.

Narasimhan, R. N. and Reddy, V. S. N. (1971). A syntax-aided recognition scheme for handprinted English letters, *Pattern Recognition* **3**, pp. 345–361.

Ney, H. (1991). Dynamic programming parsing for context-free grammars in continuous speech recognition, *IEEE Trans. Signal Processing* **39**, pp. 336–340.

Nguyen, N. T., Phung, D. Q., Venkatesh, S., and Bui, H. (2005). Learning and detecting activities from movement trajectories using the hierarchical hidden Markov models, in *Proc. 2005 IEEE Conf. on Computer Vision and Pattern Recognition* (San Diego, CA, USA), pp. 955–960.

Niggemann, O., Stein, B., Maier, A., Vodenčarević, A., and Büning, H. K. (2012). Learning behavior models for hybrid timed systems, in *Proc. 26th AAAI Conf. on Artificial Intelligence* (Toronto, Ontario, Canada), pp. 1083–1090.

Nivat, M. and Saoudi, A. (1992). Parallel recognition of high dimensional images, *International Journal of Pattern Recognition and Artificial Intelligence* **6**, pp. 285–291.

Nivat, M., Saoudi, A., Subramanian, K. G., and Dare, V. R. (1991). Puzzle grammars and context-free array grammars, *International Journal of Pattern Recognition and Artificial Intelligence* **5**, pp. 663–676.

Noord van, G. (1994). Head-corner parsing for TAG, *Computational Intelligence* **10**, pp. 525–534.

Oates, T., Desai, D., and Bhat, V. (2002). Learning k-reversible context-free grammars from positive structural examples, in *Proc. Int. Conference on Machine Learning* (San Francisco, USA), pp. 459–465.

Oates, T., Doshi, S., and Huang, F. (2003). Estimating maximum likelihood parameters for stochastic context-free graph grammars, *Lecture Notes in Artificial Intelligence* **2835**, pp. 281–298.

Ogiela, M. R. and Piekarczyk, M. (2012). Random graph languages for distorted and ambiguous patterns: single layer model, in *Proc. 6th Int. Conf. on Innovative Mobile and Internet Services in Ubiquitous Computing* (Palermo, Italy), pp. 108–113.

Ogiela, M. R. and Tadeusiewicz, R. (1999). Syntactic analysis and languages of shape feature description in computer-aided diagnosis and recognition of cancerous and inflammatory lesions of organs in selected X-ray images, *Journal of Digital Imaging* **12**, pp. 24–27.

Ogiela, M. R. and Tadeusiewicz, R. (2002). Syntactic reasoning and pattern recognition for analysis of coronary artery images, *Artificial Intelligence in Medicine* **26**, pp. 145–159.

Ogiela, M. R. and Tadeusiewicz, R. (2003). Artificial intelligence structural imaging techniques in visual pattern analysis and medical data understanding, *Pattern Recognition* **36**, pp. 2441–2452.

Ogiela, M. R., Tadeusiewicz, R., and Ogiela, L. (2006). Image languages in intelligent radiological palm diagnostics, *Pattern Recognition* **39**, pp. 2157–2165.

Okhotin, A. (2001). Conjunctive grammars, *Journal of Automata, Languages and Combinatorics* **6**, pp. 519–535.

Okhotin, A. (2003). A recognition and parsing algorithm for arbitrary conjunctive grammars, *Theoretical Computer Science* **302**, pp. 81–124.

Okhotin, A. (2004). Boolean grammars, *Information and Computation* **194**, pp. 19–48.

Okhotin, A. (2010). Fast parsing for Boolean grammars: a generalization of Valiant's algorithm, *Lecture Notes in Computer Science* **6224**, pp. 340–351.

Omlin, C. W. and Giles, C. L. (1996). Extraction of rules from discrete-time recurrent neural networks, *Neural Networks* **9**, pp. 41–52.

Oncina, J. (1996). The Cocke-Younger-Kasami algorithm for cyclic strings, in *Proc. 13th IAPR Int. Conf. on Pattern Recognition* (Vienna, Austria), pp. 413–416.

Oncina, J. and García, P. (1992). Identifying regular languages in polynomial time, in H. Bunke (ed.), *Advances in Structural and Syntactic Pattern Recognition* (World Scientific, Singapore).

Oncina, J., García, P., and Vidal, E. (1993). Learning subsequential transducers for pattern recognition interpretation tasks, *IEEE Trans. Pattern Analysis and Machine Intelligence* **15**, pp. 448–458.

Oommen, B. J. and Kashyap, R. L. (1998). A formal theory for optimal and information theoretic syntactic pattern recognition, *Pattern Recognition* **31**, pp. 1159–1177.

Oommen, B. J. and Loke, R. K. S. (1997). Pattern recognition of strings with substitutions, insertions, deletions and generalized transpositions, *Pattern Recognition* **30**, pp. 789–800.

Ozveren, C. M. and Willsky, A. S. (1990). Observability of discrete event dynamic systems, *IEEE Trans. Automatic Control* **35**, pp. 797–806.

Pachter, L., M., A., and Cawley, S. (2002). Applications of generalized pair hidden Markov models to alignment and gene finding problems, *Journal of Computational Biology* **9**, pp. 389–399.

Pagallo, G. (1998). Constrained attribute grammars for recognition of multi-dimensional objects, *Lecture Notes in Computer Science* **1451**, pp. 359–365.

Papakonstantinou, G., Skordalakis, E., and Gritzali, F. (1986). An attribute grammar for QRS detection, *Pattern Recognition* **19**, pp. 297–303.

Parikh, R. J. (1966). On context-free languages, *Journal of the Association for Computing Machinery* **13**, pp. 570–581.

Parizeau, M. and Plamondon, R. (1992). A handwriting model for syntactic recognition of cursive script, in *Proc. 11th IAPR Int. Conf. on Pattern Recognition* (The Hague, Netherlands), pp. 308–312.

Parizeau, M. and Plamondon, R. (1995). A fuzzy-syntactic approach to allograph modeling for cursive script recognition, *IEEE Trans. Pattern Analysis and Machine Intelligence* **17**, pp. 702–712.

Parizeau, M., Plamondon, R., and Lorette, G. (1992). Fuzzy-shape grammars for cursive script recognition, in *Proc. Int. Workshop on Structural, Syntactic, and Statistical Pattern Recognition* (Bern, Switzerland), pp. 320–332.

Park, S., Nie, B. X., and Zhu, S. C. (2018). Attribute And-Or grammar for joint parsing of human attributes, part and pose, *IEEE Trans. Pattern Analysis and Machine Intelligence* **40**, pp. 1555–1569.

Park, S. and Zhu, S. C. (2015). Attributed grammars for joint estimation of human attributes, parts and poses, in *Proc. 2015 IEEE Int. Conf. on Computer Vision* (Santiago, Chile), pp. 2372–2380.

Pathak, A. and Pal, S. K. (1986). Fuzzy grammars in syntactic recognition of skeletal maturity from X-rays, *IEEE Trans. Systems, Man, and Cybernetics* **16**, pp. 657–667.

Pathak, A., Pal, S. K., and King, R. A. (1984). Syntactic recognition of skeletal maturity, *Pattern Recognition Letters* **2**, pp. 193–197.

Pau, L. F. (1991). Technical analysis for portfolio trading by syntactic pattern recognition, *Journal of Economic Dynamics and Control* **15**, pp. 715–730.

Păun, G. (2000). Computing with membranes, *Journal of Computer and System Sciences* **61**, pp. 108–143.

Pavlidis, T. (1968). Analysis of set patterns, *Pattern Recognition* **1**, pp. 165–178.

Pavlidis, T. (1972a). Linear and context-free graph grammars, *Journal of the Association for Computing Machinery* **19**, pp. 11–22.

Pavlidis, T. (1972b). Representation of figures by labeled graphs, *Pattern Recognition* **4**, pp. 5–17.

Pavlidis, T. (1977). *Structural Pattern Recognition* (Springer, New York).

Pavlidis, T. (1980). Structural descriptions and graph grammars, in S. K. Chang and K. S. Fu (eds.), *Pictorial Information Systems* (Springer, Berlin - Heidelberg - New York), pp. 86–103.

Pavlidis, T. (1992). Why progress in machine vision is so slow, *Pattern Recognition Letters* **13**, pp. 221–225.

Pavlidis, T. and Ali, F. (1979). A hierarchical syntactic shape analyzer, *IEEE Trans. Pattern Analysis and Machine Intelligence* **1**, pp. 2–9.

Pearl, J. (1984). *Heuristics: Intelligent Search Strategies for Computer Problem Solving* (Addison-Wesley, Boston).

Pedersen, J. C. and Hein, J. (2003). Gene finding with a hidden Markov model of genome structure and evolution, *Bioinformatics* **19**, pp. 219–227.

Pedrycz, W. (1990). Fuzzy sets in pattern recognition: methodology and methods, *Pattern Recognition* **23**, pp. 121–146.

Pedrycz, W. and Gacek, A. (2001). Learning of fuzzy automata, *International Journal of Computational Intelligence and Applications* **1**, pp. 19–33.

Peeva, K. (1991). Fuzzy acceptors for syntactic pattern recognition, *International Journal of Approximate Reasoning* **5**, pp. 291–306.

Pei, M., Jia, Y., and Zhu, S. C. (2011). Parsing video events with goal inference and intent prediction, in *Proc. 2011 IEEE Conf. on Computer Vision* (Barcelona, Spain), pp. 487–494.

Pei, M., Si, Z., Yao, B. Z., and Zhu, S. C. (2013). Learning and parsing video events with goal and intent prediction, *Computer Vision and Image Understanding* **117**, pp. 1369–1383.

Peng, K. J., Yamamoto, T., and Aoki, Y. (1990). A new parsing scheme for plex grammars, *Pattern Recognition* **23**, pp. 393–402.

Perea, I. and López, D. (2004). Syntactic modeling and recognition of document images, *Lecture Notes in Computer Science* **3138**, pp. 416–424.

Perez-Cortes, J. C., Amengual, J. C., J. Arlandis, J., and Llobet, R. (2000). Stochastic error-correcting parsing for OCR post-processing, in *Proc. 15th IAPR Int. Conf. on Pattern Recognition* (Barcelona, Spain), pp. 405–408.

Peris, P., López, D., and Campos, M. (2008). IgTM: An algorithm to predict transmembrane domains and topology in proteins, *BMC Bioinformatics* **9**:367.

Persoon, E. and Fu, K. S. (1975). Sequential classification of strings generated by SCFGs, *International Journal of Computer and Information Sciences* **4**, pp. 205–218.

Pfaltz, J. L. (1972). Web grammars and picture description, *Computer Graphics and Image Processing* **1**, pp. 193–220.

Pfaltz, J. L. and Rosenfeld, A. (1969). Web grammars, in *Proc. First Int. Conf. Artificial Intelligence* (William Kaufmann), pp. 609–619.

Picó, D., Tomás, J., and Casacuberta, F. (2004). GIATI: A general methodology for finite-state translation using alignments, *Lecture Notes in Computer Science* **3138**, pp. 216–223.

Pollard, C. (1984). *Generalized Phrase Structure Grammars, Head Grammars, and Natural Language*, Ph.D. thesis, Stanford University, Stanford, USA.

Poller, P. (1994). Incremental parsing with LD/TLP-TAGs, *Computational Intelligence* **10**, pp. 549–562.

Prabhu, B. S. (1999). Automatic extraction of manufacturable features from CADD models using syntactic pattern recognition techniques, *International Journal of Production Research* **37**, pp. 1259–1281.

Pradella, M., Cherubini, A., and Crespi-Reghizzi, S. (2011). A unifying approach to picture grammars, *Information and Computation* **209**, pp. 1246–1267.

Pradella, M. and Crespi-Reghizzi, S. (2008). A SAT-based parser and completer for pictures specified by tiling, *Pattern Recognition* **41**, pp. 555–566.

Pratt, T. W. (1971). Pair grammars, graph languages and string-to-graph translations, *Journal of Computer and System Sciences* **5**, pp. 560–595.

Pratt, W. K. (2013). *Introduction to Digital Image Processing* (CRC Press, Boca Raton).

Prewitt, J. M. S. (1979). Graphs and grammars for histology: An introduction, in *Proc. 3rd Annual Symposium on Computer Applications in Medical Care* (Washington, D.C., USA), pp. 18–25.

Priesterjahn, S., Anderka, M., Klerx, T., and Mönks, U. (2015). Generalized ATM fraud detection, *Lecture Notes in Computer Science* **9165**, pp. 166–181.

Prophetis De, L. and Varricchio, S. (1997). Recognizability of rectangular pictures by Wang systems, *Journal of Automata, Languages and Combinatorics* **2**, pp. 269–288.

Proschak, E., Wegner, J. K., Schuller, A., Schneider, G., and Fechner, U. (2007). Molecular query language (MQL) - a context-free grammar for substructure matching, *Journal of Chemical Information and Modeling* **47**, pp. 295–301.

Przytycka, T., Srinivasan, R., and Rose, G. D. (2002). Recursive domains in proteins, *Protein Science* **11**, pp. 409–417.

Qi, S., Huang, S., Wei, P., and Zhu, S. C. (2017). Predicting human activities using stochastic grammar, in *Proc. 2017 IEEE Int. Conf. on Computer Vision* (Venice, Italy), pp. 1173–1181.

Rabin, M. O. (1963). Probabilistic automata, *Information and Control* **6**, pp. 230–245.

Rabin, M. O. (1969). Decidability of second-order theories and automata on infinite trees, *Trans. American Mathematical Society* **141**, pp. 1–35.

Rabin, M. O. and Scott, D. (1959). Finite automata and their decision problems, *IBM J. Research Development* **3**, pp. 114–125.

Rabiner, L. R. (1989). A tutorial on Hidden Markov Model and selected applications in speech recognition, *Proceedings of the IEEE* **72**, pp. 257–286.

Rabiner, L. R. and Juang, B. H. (1993). *Fundamentals of Speech Recognition* (Prentice Hall, Englewood Cliffs).

Radhakrishnan, V. and Nagaraja, G. (1987). Inference of regular grammars via skeletons, *IEEE Trans. Systems, Man, and Cybernetics* **17**, pp. 982–992.

Radhakrishnan, V. and Nagaraja, G. (1988). Inference of even linear grammars and its application to picture description languages, *Pattern Recognition* **21**, pp. 55–62.

Raisch, J. (2013). Modelling of engineering phenomena by finite automata, *Lecture Notes in Computer and Information Science* **433**, pp. 3–22.

Ramadge, P. J. and Wonham, W. M. (1987). Supervisory control of a class of discrete event processes, *SIAM Journal of Control and Optimization* **25**, pp. 206–230.

Ramamoorthy, A., Vaswani, N., Chaudhury, S., and Banerjee, S. (2003). Recognition of dynamic hand gestures, *Pattern Recognition* **36**, pp. 2069–2081.

Rangarajan, A. (2014). Revisioning the unification of syntax, semantics and statistics in shape analysis, *Pattern Recognition Letters* **43**, pp. 39–46.

Rao, K. and Balck, K. (1980). Type classification of fingerprints: a syntactic approach, *IEEE Trans. Pattern Analysis and Machine Intelligence* **2**, pp. 223–231.

Reese, M. G., Kulp, D., Tammana, H., and Haussler, D. (2000). *Genie* - gene finding in *Drosophila melanogaster*, *Genome Research* **10**, pp. 529–538.

Reisberg, D. (ed.) (2013). *The Oxford Handbook of Cognitive Psychology* (Oxford University Press, Oxford).

Rekers, J. and Schürr, A. (1997). Defining and parsing visual languages with layered graph grammars, *Journal of Visual Languages and Computing* **8**, pp. 27–55.

Rengaswamy, R. and Venkatasubramanian, V. (1995). A syntactic pattern-recognition approach for process monitoring and fault diagnosis, *Engineering Applications of Artificial Intelligence* **8**, pp. 35–51.

Resnick, P. (1992). Probabilistic tree-adjoining grammars as framework for statistical natural language processing, in *Proc. 15th Int. Conf. on Computational Linguistics* (Nantes, France), pp. 418–424.

Ribeiro, L. and Dotti, F. L. (2008). Linear ordered graph grammars: Applications to distributed systems design, *Lecture Notes in Computer Science* **5065**, pp. 133–150.

Richetin, M. and Vernadet, F. (1984). Efficient regular grammatical inference for pattern recognition, *Pattern Recognition* **17**, pp. 245–250.

Rico-Juan, J. R., Calera-Rubio, J., and Carrasco, R. C. (2005). Smoothing and compression with stochastic k-testable tree languages, *Pattern Recognition* **38**, pp. 1420–1430.

Riemenschneider, H., Krispel, U., Thaller, W., Donoser, M., Havemann, S., Fellner, D., and Bischof, H. (2012). Irregular lattices for complex shape grammar facade parsing, in *Proc. 2012 IEEE Conf. on Computer Vision and Pattern Recognition* (Providence, RI, USA), pp. 1640–1647.

Rinderle, J. R. (1991). Grammatical approaches to engineering design, Part II: Melding configuration and parametric design using attribute grammars, *Research in Engineering Design* **2**, pp. 137–146.

Ripley, B. D. (2008). *Pattern Recognition and Neural Networks* (Cambridge University Press, Cambridge).

Ripperda, N. and Brenner, C. (2007). Data driven rule proposal for grammar based façade reconstruction, *The International Archives of the Photogrammetry, Remote Sensing and Spatial Information* **36**, pp. 1–6.

Ritchings, R. T. and Colchester, A. C. F. (1986). Detection of abnormalities on carotid angiograms using syntactic techniques, *Pattern Recognition Letters* **4**, pp. 367–374.

Rivas, E. and Eddy, S. R. (2000). The language of RNA: a formal grammar that includes pseudoknots, *Bioinformatics* **16**, pp. 334–340.

Rivas, E. and Eddy, S. R. (2001). Noncoding RNA gene detection using comparative sequence analysis, *BMC Bioinformatics* **2**:8.

Rivoira, S. and Torasso, P. (1978). An isolated-word recognizer based on grammar-controlled classification processes, *Pattern Recognition* **10**, pp. 73–84.

Rivoira, S. and Torasso, P. (1982). The lexical, syntactic and semantic processing of a speech recognition system, *International Journal of Man-Machine Studies* **16**, pp. 39–63.

Rosenblueth, D. A., Thieffry, D., Huerta, A. M., Salgado, H., and Collado-Vides, J. (1996). Syntactic recognition of regulatory regions in *Escherichia coli*, *Computer Applications in the Biosciences* **12**, pp. 15–22.

Rosenfeld, A. (1971). Isotonic grammars, parallel grammars, and picture generation, in B. Meltzer and E. Michie (eds.), *Machine Intelligence 6* (Edinburgh University Press, Edinburgh), pp. 281–294.

Rosenfeld, A. (1973). Array grammar normal forms, *Information and Control* **23**, pp. 173–182.

Rosenfeld, A. (1976). Some notes on finite-state picture languages, *Information and Control* **31**, pp. 177–184.

Rosenfeld, A. (1979). *Picture Languages - Formal Models for Picture Recognition* (Academic Press, New York).

Rosenfeld, A. (1989). Coordinate grammars revisited: generalized isometric grammars, in P. S. P. Wang (ed.), *Array Grammars, Patterns and Recognizers* (World Scientific, Singapore - New Jersey - London), pp. 157–166.

Rosenfeld, A. and Kak, A. (1982). *Digital Picture Processing* (Academic Press, New York).

Rosenfeld, A. and Milgram, D. L. (1972). Web automata and web grammars, in B. Meltzer and E. Michie (eds.), *Machine Intelligence 7* (Edinburgh University Press, Edinburgh), pp. 307–324.

Rosenkrantz, D. J. (1969). Programmed grammars and classes of formal languages, *Journal of the Association for Computing Machinery* **16**, pp. 107–131.

Rosenkrantz, D. J. and Stearns, R. E. (1970). Properties of deterministic top-down grammars, *Information and Control* **17**, pp. 226–256.

Rosselló, F. and Valiente, G. (2005). Chemical graphs, chemical reaction graphs, and chemical graph transformation, *Electronic Notes in Theoretical Computer Science* **127**, pp. 157–166.

Rothrock, B., Park, S., and Zhu, S. C. (2013). Integrating grammar and segmentation for human pose estimation, in *Proc. 2013 IEEE Conf. on Computer Vision and Pattern Recognition* (Portland, OR, USA), pp. 3214–3221.

Rounds, W. (1968). *Trees, transducers and transformations*, Ph.D. thesis, Stanford University, Stanford, USA.

Rounds, W. C. (1970). Mappings and grammars on trees, *Mathematical Systems Theory* **4**, pp. 257–287.

Rozenberg, G. (ed.) (1997). *Handbook of Graph Grammars and Computing by Graph Transformation, Vol. 1: Foundations* (World Scientific, Singapore).

Rozenberg, G. and Salomaa, A. (eds.) (1997). *Handbook of Formal Languages, vol. I, II, III* (Springer, Berlin-Heidelberg).

Rozenberg, G. and Welzl, E. (1986). Boundary NLC graph grammars - basic definitions, normal forms, and complexity, *Information and Control* **69**, pp. 136–167.

Rulot, H. and Vidal, E. (1988). An efficient algorithm for the inference of circuit-free automata, in G. Ferrate, T. Pavlidis, A. Sanfeliu, and H. Bunke (eds.), *Syntactic and Structural Pattern Recognition* (Springer, Berlin-Heidelberg), pp. 173–184.

Russell, S. J. and Norvig, P. (2009). *Artificial Intelligence. A Modern Approach* (Prentice Hall, Englewood Cliffs).

Ryoo, M. S. and Aggarwal, J. K. (2006). Recognition of composite human activities through context-free grammar based representation, in *Proc. 2006 IEEE Conf. on Computer Vision and Pattern Recognition* (New York, NY, USA), pp. 1709–1718.

Sadeghipour, A. and Kopp, S. (2014). A hybrid grammar-based approach for learning and recognizing natural hand gestures, in *Proc. 28th AAAI Conference on Artificial Intelligence* (Quebec City, Canada), pp. 2069–2077.

Sagar, S. and Sidorova, J. (2016). Sequence retriever for known, discovered, and user-specified molecular fragments, *Advances in Intelligent Systems and Computing* **477**, pp. 51–58.

Sainz, M. and Alquezar, R. (1996). Learning bidimensional context-dependent models using a context-sensitive language, in *Proc. 13th IAPR Int. Conf. on Pattern Recognition* (Vienna, Austria), pp. 565–569.

Sakakibara, Y. (1990). Learning context-free grammars from structural data in polynomial time, *Theoretical Computer Science* **76**, pp. 223–242.

Sakakibara, Y. (1992). Efficient learning of context-free grammars from positive structural examples, *Information and Computation* **97**, pp. 23–60.

Sakakibara, Y. (1997). Recent advances of grammatical inference, *Theoretical Computer Science* **185**, pp. 15–45.

Sakakibara, Y. (2005a). Grammatical inference in bioinformatics, *IEEE Trans. Pattern Analysis and Machine Intelligence* **27**, pp. 1051–1062.

Sakakibara, Y. (2005b). Learning context-free grammars using tabular representations, *Pattern Recognition* **38**, pp. 1372–1383.

Sakakibara, Y., Brown, M., Hughley, R., Mian, I., Sjölander, K., Underwood, R., and Haussler, D. (1994). Stochastic context-free grammars for tRNA modeling, *Nuclear Acids Research* **22**, pp. 5112–5120.

Salomaa, A. (1969). Probabilistic and weighted grammars, *Information and Control* **15**, pp. 529–544.

Salomaa, A. (1972). Matrix grammars with a leftmost restriction, *Information and Control* **20**, pp. 143–149.

Sampath, M., Sengupta, R., Lafortune, S., Sinnamohideen, K., and Teneketzis, D. (1995). Diagnosability of discrete-event systems, *IEEE Trans. Automatic Control* **40**, pp. 1555–1575.

Sampath, M., Sengupta, R., Lafortune, S., Sinnamohideen, K., and Teneketzis, D. C. (1996). Failure diagnosis using discrete-event models, *IEEE Trans. Control Systems Technology* **4**, pp. 105–124.

Samuelsson, C. (2000). Theory of stochastic grammars, *Lecture Notes in Computer Science* **1835**, pp. 95–105.

Sánchez, G., Lladós, J., and Tombre, K. (2002). An error-correction graph grammar to recognize texture symbols, *Lecture Notes in Computer Science* **2390**, pp. 128–138.

Sánchez, J. A. and Benedí, J. M. (1997). Consistency of stochastic context-free grammars from probabilistic estimation based on growth transformations, *IEEE Trans. Pattern Analysis and Machine Intelligence* **19**, pp. 1052–1055.

Sánchez, J. A., Benedí, J. M., and Casacuberta, F. (1996). Comparison between the Inside-Outside algorithm and the Viterbi algorithm for stochastic context-free grammars, *Lecture Notes in Computer Science* **1121**, pp. 50–59.

Sánchez, J. A., Rocha, M. A., Romero, V., and Villegas, M. (2018). On the derivational entropy of left-to-right probabilistic finite-state automata and hidden Markov models, *Computational Linguistics* **44**, pp. 17–37.

Sands, O. S. and Garber, F. D. (1990). Pattern representations and syntactic classification of radar measurements of commercial aircraft, *IEEE Trans. Pattern Analysis and Machine Intelligence* **12**, pp. 204–211.

Sanfeliu, A. (1984). A distance measure based on tree-graph-grammars: A way of recognizing hidden and deformed 3-D complex objects, in *Proc. 7th Int. Conf. on Pattern Recognition* (Montreal, Canada), pp. 739–741.

Sanfeliu, A. (1988). Combining logic based and syntactic techniques: A powerful approach, in G. Ferraté, T. Pavlidis, A. Sanfeliu, and H. Bunke (eds.), *Syntactic and Structural Pattern Recognition* (Springer, Berlin - Heidelberg), pp. 395–429.

Sanfeliu, A. and Alquézar, R. (1995a). Active grammatical inference: a new learning methodology, in D. Dori and A. Bruckstein (eds.), *Shape and Structure in Pattern Recognition* (World Scientific, Singapore), pp. 191–200.

Sanfeliu, A. and Alquézar, R. (1995b). Incremental grammatical inference from positive and negative data using unbiased finite state automata, in D. Dori and A. Bruckstein (eds.), *Shape and Structure in Pattern Recognition* (World Scientific, Singapore), pp. 291–300.

Sanfeliu, A. and Alquézar, R. (1996). Efficient recognition of a class of context-sensitive languages described by Augmented Regular Expressions, *Lecture Notes in Computer Science* **1121**, pp. 1–10.

Sanfeliu, A. and Fu, K. S. (1983a). A distance measure between attributed relational graphs for pattern recognition, *IEEE Trans. Systems, Man, and Cybernetics* **13**, pp. 353–362.

Sanfeliu, A. and Fu, K. S. (1983b). Tree-graph grammars for pattern recognition, *Lecture Notes in Computer Science* **153**, pp. 349–368.

Sanfeliu, A. and Sainz, M. (1996). Automatic recognition of bidimensional models learned by grammatical inference in outdoor scenes, *Lecture Notes in Computer Science* **1121**, pp. 160–169.

Sanroma, G., Burghouts, G. J., and Schutte, K. (2012). Recognition of long-term behaviors by parsing sequences of short-term actions with a stochastic regular grammar, *Lecture Notes in Computer Science* **7626**, pp. 225–233.

Sanroma, G., Patino, L., Burghouts, G. J., Schutte, K., and Ferryman, J. (2014). A unified approach to the recognition of complex actions from sequences of zone-crossings, *Image and Vision Computing* **32**, pp. 363–378.

Santos, E. S. (1968). Maximin automata, *Information and Control* **13**, pp. 363–377.

Santos, E. S. (1974). Context-free fuzzy languages, *Information and Control* **26**, pp. 1–11.

Santos, E. S. (1976). Fuzzy automata and languages, *Information Sciences* **10**, pp. 193–197.

Saoudi, A. (1992). Parallel recognition of multidimensional images using regular tree grammars, *Lecture Notes in Computer Science* **654**, pp. 231–239.

Sass, L. (2008). A physical design grammar: A production system for layered manufacturing machines, *Automation in Construction* **17**, pp. 691–704.

Sastry, P. S. and Thathachar, M. A. L. (1994). Analysis of stochastic automata algorithm for relaxation labelling, *IEEE Trans. Pattern Analysis and Machine Intelligence* **16**, pp. 538–543.

Satta, G. (1993). Tree adjoining grammar parsing and Boolean matrix multiplication, *Computational Linguistics* **20**, pp. 173–191.

Schabes, Y. and Joshi, A. K. (1988). An Earley-type parsing algorithm for Tree Adjoining Grammars, in *Proc. 26th Meeting of the Association for Computational Linguistics* (Buffalo, NY, USA), pp. 258–269.

Schabes, Y. and Vijay-Shanker, K. (1990). Deterministic left to right parsing of tree adjoining languages, in *Proc. 28th Meeting of the Association for Computational Linguistics* (Pittsburgh, PA, USA), pp. 276–283.

Schabes, Y. and Waters, R. C. (1995). Tree insertion grammar: A cubic-time parsable formalism that lexicalizes context-free grammars without changing the trees produced, *Computational Linguistics* **21**, pp. 479–513.

Schalkoff, R. (2005). *Pattern Recognition: Statistical, Structural and Neural Approaches* (Wiley, New York).

Schimpf, K. M. (1982). *A Parsing Method for Context-free Tree Languages*, Ph.D. thesis, University of Pennsylvania, Philadelphia, USA.

Schimpf, K. M. and Gallier, J. H. (1985). Tree pushdown automata, *Journal of Computer and System Sciences* **30**, pp. 25–40.

Schlenzig, J., Hunter, E., and Jain, R. (1994). Recursive identification of gesture inputs using hidden Markov models, in *Proc. 1994 IEEE Workshop on Applications of Computer Vision* (Sarasota, FL, USA), pp. 187–194.

Schmidt, J. and Kramer, S. (2014). Online induction of probabilistic real-time automata, *Journal of Computer Science and Technology* **29**, pp. 345–360.

Schmuck, A. K., Schneider, S., Raisch, J., and Nestmann, U. (2014). Extending supervisory controller synthesis to deterministic pushdown automata - Enforcing controllability least restrictively, in *Proc. 12th IFAC IEEE Workshop on Discrete Event Systems* (Cachan, France), pp. 286–293.

Schmuck, A. K., Schneider, S., Raisch, J., and Nestmann, U. (2016). Supervisory control synthesis for deterministic context free specification languages, *Discrete Event Dynamic Systems* **26**, pp. 5–32.

Schneider, S., Schmuck, A. K., Nestmann, U., and Raisch, J. (2014). Reducing an operational supervisory control problem by decomposition for deterministic pushdown automata, in *Proc. 12th IFAC IEEE Workshop on Discrete Event Systems* (Cachan, France), pp. 214–221.

Schützenberger, M. P. (1963). Context-free languages and pushdown automata, *Information and Control* **6**, pp. 246–264.

Searls, D. B. (1992). The linguistics of DNA, *American Scientist* **80**, pp. 579–591.

Searls, D. B. (1993). The computational linguistics of biological sequences, in L. Hunter (ed.), *Artificial Intelligence and Molecular Biology* (AAAI/MIT Press, Menlo Park, CA), pp. 47–120.

Searls, D. B. (1995). String Variable Grammar: a logic grammar formalism for DNA sequences, *The Journal of Logic Programming* **24**, pp. 73–102.

Searls, D. B. (1997). Linguistic approaches to biological sequences, *Computer Applications in the Biosciences* **13**, pp. 333–344.

Searls, D. B. (2001). Reading the book of life, *Bioinformatics* **17**, pp. 579–580.

Searls, D. B. (2002). The language of genes, *Nature* **420**, pp. 211–217.

Sebesta, R. W. (1989). On context-free programmed grammars, *Computer Languages* **14**, pp. 99–108.

Segarra, E., Galiano, I., and Casacuberta, F. (1992). A semi-continuous extension of the morphic generator grammatical inference methodology, in *Proc. Int. Workshop on Structural and Syntactic Pattern Recognition* (Bern, Switzerland), pp. 184–193.

Seifert, S. and Fischer, I. (2004). Parsing string generating hypergraph grammars, *Lecture Notes in Computer Science* **3256**, pp. 352–367.

Sempere, J. M. (2000). On a class of regular-like expressions for linear languages, *Journal of Automata, Languages and Combinatorics* **3**, pp. 343–354.

Sempere, J. M. and García, P. (1994). A characterisation of even linear languages and its application to the learning problem, in C. Carrasco and J. Oncina (eds.), *Grammatical Inference and Applications* (Springer, Berlin-Heidelberg), pp. 38–44.

Sempere, J. M. and López, D. (2003). Learning decision trees and tree automata for a syntactic pattern recognition task, *Lecture Notes in Computer Science* **2652**, pp. 943–950.

Seneff, S. (1992). TINA: A probabilistic syntactic parser for speech understanding systems, in P. Laface and R. Mori De (eds.), *Speech Recognition and Understanding: Recent Advances, Trends and Applications* (Springer, Berlin-Heidelberg), pp. 403–414.

Senin, P., Lin, J., Wang, X., Oates, T., Gandhi, S., Boedihardjo, A. P., Chen, C., and Frankenstein, S. (2015). Time series anomaly discovery with grammar-based compression, in *Proc. 18th Int. Conf. on Extending Database Technology* (Brussels, Belgium), pp. 481–492.

Shah, A. N. (1974). Pebble automata on arrays, *Computer Graphics and Image Processing* **3**, pp. 236–246.

Shannon, C. E. (1948). A mathematical theory of communication, *The Bell System Technical Journal* **27**, pp. 379–423.

Shapiro, L. G. (1980). A structural model of shape, *IEEE Trans. Pattern Analysis and Machine Intelligence* **2**, pp. 111–126.

Shapiro, L. G. and Stockman, G. C. (2001). *Computer Vision* (Prentice-Hall, Upper Saddle River, NJ).

Sharman, R., Jelinek, E., and Mercer, R. (1990). Generating a grammar for statistical training, in *Proc. Workshop on Speech and Natural Language* (Hidden Valley, PA, USA), pp. 267–274.

Shaw, A. C. (1968). The formal description and parsing of pictures, Tech. Rep. SLAC 84, Stanford Linear Accelerator Center, Stanford, CA.

Shaw, A. C. (1969). A formal picture description scheme as a basis for picture processing systems, *Information and Control* **14**, pp. 9–52.

Shaw, A. C. (1970). Parsing of graph-representable pictures, *Journal of the Association for Computing Machinery* **17**, pp. 453–487.

Shen, X. and Vikalo, H. (2012). ParticleCall: A particle filter for base calling in next-generation sequencing systems, *BMC Bioinformatics* **13**:160.

Shi, Q. Y. and Fu, K. S. (1982). Efficient error-correcting parsing for (attributed and stochastic) tree grammars, *Information Sciences* **26**, pp. 159–188.

Shi, Q. Y. and Fu, K. S. (1983). Parsing and translation of attributed expansive graph languages for scene analysis, *IEEE Trans. Pattern Analysis and Machine Intelligence* **5**, pp. 472–485.

Shieber, S. M. and Schabes, Y. (1990). Synchronous tree-adjoining grammars, in *Proc. 13th Int. Conf. on Computational Linguistics* (Helsinki, Finland), pp. 253–258.

Shimizu, T., Monzen, S., Singer, H., and Matsunaga, S. (1995). Time-synchronous continuous speech recognition driven by a context-free grammar, in *Proc. 1995 Int. Conf. on Acoustics, Speech, and Signal Processing* (Detroit, MI, USA), pp. 584–587.

Shridhar, M. and Badreldin, A. (1985). A high-accuracy syntactic recognition algorithm for handwritten numerals, *IEEE Trans. Systems, Man, and Cybernetics* **15**, pp. 152–158.

Sidorova, J. and Anisimova, M. (2014). NLP-inspired structural pattern recognition in chemical application, *Pattern Recognition Letters* **45**, pp. 11–16.

Sidorova, J. and Garcia, J. (2015). Bridging from syntactic to statistical methods: Classification with automatically segmented features from sequences, *Pattern Recognition* **48**, pp. 3749–3756.

Simistira, F., Katsouros, V., and Carayannis, G. (2015). Recognition of online handwritten mathematical formulas using probabilistic SVMs and stochastic context free grammars, *Pattern Recognition Letters* **53**, pp. 85–92.

Simon, L., Teboul, O., Koutsourakis, P., Gool Van, L., and Paragios, N. (2012). Parameter-free/Pareto-driven procedural 3D reconstruction of buildings from ground-level sequences, in *Proc. 2012 IEEE Conf. on Computer Vision and Pattern Recognition* (Providence, RI, USA), pp. 518–525.

Singh, P., Bandyopadhyay, P., Bhattacharya, S., Krishnamachari, A., and Sengupta, S. (2009). Riboswitch detection using profile hidden Markov models, *BMC Bioinformatics* **10**:325.

Siromoney, G., Siromoney, R., and Krithivasan, K. (1972). Abstract families of matrices and picture languages, *Computer Graphics and Image Processing* **1**, pp. 234–307.

Siromoney, G., Siromoney, R., and Krithivasan, K. (1973). Picture languages with array rewriting rules, *Information and Control* **22**, pp. 447–470.

Siromoney, G., Siromoney, R., and Subramanian, K. G. (1982). Stochastic table arrays, *Computer Graphics and Image Processing* **18**, pp. 202–211.

Siromoney, R. (1969). On equal matrix languages, *Information and Control* **14**, pp. 135–151.

Siromoney, R., Huq, A., Chandrasekaran, M., and Subramanian, K. G. (1992). Stochastic puzzle grammars, *International Journal of Pattern Recognition and Artificial Intelligence* **6**, pp. 572–273.

Siromoney, R., Subramanian, K. G., Dare, V. R., and Thomas, D. G. (1999). Some results on picture languages, *Pattern Recognition* **32**, pp. 295–304.

Siskind, J. M., Sherman, J., Pollak, I., Harper, M. P., and Bouman, C. A. (2007). Spatial random tree grammars for modeling hierarchical structure in images with regions of arbitrary shape, *IEEE Trans. Pattern Analysis and Machine Intelligence* **29**, pp. 1504–1519.

Skomorowski, M. (1999). Use of random graph parsing for scene labelling by probabilistic relaxation, *Pattern Recognition Letters* **20**, pp. 949–956.

Skomorowski, M. (2007). Syntactic recognition of distorted patterns by means of random graph parsing, *Pattern Recognition Letters* **28**, pp. 572–581.

Skordalakis, E. (1986). Syntactic ECG processing: A review, *Pattern Recognition* **19**, pp. 305–313.

Slagle, J. R. (1963). A heuristic program that solves symbolic integration problems in freshman calculus, *Journal of the Association for Computing Machinery* **10**, pp. 507–520.

Slagle, J. R. (1971). *Artificial Intelligence: The Heuristic Programming Approach* (McGraw-Hill, New York).

Slisenko, A. O. (1982). Context-free grammars as a tool for describing polynomial-time subclasses of hard problems, *Information Processing Letters* **14**, pp. 52–56.

Smith, E. G. and Baker, P. A. (1975). *The Wiswesser Line-Formula Chemical Notation (WLN)* (Chemical Information Management, Cherry Hill, NJ, USA).

Smoly, I., Carmel, A., Shemer-Avni, Y., Yeger-Lotem, E., and Ziv-Ukelson, M. (2016). Algorithms for regular tree grammar network search and their application to mining human-viral infection patterns, *Journal of Computational Biology* **23**, pp. 165–179.

Sonka, M., Hlavac, V., and Boyle, R. (2015). *Image Processing, Analysis, and Machine Vision* (Cengage Learning, Stamford, CT).

Sproat, R., Shih, C., Gale, W., and Chang, N. (1996). A stochastic finite-state word-segmentation algorithm for Chinese, *Computational Linguistics* **22**, pp. 377–404.

Srinivasan, R., Liu, C. R., and Fu, K. S. (1985). Extraction of manufacturing details from geometric models, *Computers and Industrial Engineering* **9**, pp. 125–133.

Srivastava, P. K., Desai, D. K., Nandi, S., and Lynn, A. M. (2007). HMM-ModE-improved classification using profile hidden Markov models by optimising the discrimination threshold and modifying emission probabilities with negative training sequences, *BMC Bioinformatics* **8**:104.

Staley, S. M., Henderson, M. R., and Anderson, D. C. (1983). Using syntactic pattern recognition to extract feature information from a solid geometric data base, *Computers in Mechanical Engineering* **2**, pp. 61–66.

Starner, T. E., Weaver, J., and Pentland, A. P. (1998). Real-time American Sign Language recognition using desk and wearable computer based video, *IEEE Trans. Pattern Analysis and Machine Intelligence* **20**, pp. 1371–1375.

Staudacher, P. (1993). New frontiers beyond context-freeness: DI-grammars and DI-automata, in *Proc. 6th Conf. European Chapter of the Association for Computational Linguistics* (Utrecht, The Netherlands), pp. 358–367.

Steedman, M. (1987). Combinatory grammars and parasitic gaps, *Natural Language and Linguistic Theory* **5**, pp. 403–439.

Steedman, M. (2000). *The Syntactic Process* (MIT Press, Cambridge, MA).

Steedman, M. (2013). *Combinatory Categorical Grammars for Robust Natural Language Processing* (Morgan and Claypool, San Rafael, CA).

Steger, C., Ulrich, M., and Wiedemann, C. (2018). *Machine Vision Algorithms and Applications* (Wiley-VCH, Weinheim, Germany).

Stiny, G. (1975). *Pictorial and Formal Aspects of Shape and Shape Grammars* (Birkhäuser Verlag, Basel).

Stiny, G. (1980). Introduction to shape and shape grammars, *Environment and Planning B* **7**, pp. 343–351.

Stiny, G. (1982). Spatial relations and grammars, *Environment and Planning B* **9**, pp. 113–114.

Stiny, G. (2006). *Shape* (MIT Press, Cambridge, MA).

Stiny, G. and Gips, J. (1972). Shape grammars and the generative specification of painting and sculpture, in C. V. Freiman (ed.), *Proc. International Federation for Information Processing (IFIP) Congress* (Ljubljana, Yugoslavia), pp. 1460–1465.

Stiny, G. and Mitchell, W. J. (1978). The palladian grammar, *Environment and Planning B* **5**, pp. 5–18.

Stockman, G. and Kanal, L. N. (1983). Problem reduction representation for the linguistic analysis of waveforms, *IEEE Trans. Pattern Analysis and Machine Intelligence* **5**, pp. 287–298.

Stockman, G., Kanal, L. N., and Kyle, M. C. (1976). Structural pattern recognition of carotid pulse waves using a general waveform parsing system, *Communications of the Association for Computing Machinery* **19**, pp. 688–695.

Stolcke, A. (1995). An efficient probabilistic context-free parsing algorithm that computes prefix probabilities, *Computational Linguistics* **21**, pp. 165–201.

Stringa, L. (1990). A new set of constraint-free character recognition grammars, *IEEE Trans. Pattern Analysis and Machine Intelligence* **12**, pp. 1210–1217.

Su, R., Wonham, W. M., and Rogers, E. S. (2004). Supervisor reduction for discrete-event systems, *Discrete Event Dynamic Systems* **14**, pp. 31–53.

Subramanian, K. G., Ali, R. M., Geethalakshmi, M., and Nagar, A. K. (2009). Pure 2D picture grammars and languages, *Discrete Applied Mathematics* **157**, pp. 3401–3411.

Subramanian, K. G., Revathi, L., and Siromoney, R. (1989). Siromoney array grammars and applications, *International Journal of Pattern Recognition and Artificial Intelligence* **3**, pp. 333–352.

Subramanian, K. G., Siromoney, R., and Dare, V. R. (1995). Basic puzzle grammars, *International Journal of Pattern Recognition and Artificial Intelligence* **9**, pp. 763–775.

Subramanian, K. G., Thomas, D. G., Chandra, P. H., and Hoeberechts, M. (2001). Basic puzzle grammars and generation of polygons, *Journal of Automata, Languages and Combinatorics* **6**, pp. 555–568.

Supavatanakul, P., Lunze, J., Puig, V., and Quevedo, J. (2006). Diagnosis of timed automata: Theory and application to the DAMADICS actuator benchmark problem, *Control Engineering Practice* **14**, pp. 609–619.

Swain, P. H. and Fu, K. S. (1972). Stochastic programmed grammars for syntactic pattern recognition, *Pattern Recognition* **4**, pp. 83–100.

Szeliski, R. (2011). *Computer Vision: Algorithms and Applications* (Springer, London).

Tadeusiewicz, R. and Ogiela, M. R. (2004). *Medical Image Understanding Technology* (Springer, Berlin-Heidelberg-New York).

Tai, J. W. and Fu, K. S. (1982). Inference of a class of CFPG by means of semantic rules, *International Journal of Computer and Information Sciences* **11**, pp. 1–23.

Takada, Y. (1988). Grammatical inference for even linear languages based on control sets, *Information Processing Letters* **28**, pp. 193–199.

Takada, Y. (1995). A hierarchy of language families learnable by regular language learning, *Information and Computation* **123**, pp. 138–145.

Takeda, K. (1996). Pattern-based context-free grammars for machine translation, in *Proc. 34th Annual Meeting of Association for Computational Linguistics* (Santa Cruz, CA, USA), pp. 144–151.

Tamura, S. and Tanaka, K. (1973). Learning of fuzzy formal language, *IEEE Trans. Systems, Man, and Cybernetics* **3**, pp. 98–102.

Tanaka, E. (1995). Theoretical aspects of syntactic pattern recognition, *Pattern Recognition* **28**, pp. 1053–1061.

Tanaka, E. and Fu, K. S. (1978). Error-correcting parsers for formal languages, *IEEE Trans. Computers* **27**, pp. 605–616.

Tanaka, E., Ikeda, M., and Ezure, K. (1986). Direct parsing, *Pattern Recognition* **19**, pp. 315–323.

Tang, C. Y. and Huang, T. S. (1979). A syntactic-semantic approach to image understanding and creation, *IEEE Trans. Pattern Analysis and Machine Intelligence* **1**, pp. 135–144.

Tauber, S. J. and Rankin, K. (1972). Valid structure diagrams and chemical gibberish, *Journal of Chemical Documentation* **12**, pp. 30–34.

Teboul, O., Kokkinos, L., I. Simon, Koutsourakis, P., and Paragios, N. (2013). Parsing facades with shape grammars and reinforcement learning, *IEEE Trans. Pattern Analysis and Machine Intelligence* **35**, pp. 1744–1756.

Thatcher, J. W. (1970). Generalized sequential machine maps, *Journal of Computer and System Sciences* **4**, pp. 339–367.

Thatcher, J. W. and Wright, J. B. (1968). Generalized finite automata theory with an application to a decision problem of second-order logic, *Mathematical Systems Theory* **2**, pp. 57–81.

Thomas, D. G., Sweety, F., and Kalyani, T. (2008). Results on hexagonal tile rewriting grammars, *Lecture Notes in Computer Science* **5358**, pp. 945–952.

Thomason, M. G. (1973). Finite fuzzy automata, regular fuzzy languages and pattern recognition, *Pattern Recognition* **5**, pp. 383–390.

Thomason, M. G. (1974a). Errors in regular languages, *IEEE Trans. Computers* **23**, pp. 597–602.

Thomason, M. G. (1974b). Fuzzy syntax-directed translation, *Journal of Cybernetics* **24**, pp. 87–94.

Thomason, M. G. (1975). Stochastic syntax-directed translation schemata for correction of errors in context-free languages, *IEEE Trans. Computers* **24**, pp. 1211–1216.

Thomason, M. G. (1981). Stochastic syntax-directed translations in syntactic pattern processing, *Pattern Recognition* **14**, pp. 187–190.

Thomason, M. G. (1982). Syntactic/semantic techniques in pattern recognition: a survey, *International Journal of Computer and Information Sciences* **11**, pp. 75–100.

Thomason, M. G. (1990a). Generating functions for stochastic context-free grammars, *International Journal of Pattern Recognition and Artificial Intelligence* **4**, pp. 553–572.

Thomason, M. G. (1990b). Introduction and overview, in H. Bunke and A. Sanfeliu (eds.), *Syntactic and Structural Pattern Recognition - Theory and Applications* (World Scientific, Singapore), pp. 3–28.

Thomason, M. G. and Gonzales, R. C. (1975). Syntactic recognition of imperfectly specified patterns, *IEEE Trans. Computers* **24**, pp. 93–95.

Thomason, M. G. and Marinos, P. N. (1974). Deterministic acceptors of regular fuzzy languages, *IEEE Trans. Systems, Man, and Cybernetics* **4**, pp. 228–230.

Thompson, G. R. and Flynn, L. A. (2007). Polymorphic malware detection and identification via context-free grammar homomorphism, *Bell Labs Technical Journal* **12**, pp. 139–147.

Thompson, S. F. and Rosenfeld, A. (1999). Parallel array grammars as models for the growth of planar patterns, *Pattern Recognition* **32**, pp. 255–2967.

Tombre, K. (1996). Structural and syntactic methods in line drawing analysis: to which extent do they work? *Lecture Notes in Computer Science* **1121**, pp. 310–321.

Tomita, M. (1982). Dynamic construction of finite-state automata from examples using hill-climbing, in *Proc. Fourth Annual Cognitive Science Conference* (University of Michigan, Ann Arbor, USA), pp. 105–108.

Tomita, M. (1985). *Efficient Parsing for Natural Language: A Fast Algorithm for Practical Systems* (Kluwer Academic Publishers, Boston, MA).

Tomita, M. (1987). An efficient augmented-context-free parsing algorithm, *Computational Linguistics* **13**, pp. 31–46.

Torre La, S., Mukhopadhyay, S., and Murano, A. (2002). Optimal-reachability and control for acyclic weighted timed automata, in *Proc. IFIP 17th World Computer Congress* (Montreal, Quebec, Canada), pp. 485–497.

Toshev, A., Mordohai, P., and Taskar, B. (2010). Detecting and parsing architecture at city scale from range data, in *Proc. 2010 IEEE Conf. on Computer Vision and Pattern Recognition* (San Francisco, CA, USA), pp. 398–405.

Trahanias, P. and Skordalakis, E. (1990). Syntactic pattern recognition of the ECG, *IEEE Trans. Pattern Analysis and Machine Intelligence* **12**, pp. 648–657.

Trahanias, P., Skordalakis, E., and Papaconstantinou, G. (1989). A syntactic method for the classification of the QRS patterns, *Pattern Recognition Letters* **9**, pp. 13–18.

Trakhtenbrot, B. A. and Barzdin', Y. M. (1970). *Finite Automata: Behaviour and Synthesis (in Russian)* (Nauka, Moscow, English transl.: North-Holland, Amsterdam, 1973).

Tripakis, S. (2002). Fault diagnosis for timed automata, *Lecture Notes in Computer Science* **2469**, pp. 205–221.

Trzupek, M. and Ogiela, M. R. (2013). Cognitive analysis system for description and recognition of pathological changes in coronary arteries structure, *Mathematical and Computer Modelling* **58**, pp. 1441–1448.

Tsafnat, G., Schaeffer, J., Clayphan, A., Iredell, J. R., Partridge, S. R., and Coiera, E. (2011). Computational inference of grammars for larger-than-gene structures from annotated gene sequences, *Bioinformatics* **27**, pp. 791–796.

Tsai, W. H. and Fu, K. S. (1979). A pattern deformational model and Bayes error-correcting recognition system, *IEEE Trans. Systems, Man, and Cybernetics* **9**, pp. 745–756.

Tsai, W. H. and Fu, K. S. (1980). Attributed grammar - a tool for combining syntactic and statistical approaches to pattern recognition, *IEEE Trans. Systems, Man, and Cybernetics* **10**, pp. 873–885.

Tsatsoulis, C. and Fu, K. S. (1985). Modeling rule-based systems by stochastic programmed production systems, *Information Sciences* **36**, pp. 207–230.

Tucci, M., Vitiello, G., and Costagliola, G. (1994). Parsing nonlinear languages, *IEEE Trans. Software Engineering* **20**, pp. 720–739.

Tümer, M. B., Belfore, L. A., and Ropella, K. M. (2003). A syntactic methodology for automatic diagnosis by analysis of continuous time measurements using hierarchical signal representations, *IEEE Trans. Systems, Man, and Cybernetics, Part B: Cybernetics* **33**, pp. 951–965.

Turakainen, P. (1968). On stochastic languages, *Information and Control* **12**, pp. 304–313.

Turan, G. (1982). On the complexity of graph grammars, Rep. Automata Theory Research Group, Szeged, Hungary.

Turing, A. M. (1937). On computable numbers, with an application to the Entscheidungsproblem, *Proc. London Mathematical Society - Series 2* **42**, pp. 230–265.

Turnbaugh, M. A., Bauer, K. W., Oxley, M. E., and Miller, J. O. (2008). HRR signature classification using syntactic pattern recognition, in *Proc. 2008 IEEE Conf. on Aerospace* (Big Sky, MT, USA), pp. 1–9.

Udupa, J. and Murthy, I. S. N. (1980). Syntactic approach to ECG rhythm analysis, *IEEE Trans. Biomedical Engineering* **27**, pp. 370–375.

Uemura, Y., Hasegawa, A., Kobayashi, S., and Yokomori, T. (1999). Tree adjoining grammars for RNA structure prediction, *Theoretical Computer Science* **210**, pp. 277–303.

Vafaie, H. and Bourbakis, N. G. (1988). A tree grammar scheme for generation and recognition of simple texture paths in pictures, in *Proc. 1988 IEEE Int. Symposium on Intelligent Control* (Arlington, VA, USA), pp. 201–206.

Valiant, L. G. (1984). A theory of the learnable, *Communications of the Association for Computing Machinery* **27**, pp. 1134–1142.

Vanegas, C. A., Aliaga, D. G., and Beneš, B. (2010). Building reconstruction using

Manhattan-world grammars, in *Proc. 2010 IEEE Conf. on Computer Vision and Pattern Recognition* (San Francisco, CA, USA), pp. 358–365.

Vapnik, V. (1998). *Statistical Learning Theory* (Wiley, New York).

Varona, A. and Torres, M. I. (2000). Evaluating pruned k-TSS language models: perplexity and word recognition rates, in M. I. Torres and A. Sanfeliu (eds.), *Pattern Recognition and Applications* (IOS Press, Amsterdam), pp. 193–202.

Venugopal, A., Zollmann, A., and Vogel, S. (2007). An efficient two-pass approach to Synchronous-CFG driven statistical MT, in *Proc. North American Association for Computational Linguistics Conference on Human Language Technology* (Rochester, NY, USA), pp. 500–507.

Verdú-Mas, J. L., Carrasco, R. C., and Calera-Rubio, J. (2005). Parsing with probabilistic strictly locally testable tree languages, *IEEE Trans. Pattern Analysis and Machine Intelligence* **27**, pp. 1040–1050.

Verdú-Mas, J. L., Forcada, M. L., Carrasco, R. C., and Calera-Rubio, J. (2002). Tree k-grammar models for natural language modelling and parsing, *Lecture Notes in Computer Science* **2396**, pp. 56–63.

Vernadat, F., Richetin, M., and Gros, J. B. (1982). Characterization of dynamical systems via syntactic pattern recognition, *IFAC Proceedings* **15**, pp. 343–348.

Verwer, S., Weerdt de, M., and Witteveen, C. (2011). Learning driving behavior by timed syntactic pattern recognition, in *Proc. 22nd Int. Joint Conf. on Artificial Intelligence* (Barcelona, Spain), pp. 1529–1534.

Verwer, S., Weerdt de, M., and Witteveen, C. (2012). Efficiently identifying deterministic real-time automata from labeled data, *Machine Learning* **86**, pp. 295–333.

Vidal, E., Casacuberta, F., Sanchis, E., and Benedí, J. M. (1985). A general fuzzy-parsing scheme for speech recognition, in R. Mori De and C. Y. Suen (eds.), *New Systems and Architectures for Automatic Speech Recognition and Synthesis* (Springer, Berlin-Heidelberg), pp. 427–446.

Vidal, E., Rulot, H., Valiente, J. M., and Andreu, G. (1992). Font-independent mixed-size digit recognition through error-correcting grammatical inference (ECGI), in *Proc. 11th IAPR Int. Conf. on Pattern Recognition* (The Hague, Netherlands), pp. 334–337.

Vidal, E., Thollard, F., Higuera de la, C., Casacuberta, F., and Carrasco, R. (2005a). Probabilistic finite-state machines - part I, *IEEE Trans. Pattern Analysis and Machine Intelligence* **27**, pp. 1013–1025.

Vidal, E., Thollard, F., Higuera de la, C., Casacuberta, F., and Carrasco, R. (2005b). Probabilistic finite-state machines - part II, *IEEE Trans. Pattern Analysis and Machine Intelligence* **27**, pp. 1026–1039.

Vijay-Shanker, K. (1992). Using description of trees in a tree-adjoining grammar, *Computational Linguistics* **18**, pp. 481–517.

Vijay-Shanker, K. and Joshi, A. K. (1985). Some computational properties of tree adjoining grammars, in *Proc. 23rd Meeting of the Association for Computational Linguistics* (Chicago, IL, USA), pp. 82–93.

Vijay-Shanker, K. and Weir, D. J. (1994a). The equivalence of four extensions of context-free grammars, *Mathematical Systems Theory* **27**, pp. 511–546.

Vijay-Shanker, K. and Weir, D. J. (1994b). Parsing some constrained grammar formalisms, *Computational Linguistics* **19**, pp. 591–636.

Vinciarelli, A., Bengio, S., and Bunke, H. (2004). Offline recognition of unconstrained handwritten texts using HMMs and statistical language models, *IEEE Trans. Pattern Analysis and Machine Intelligence* **26**, pp. 709–720.

Visnevski, N., Krishnamurthy, V., Wang, A., and Haykin, S. (2007). Syntactic modeling and signal processing of multifunction radars: A stochastic context-free grammar approach, *Proceedings of the IEEE* **95**, pp. 1000–1025.

Viterbi, A. J. (1967). Error bounds for convolutional codes and an asymptotically optimum decoding algorithm, *IEEE Trans. Information Theory* **13**, pp. 260–269.

Vogler, C. and Metaxas, D. (2001). A framework for recognizing the simultaneous aspects of American Sign Language, *Computer Vision and Image Understanding* **81**, pp. 358–384.

Vogler, W. (1991). Recognizing edge replacement graph languages in cubic time, *Lecture Notes in Computer Science* **532**, pp. 676–687.

Waez, M. T. B., Dingel, J., and Rudie, K. (2013). A survey of timed automata for the development of real-time systems, *Computer Science Review* **9**, pp. 1–26.

Waltz, D. (1975). Understanding line drawings with shadows, in P. H. Winston (ed.), *The Psychology of Computer Vision* (McGraw–Hill, New York), pp. 19–91.

Wang, A. and Krishnamurthy, V. (2008). Signal interpretation of multifunction radars: modeling and statistical signal processing with stochastic context free grammar, *IEEE Trans. Signal Processing* **56**, pp. 1106–1119.

Wang, A., Krishnamurthy, V., and Balaji, B. (2011). Intent inference and syntactic tracking with GMTI measurements, *IEEE Trans. Aerospace and Electronic Systems* **47**, pp. 2824–2843.

Wang, H. (1960). Proving theorems by pattern recognition I, *Communications of the Association for Computing Machinery* **3**, pp. 220–234.

Wang, H. (1961). Proving theorems by pattern recognition II, *The Bell System Technical Journal* **40**, pp. 1–42.

Wang, H., Leu, M. C., and Oz, C. (2006a). American Sign Language recognition using multi-dimensional Hidden Markov Models, *Journal of Information Science and Engineering* **22**, pp. 1109–1123.

Wang, H. Q., Ritchings, R. T., and Colchester, A. C. F. (1987). Image understanding system for carotid angiograms, *Image and Vision Computing* **5**, pp. 79–83.

Wang, J., Keightley, P. D., and Johnson, T. (2006b). MCALIGN2: faster, accurate global pairwise alignment of non-coding DNA sequences based on explicit models of indel evolution, *BMC Bioinformatics* **7**:292.

Wang, L., Wang, Y., and Gao, W. (2010). Mining layered grammar rules for action recognition, *International Journal of Computer Vision* **93**, pp. 162–182.

Wang, P. S. P. (1984). An application of array grammars to clustering analysis for syntactic patterns, *Pattern Recognition* **17**, pp. 441–451.

Wang, P. S. P. (1989). *Array Grammars, Patterns and Recognizers* (World Scientific, Singapore - New Jersey - London).

Watrous, R. L. and Kuhn, G. M. (1992). Induction of finite-state languages using second-order recurrent networks, *Neural Computation* **4**, pp. 406–414.

Webb, A. R. and Copsey, K. D. (2011). *Statistical Pattern Recognition* (Wiley, New York).

Wee, W. G. and Fu, K. S. (1969). A formulation of fuzzy automata and its application as a model of learning systems, *IEEE Trans. Systems Science and Cybernetics* **5**, pp. 215–223.

Weinberg, Z. and Ruzzo, W. L. (2006). Sequence-based heuristics for faster annotation of non-coding RNA families, *Bioinformatics* **22**, pp. 35–39.

Weininger, D. (1988). SMILES, a chemical language and information system. 1. Introduction to methodology and encoding rules, *Journal of Chemical Information and Computer Sciences* **28**, pp. 31–36.

Weininger, D. (2003). SMILES - a language for molecules and reactions, in J. Gasteiger (ed.), *Handbook of Chemoinformatics, Vol. 1* (Wiley - VCH, Weinheim, Germany), pp. 80–102.

Weissenberg, J. (2014). *Inverse Procedural Modelling and Applications*, Ph.D. thesis, ETH, Zürich, Switzerland.

Welford, S. M., Lynch, M. F., and Barnard, J. M. (1981). Computer storage and retrieval of generic chemical structures in patents, 3. Chemical grammars and their role in the manipulation of chemical structures, *Journal of Chemical Information and Computer Sciences* **21**, pp. 161–168.

Wieczorek, W. (2017). *Grammatical Inference - Algorithms, Routines and Applications* (Springer International, Switzerland).

Wieczorek, W. and Unold, O. (2016). Use of a novel grammatical inference approach in classification of amyloidogenic hexapeptides, *Computational and Mathematical Methods in Medicine* **2016**:1782732.

Wills, L. M. (1996). Using attributed graph parsing to recognize clichés in programs, *Lecture Notes in Computer Science* **1073**, pp. 170–184.

Wilson, A. D. and Bobick, A. F. (1995). Learning visual behavior for gesture analysis, in *Proc. Int. Symposium on Computer Vision* (Coral Gables, FL, USA), pp. 229–234.

Winston, P. H. (1993). *Artificial Intelligence* (Addison-Wesley, Reading, MA).

Wirth, N. and Weber, H. (1966). EULER: A generalization of ALGOL and its formal definition, *Communications of the Association for Computing Machinery* **9**, pp. 13–25.

Wistrand, M. and Sonnhammer, E. L. (2004). Improving profile HMM discrimination by adapting transition probabilities, *Journal of Molecular Biology* **338**, pp. 847–854.

Wiswesser, W. J. (1982). How the WLN began in 1949 and how it might be in 1999, *Journal of Chemical Information and Computer Sciences* **22**, pp. 88–93.

Wittenburg, K. (1992). Earley-style parsing for relational grammars, in *Proc. IEEE Workshop on Visual Languages* (Seattle, WA, USA), pp. 192–199.

Wittenburg, K. (1993). Adventures in multidimensional parsing: cycles and disorders, in *Proc. Int. Workshop on Parsing Technologies* (Tilburg, The Netherlands), pp. 333–348.

Wittenburg, K. and Weitzman, L. (1990). Visual grammars and incremental parsing for interface languages, in *Proc. IEEE Workshop on Visual Languages* (Skokie, IL, USA), pp. 111–118.

Wittenburg, K., Weitzman, L., and Talley, J. (1991). Unification-based grammars and tabular parsing for graphical languages, *Journal of Visual Languages and Computing* **2**, pp. 347–370.

Wittenburg, K. and Weitzman, L. M. (1998). Relational grammars: theory and practice in a visual language interface for process modeling, in K. Marriott and B. Meyer (eds.), *Visual Language Theory* (Springer, New York), pp. 193–217.

Wojnicki, I. and Kotulski, L. (2018). Improving control efficiency of dynamic street lighting by utilizing the dual graph grammar concept, *Energies* **11**, pp. 1–15.

Wolberg, G. (1987). A syntactic omni-font character recognition system, *International Journal of Pattern Recognition and Artificial Intelligence* **1**, pp. 303–322.

Won, K. J., Hamelryck, T., Prügel-Bennett, A., and Krogh, A. (2007). An evolutionary method for learning HMM structure: prediction of protein secondary structure, *BMC Bioinformatics* **8**:357.

Wonka, P., Wimmer, M., Sillion, F. X., and Ribarsky, W. (2003). Instant architecture, *ACM Trans. on Graphics* **22**, pp. 669–677.

Wright, J. (1990). LR parsing of probabilistic grammars with input uncertainty for speech recognition, *Computer Speech and Language* **4**, pp. 297–323.

Wright, J. and Wrigley, E. (1989). Probabilistic LR parsing for speech recognition, in *Proc. 1st Int. Workshop on Parsing Technologies* (Pittsburgh, PA, USA), pp. 193–202.

Wu, D. (1997). Stochastic inversion transduction grammars and bilingual parsing of parallel corpora, *Computational Linguistics* **23**, pp. 377–404.

Wu, F., Yan, D. M., Dong, W., Zhang, X., and Wonka, P. (2014). Inverse procedural modeling of facade layouts, *ACM Trans. on Graphics* **33**:121.

Xu, X. and Man, H. (2015). Interpreting sports tactic based on latent context-free grammar, in *Proc. 2015 IEEE International Conference on Image Processing* (Quebec City, QC, Canada), pp. 4072–4076.

Yager, N. and Amin, A. (2004). Fingerprint classification: a review, *Pattern Analysis and Applications* **7**, pp. 77–93.

Yamada, H. and Amoroso, S. (1969). Tessellation automata, *Information and Control* **14**, pp. 299–317.

Yamamoto, Y., Morita, K., and Sugata, K. (1989). Context-sensitivity of two-dimensional regular array grammars, *International Journal of Pattern Recognition and Artificial Intelligence* **3**, pp. 295–319.

Yamato, J., Ohya, J., and Ishii, K. (1992). Recognizing human action in time-sequential images using hidden Markov model, in *Proc. IEEE Conf. on Computer Vision and Pattern Recognition* (Champaign, IL, USA), pp. 379–385.

Yan, Y., Dague, P., Pencolé, Y., and Cordier, M. O. (2009). A model-based approach for diagnosing faults in Web service processes, *International Journal of Web Services Research* **6**, pp. 87–110.

Yandell, M. D. and Majoros, W. H. (2002). Genomics and natural language processing, *Nature Reviews Genetics* **3**, pp. 601–610.

Yang, C., Han, T., Quan, L., and Tai, C. L. (2012). Parsing façade with rank-one approximation, in *Proc. 2012 IEEE Conf. on Computer Vision and Pattern Recognition* (Providence, RI, USA), pp. 1720–1727.

Yang, G. (1988). A syntactic approach for building a knowledge-based pattern recognition system, in *Proc. 9th IAPR Conf. on Pattern Recognition* (Rome, Italy), pp. 1236–1238.

Yang, G. (1991). On the knowledge-based pattern recognition using syntactic approach, *Pattern Recognition* **24**, pp. 185–193.

Yang, G. (1993). The search algorithms stimulated by premise set in the syntactic knowledge system, *Pattern Recognition* **26**, pp. 17–22.

Yokomori, T. (1988). Inductive inference of context-free languages based on context-free expressions, *International Journal of Computer Mathematics* **24**, pp. 115–140.

Yokomori, T. (2003). Polynomial-time identification of very simple grammars from positive data, *Theoretical Computer Science* **298**, pp. 179–206.

Yokomori, T. and Kobayashi, S. (1998). Learning local languages and their application to DNA sequence analysis, *IEEE Trans. Pattern Analysis and Machine Intelligence* **20**, pp. 1067–1079.

Yoon, B. J. (2009). Hidden Markov models and their applications in biological sequence analysis, *Current Genomics* **10**, pp. 402–415.

Yoon, B. J. and Vaidyanathan, P. P. (2008). Structural alignment of RNAs using profile-csHMMs and its application to RNA homology search: Overview and new results, *IEEE Trans. Automatic Control* **53**, pp. 10–25.

Yoon, H. S., Soh, J., Bae, Y. J., and Yang, H. S. (2001). Hand gesture recognition using combined features of location, angle and velocity, *Pattern Recognition* **34**, pp. 1491–1501.

You, K. C. and Fu, K. S. (1979). A syntactic approach to shape recognition using attributed grammars, *IEEE Trans. Systems, Man, and Cybernetics* **9**, pp. 334–345.

You, K. C. and Fu, K. S. (1980). Distorted shape recognition using attributed grammars and error-correcting techniques, *Computer Graphics and Image Processing* **13**, pp. 1–16.

Younger, D. (1967). Recognition of parsing and context-free languages in time $n^3$, *Information and Control* **10**, pp. 189–208.

Yu, C., Liu, X. B., and Zhu, S. C. (2017). Single-image 3D scene parsing using geometric commonsense, in *Proc. 26th Int. Joint Conf. on Artificial Intelligence* (Melbourne, Australia), pp. 4655–4661.

Zadeh, L. A. (1965). Fuzzy sets, *Information and Control* **8**, pp. 338–353.

Zadeh, L. A. (1969). Note on fuzzy languages, *Information Sciences* **1**, pp. 421–434.

Zarchi, M. S., Tan, R. T., Gemeren van, C., Monadjemi, A., and Veltkamp, R. C. (2016). Understanding image concepts using ISTOP model, *Pattern Recognition* **53**, pp. 174–183.

Zeng, Z., Goodman, R., and Smyth, P. (1994). Discrete recurrent neural networks for grammatical inference, *IEEE Trans. Neural Networks* **5**, pp. 320–330.

Zhan, Z., Tan, T., and Huang, K. (2011). An extended grammar system for learning and recognizing complex visual events, *IEEE Trans. Pattern Analysis and Machine Intelligence* **33**, pp. 240–255.

Zhang, D. Q., Zhang, K., and Cao, J. (2001). A context-sensitive graph grammar formalism for the specification of visual languages, *The Computer Journal* **44**, pp. 186–200.

Zhang, J., Wang, Y., Wang, C., and M., Z. (2018). Fast variable structure stochastic automaton for discovering and tracking spatiotemporal event patterns, *IEEE Trans. Cybernetics* **48**, pp. 890–903.

Zhang, S., Borovok, I., Aharonowitz, Y., Sharan, R., and Bafna, V. (2006). A sequence-based filtering method for ncRNA identification and its application to searching for riboswitch elements, *Bioinformatics* **22**, pp. e557–e565.

Zhang, Y., Lin, Q., Wang, J., and Verwer, S. (2017). Car-following behavior model learning using timed automata, in *Proc. 20th World Congress of the International Federation of Automatic Control* (Toulouse, France), pp. 2353–2358.

Zhao, M. (1990). Two-dimensional extended attribute grammar method for the recognition of hand-printed Chinese characters, *Pattern Recognition* **23**, pp. 685–695.

Zhao, Y. and Zhu, S. C. (2011). Image parsing with stochastic scene grammar, in J. Shawe-Taylor, R. S. Zemel, P. L. Bartlett, F. Pereira, and K. Q. Weinberger (eds.), *Advances in Neural Information Processing Systems 24* (Curran Associates, Inc.), pp. 73–81.

Zhu, L., Chen, Y., and Yuille, A. (2009). Unsupervised learning of probabilistic grammar-Markov models for object categories, *IEEE Trans. Pattern Analysis and Machine Intelligence* **31**, pp. 114–128.

Zhu, S. C. (2003). Statistical modeling and conceptualization of visual patterns, *IEEE Trans. Pattern Analysis and Machine Intelligence* **25**, pp. 691–712.

Zhu, S. C. and Mumford, D. (2006). A stochastic grammar of images, *Foundations and Trends in Computer Graphics and Vision* **2**, pp. 259–362.

Zieliński, B., Skomorowski, M., Wojciechowski, W., Korkosz, M., and Sprężak, K. (2015). Computer aided erosions and osteophytes detection based on hand radiographs, *Pattern Recognition* **48**, pp. 2304–2317.

Zimmermann, M., Chappelier, J. C., and Bunke, H. (2006). Offline grammar-based recognition of handwritten sentences, *IEEE Trans. Pattern Analysis and Machine Intelligence* **28**, pp. 818–821.

# Index

Printed in the United States
By Bookmasters